Retinal Dystrophy Gene Atlas

Sarwar Zahid • Kari Branham • Dana Schlegel
Mark E. Pennesi • Michel Michaelides
John Heckenlively • Thiran Jayasundera

Retinal Dystrophy Gene Atlas

Springer

Sarwar Zahid, MS, MD
Kellogg Eye Center
University of Michigan
Ann Arbor, Michigan, USA

Dana Schlegel, MS, MPH, CGC
Kellogg Eye Center
University of Michigan
Ann Arbor, Michigan, USA

Michel Michaelides, MB, MD
Institute of Ophthalmology
Moorfields Eye Hospital UCL
London, UK

Thiran Jayasundera, MD
Kellogg Eye Center
University of Michigan
Ann Arbor, Michigan, USA

Kari Branham, MS, CGC
Kellogg Eye Center
University of Michigan
Ann Arbor, Michigan, USA

Mark E. Pennesi, MD, PhD
Casey Eye Institute
Oregon Health & Science University
Portland, Oregon, USA

John Heckenlively, MD
Kellogg Eye Center
University of Michigan
Ann Arbor, Michigan, USA

ISBN 978-3-030-13234-7 ISBN 978-3-319-10867-4 (eBook)
DOI 10.1007/978-3-319-10867-4

Softcover re-print of the Hardcover 1st edition 2018

Printed on acid-free paper

This Springer imprint is published by the registered company Springer International Publishing AG part of Springer Nature.
The registered company address is: Gewerbestrasse 11, 6330 Cham, Switzerland

We are forever indebted to the individuals whose efforts have transformed the field of retinal dystrophies into the dynamic and growing field it is today. We dedicate this work to the spirit of collaboration critical to achieving major breakthroughs in genetic diagnosis and treatments.

Sarwar Zahid

Preface

Although the practice of medicine has changed over the centuries, the core principle of "First, do no harm" laid down by Hippocrates remains a central tenet. As the field of genetic testing has rapidly advanced into next-generation sequencing and to whole exome and whole genome sequencing, there has been a rapid proliferation of information available to patients and physicians. However, as a profession, we must exercise caution when giving patients genetic diagnoses. We hope that this book will help health-care professionals make genotype-phenotype correlations. When we encounter genetic variants that were previously unreported or that are of unknown significance, we encourage physicians and genetic counselors to refer to the relevant chapters in this book to gain an understanding of variable expression of these inherited retinal diseases.

Writing and collecting images for this book has been a team effort. Physicians, genetic counselors, and researchers from three institutions (Oregon Health & Science University, Casey Eye Institute; Moorfields Eye Hospital; and University of Michigan, Kellogg Eye Center) came together through friendship to complete the colossal task of compiling these book chapters, with the shared goal of helping physicians and patients better understand these conditions.

In Shakespeare's *King Lear*, Gloucester, who has been blinded and thrown out of the kingdom, hides, stripped of all his dignities, and Edgar, his banished son, comes to save him from his misery. This is not just an act of saving a blind individual but an act of love and obligation. We are all Edgars in medicine—we love our patients and our profession, and we are obligated to our patients from the day we decide to practice medicine.

It is only by working together that we can advance this field of "orphan" diseases. As therapeutic clinical trials are initiated, let us collaborate to share our precious patients as subjects in the trials that show the most promise. Let us stand united in protecting our patients, while also informing them of opportunities to partake in therapeutic trials. We must carefully weigh the risks and benefits for each patient rather than our obligations to companies running particular clinical trials.

Let us keep in perspective the reason for participating in these trials in the first place—the improvement of vision or halting of progressive loss of vision in patients affected by inherited retinal diseases. We want to be able to encourage children and adults newly diagnosed with retinal dystrophies that treatments for these conditions are in the not-too-distant future.

Ann Arbor, MI, USA
August 2017

Thiran Jayasundera

Acknowledgment

The volume editors would like to acknowledge contributions throughout the atlas by Naheed Khan, PhD (University of Michigan, Kellogg Eye Center), Fernanda Abalem, MD (University of Michigan, Kellogg Eye Center), and Mahdi Mahmood (New York, NY).

Contents

1 ABCA4

ABCA4 encodes an ATP-binding cassette transporter expressed in cone and rod photoreceptors that is responsible for the transport of N-retinyl-phosphatidyl-ethanolamine and all-trans-retinaldehyde as part of the visual cycle. Recessively inherited mutations can cause a variety of *ABCA4*-related retinopathies that includes Stargardt disease, fundus flavimaculatus, retinitis pigmentosa (rod-cone dystrophy)-like phenotype, cone dystrophy, and cone-rod dystrophy [1–3].

Patients with Stargardt disease (STGD) typically present with central visual dysfunction (reduced visual acuity, dyschromatopsia, and reduced contrast sensitivity) in the first-to-second decades. A second common presentation is in early adulthood with less rapidly progressive disease than in those with the childhood-onset form. A minority of patients present in later life, in their 40s through 60s, with relatively stable visual acuity, and relatively preserved foveal structure and function – 'foveal sparing STGD' [4]. The extent of visual acuity deterioration is often variable and reflects involvement of the fovea, ranging from better than 20/40 to worse than 20/200. Patients who present later are more likely to maintain acuity better than 20/200 than those who present with childhood onset disease [5]. The degree of photosensivity or night blindness/peripheral visual field loss is variable, ranging from unaffected to severely affected, and can be determined with electrophysiological assessment (see below).

Typical fundus findings include central macular atrophy and yellow-white flecks at the posterior pole, primarily at the level of the RPE (Figs. 1.1a, 1.2b, 1.3a, 1.4a, and 1.5a). There is, however, considerable phenotypic heterogeneity, including the presence/absence, distribution, and extent of flecks and retinal pigmentary changes (Fig. 1.2a), and the degree of macular atrophy, which can also have a bull's-eye maculopathy (BEM)-like pattern (Fig. 1.3a, b). Approximately a third of patients with non-toxic BEM harbor disease-causing variants in *ABCA4* [6]. Before the identification of the gene *ABCA4*, fundus flavimaculatus (FFM) was used to describe patients with retinal flecks but no ophthalmoscopic evidence of macular atrophy; following the discovery that *ABCA4* mutations cause both STGD and FFM, the term FFM is now rarely used.

Three electrophysiological phenotypes with prognostic implications have been identified in STGD [7, 8]. Patients in group 1 have dysfunction confined to the macula; group 2 have macular and generalized cone system dysfunction; and group 3 have macular, generalized cone, and generalized rod system dysfunction. A longitudinal study of patients with STGD found that all patients with initial rod dysfunction on electroretinography (ERG) demonstrated clinically significant electrophysiologic deterioration; only 20% of patients with normal full-field ERGs at baseline showed clinically significant progression [8]. Patients with group 3 STGD have central scotomata on Goldmann visual field (GVF), in keeping with all patients with STGD, with progressively constricting peripheral fields, and thereby experience more severe visual impairment [9].

Fundus autofluorescence (FAF) can identify a characteristic pattern of areas of increased and decreased autofluorescence (AF) at the posterior pole, with centrally reduced AF corresponding with macular atrophy, which can aid diagnosis, especially in childhood. In advanced disease, peripapillary sparing of AF can be helpful in suggesting *ABCA4*-related disease [10, 11]. In addition, FAF has a role in monitoring progression by determining changes in AF over time (Figs. 1.1b and 1.5b) [8, 12]. A longitudinal study of FAF in STGD found that the AF pattern at baseline influences the enlargement of macular atrophy over time and has genetic correlates [8]. Fluorescein angiography (FA) may reveal a "dark choroid" (Fig. 1.4b), but this is less commonly seen since the advent of FAF and increasing accessibility of genetic testing have made FA less crucial to diagnosis [13]. If extensive atrophy precludes visualization of a dark choroid, the diagnosis may be suggested by the presence of a peripapillary hypofluorescent ring on FA (peripapillary dark choroid ring), also seen as a preserved area on FAF imaging [14]. However, absence of a dark choroid does not exclude *ABCA4*-associated disease; some patients with less extensive disease may not exhibit a dark choroid [2]. Additionally, auto-contrast features on modern fundus cameras may render a dark choroid difficult to visualize.

S. Zahid et al., *Retinal Dystrophy Gene Atlas*, https://doi.org/10.1007/978-3-319-10867-4_1

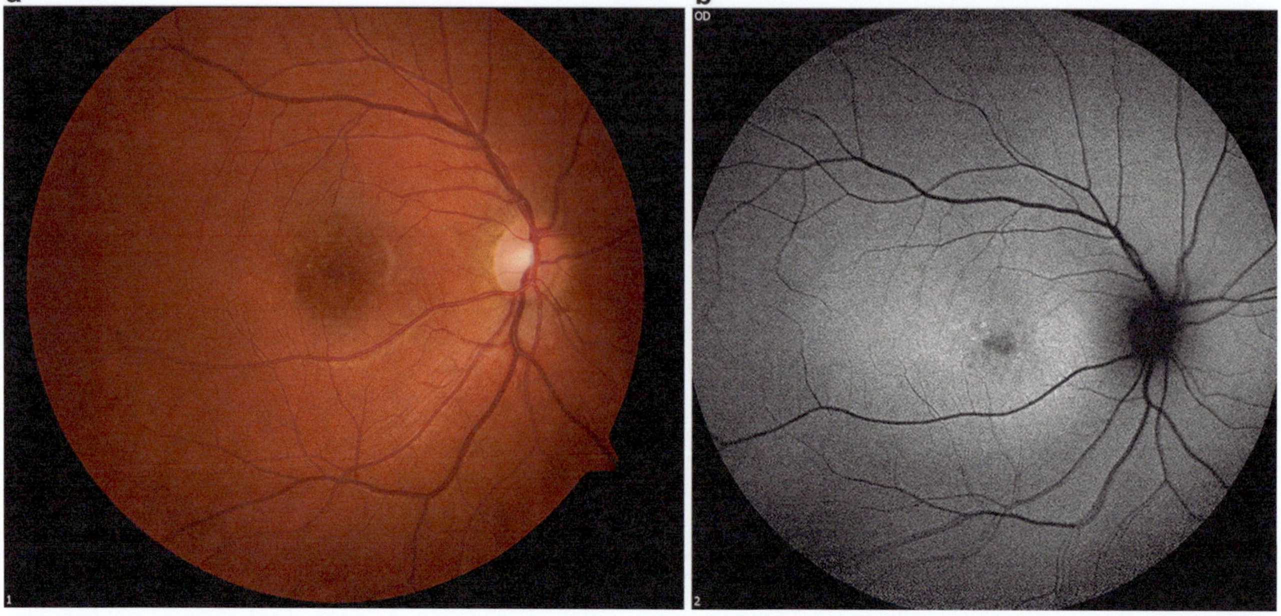

Fig. 1.1 Case summary: 21-year-old female with Stargardt disease. (**a**) Color fundus photograph of the right eye showing minimal macular flecks with an area of central macular atrophy. (**b**) Fundus autofluorescence of the right eye showing increased macular autofluorescence with hyperautofluorescent small flecks. There is also central hypoautofluorescence in the area of macular atrophy, which is better visualized with autofluorescence imaging.

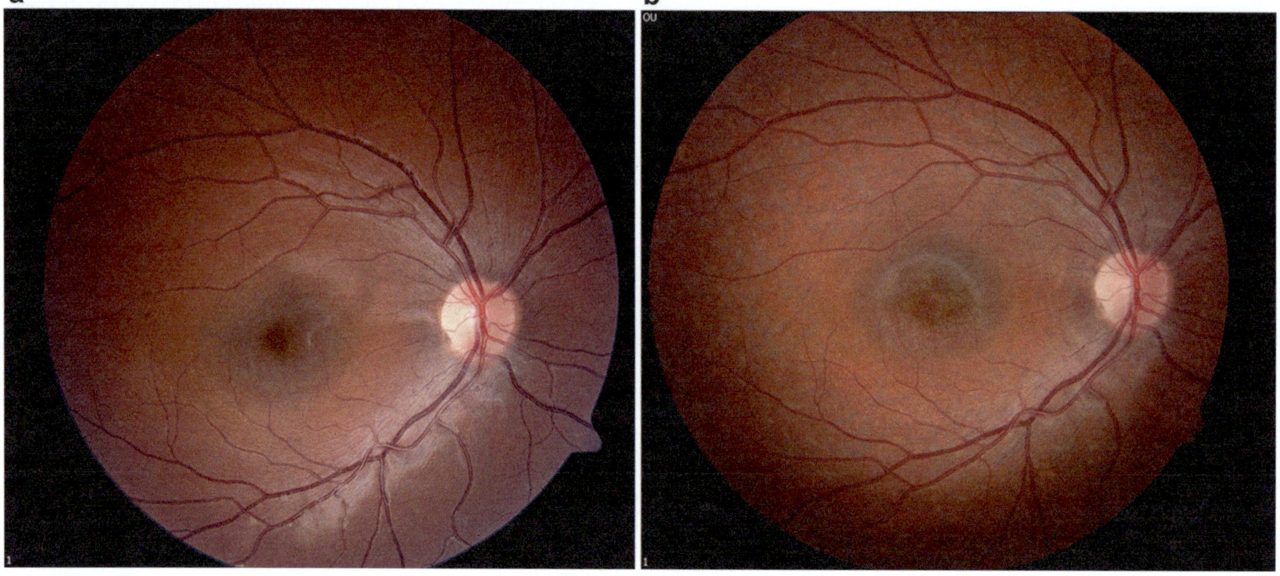

Fig. 1.2 Case summary: 8-year-old with mutations in *ABCA4*. (**a**) Color fundus photograph at age 8 years showing a normal-appearing fundus except for an occasional fleck-like lesion in the macula in the right eye, despite 20/200 visual acuity. There was an identical visual acuity and fundus appearance in the left eye. (**b**) Color fundus photograph at age 11 years, showing the development of foveal atrophy and increased flecks in the posterior pole.

Bull's-eye maculopathy (BEM) is characterized by a distinct lesion at the macula (Fig. 1.3a, b) [6]. Three distinct FAF phenotypes have been described by Kurz-Levin et al. depending on relative hyper- or hypoautofluorescence inside and outside the bull's-eye lesion [15]. BEM associated with *ABCA4* mutations may be observed in the context of cone-rod dystrophy or STGD. *ABCA4* has been implicated in at least 30% of recessive cone-rod dystrophy [16]. These patients usually present in their first-to-second decades with blurred vision and reduced visual acuity; night blindness and

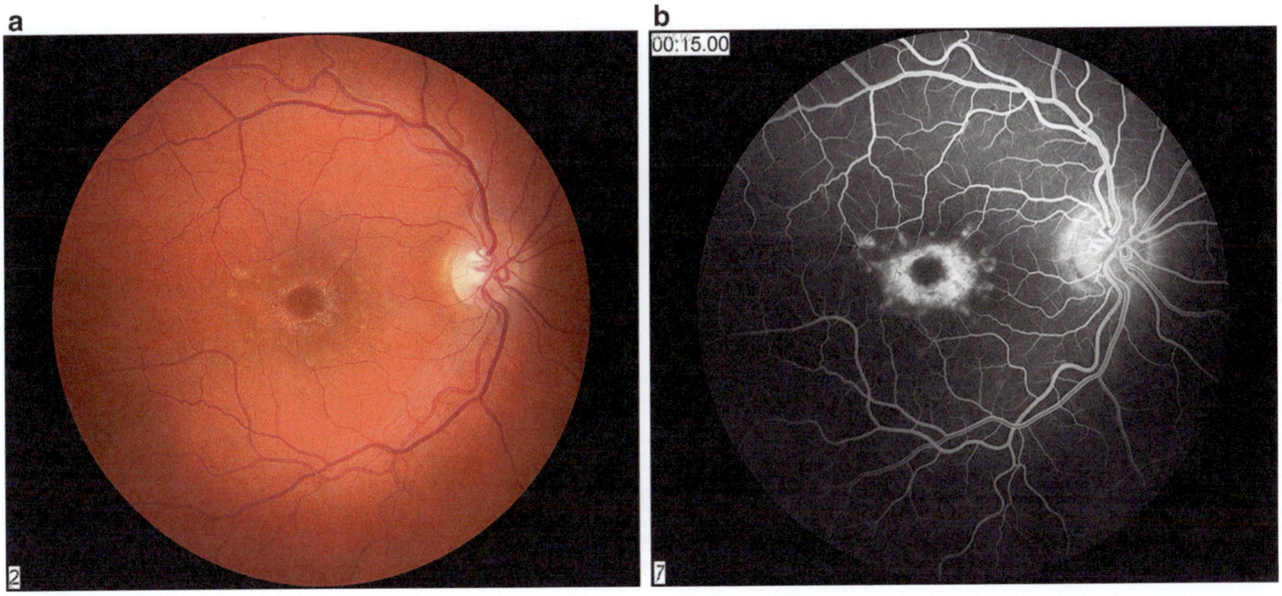

Fig. 1.3 Case summary: 29-year-old male with bull's-eye maculopathy. (**a**) Color fundus photograph of the right eye showing a bull's-eye atrophy lesion in the macula surrounded by retinal deposits. (**b**) Fluorescein angiography of the right eye (AV-transit phase) showing a window defect in the area of bull's eye atrophy. The deposits exhibit hyperfluorescent staining.

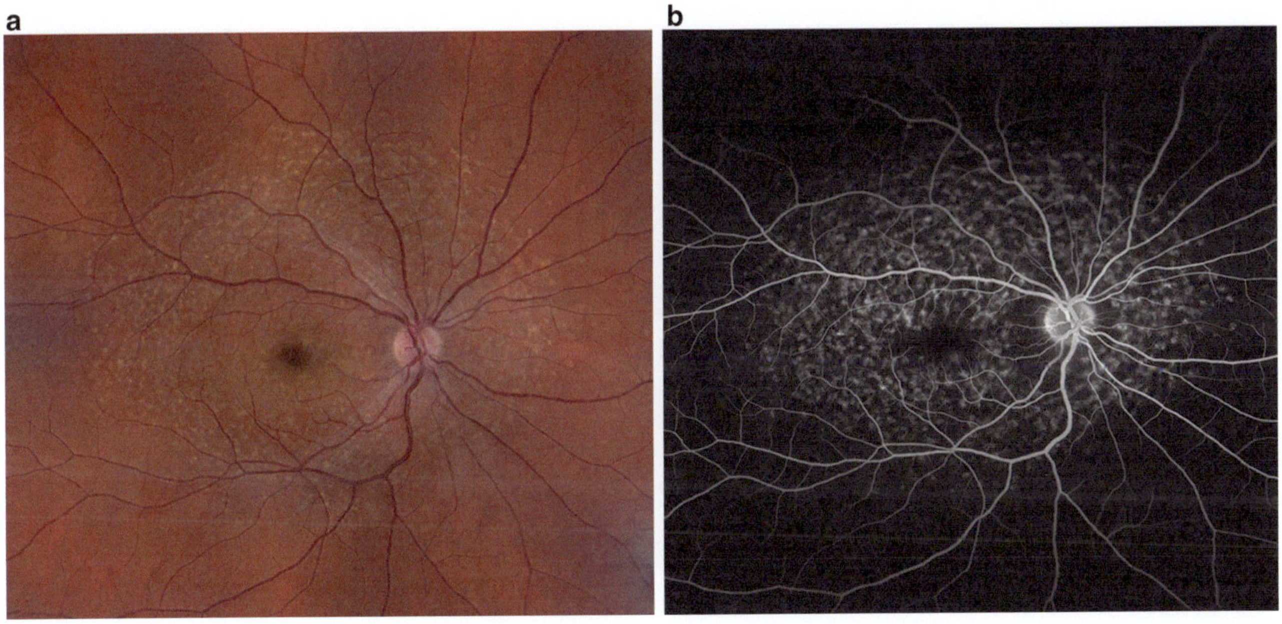

Fig. 1.4 Case summary: 24-year-old female with mutations in *ABCA4*. (**a**) Wide-field color fundus photograph of the right eye showing diffuse pisciform flecks throughout the posterior pole without any associated atrophy. (**b**) Wide-field fluorescein angiography (AV-transit phase) showing hyperfluorescent staining of the flecks on the background of a dark choroid.

peripheral visual field loss typically occur later [17]. Visual acuity may range from 20/30 in children to worse than 20/200 to LP late in the disease process, but there is marked variability [17]. Some groups have also described individual patients with certain solitary heterozygous mutations and milder, later-onset disease, but it is unclear if the single *ABCA4* mutation in these patients is causative [18, 19].

Mutations in *ABCA4* have rarely been reported to cause an autosomal recessive retinitis pigmentosa (RP)-like phenotype. These patients usually present with night blindness in the first-to-second decade with very poor visual acuity. Fundus findings include the classical findings of RP, such as optic disc pallor, attenuated vessels, and bone-spicule pigment deposits, as well as posterior pole atrophy [20].

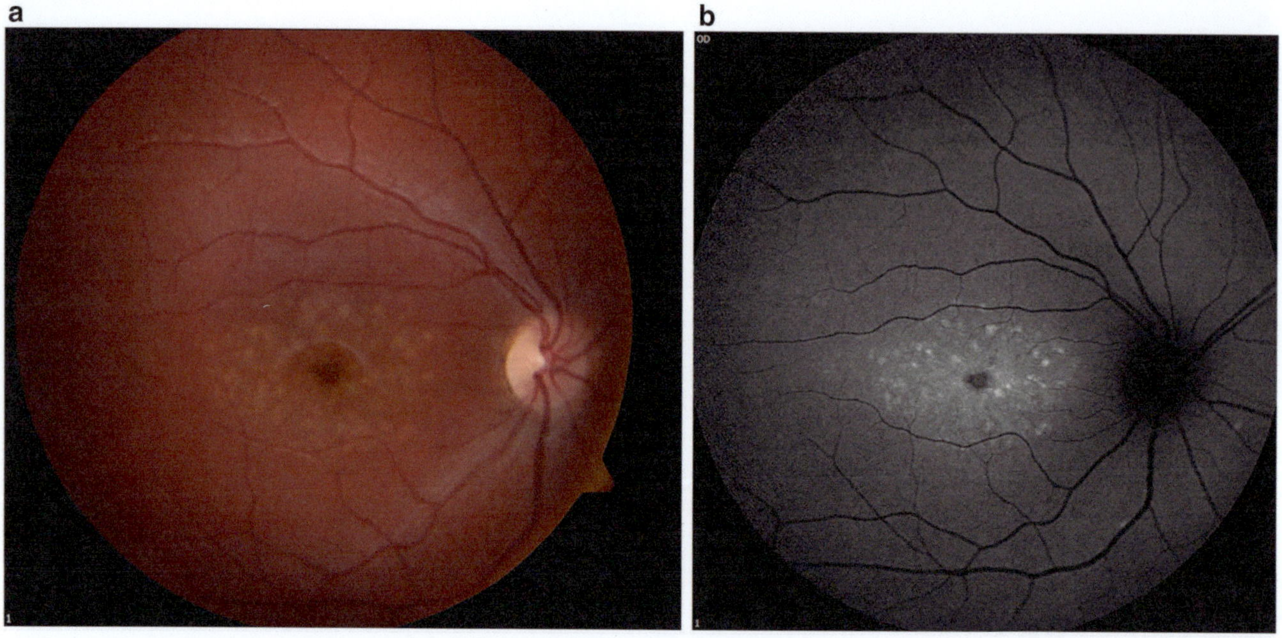

Fig. 1.5 Case summary: 13-year-old girl with Stargardt disease. (**a**) Color fundus photograph of the right eye showing flecks throughout the macula without any obvious macular atrophy. (**b**) Fundus autofluorescence of the right eye showing hyperautofluorescence of the flecks on a background of increased macular autofluorescence. There is a central focus of hypoautofluorescence suggestive of atrophy that is not obvious on fundus photography.

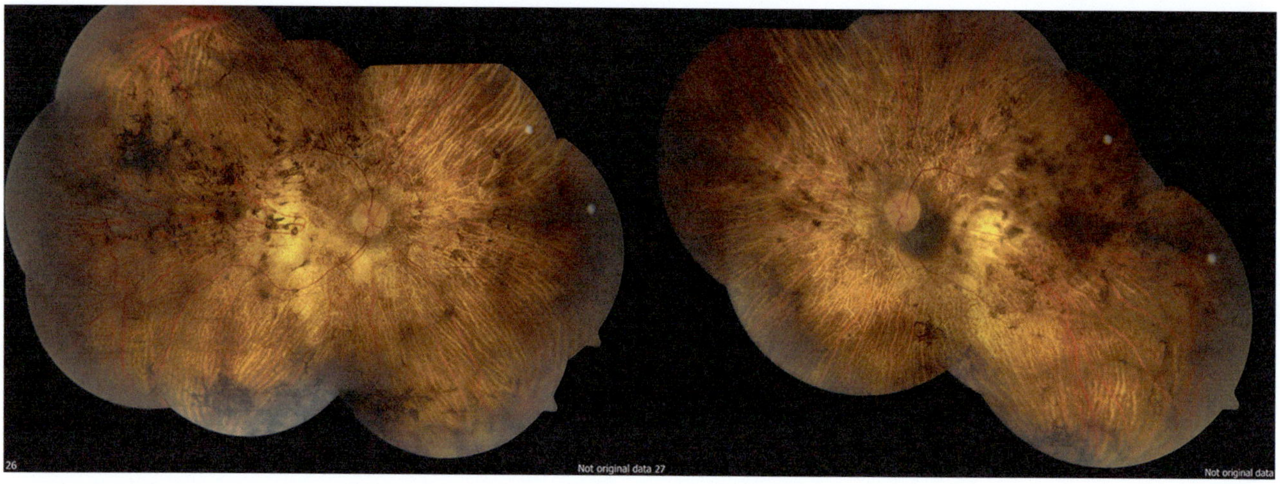

Fig. 1.6 Wide-field fundus photographs of the right and left eyes from a 64-year-old male with a rod-cone dystrophy-like phenotype with diffuse bone spicule pigment deposition and atrophy with a non-recordable ERG and with peripheral islands of remaining visual fields on Goldmann Visual Field testing.

ERG and GVF usually reveal a rod-cone pattern of degeneration (Fig. 1.6).

The carrier frequency of likely pathogenic *ABCA4* alleles has been reported to be as high as 1:20, and over 700 *ABCA4* variants have so far been identified. The high allelic heterogeneity makes molecular genetic analyses of *ABCA4*-associated retinal disease very challenging. It has been reported that direct Sanger sequencing of the entire *ABCA4* coding region (50 exons) detects between 66% and 80% of disease-causing alleles; however, this approach has significant limitations in large patient cohorts due to the prohibitive time and cost implications [21].

Since the development of the *ABCA4* genotyping microarray using arrayed primer extension (APEX) technology, systematic screening of all known previously reported *ABCA4* variants has been available; APEX detects approximately 65–75% of all disease-associated alleles. However, by definition, novel variants are not detected by APEX technology, necessitating the use of other methodologies for high-throughput systematic screening of the entire coding region, especially in cases where one or both disease-causing alleles have not been identified by the array.

Zernant et al. reported the capability of a next-generation sequencing (NGS) strategy to detect new *ABCA4* variants that were not included on the APEX array; all 50 *ABCA4* exons of 168 patients were amplified in parallel using an amplicon tagging polymerase chain reaction (PCR) protocol, and NGS was applied to the resulting amplicons [22]. This NGS strategy has been repeated in another cohort with similar findings, identifying the second disease-causing allele in 48% of the cohort in whom only one allele had been previously found with APEX [8]. These findings suggest that many disease-associated mutations in the *ABCA4* gene are very rare and yet unknown, supporting the validity of the PCR-enrichment-based NGS method either as the screening method of choice or as an additional screening method for patients in whom APEX does not reveal two variants.

References

1. Klevering BJ, Blankenagel A, Maugeri A, Cremers FP, Hoyng CB, Rohrschneider K. Phenotypic spectrum of autosomal recessive cone-rod dystrophies caused by mutations in the ABCA4 (ABCR) gene. Invest Ophthalmol Vis Sci. 2002;43(6):1980–5.
2. Burke TR, Tsang SH. Allelic and phenotypic heterogeneity in ABCA4 mutations. Ophthalmic Genet. 2011;32(3):165–74.
3. Martinez-Mir A, Paloma E, Allikmets R, Ayuso C, del Rio T, Dean M, et al. Retinitis pigmentosa caused by a homozygous mutation in the Stargardt disease gene ABCR. Nat Genet. 1998;18(1):11–2.
4. Noble KG, Carr RE. Stargardt's disease and fundus flavimaculatus. Arch Ophthalmol. 1979;97(7):1281–5.
5. Rotenstreich Y, Fishman GA, Anderson RJ. Visual acuity loss and clinical observations in a large series of patients with Stargardt disease. Ophthalmology. 2003;110(6):1151–8.
6. Michaelides M, Chen LL, Brantley MA Jr, Andorf JL, Isaak EM, Jenkins SA, et al. ABCA4 mutations and discordant ABCA4 alleles in patients and siblings with bull's-eye maculopathy. Br J Ophthalmol. 2007;91(12):1650–5.
7. Lois N, Holder GE, Bunce C, Fitzke FW, Bird AC. Phenotypic subtypes of Stargardt macular dystrophy-fundus flavimaculatus. Arch Ophthalmol. 2001;119(3):359–69.
8. Fujinami K, Lois N, Mukherjee R, McBain VA, Tsunoda K, Tsubota K, et al. A longitudinal study of Stargardt disease: quantitative assessment of fundus autofluorescence, progression, and genotype correlations. Invest Ophthalmol Vis Sci. 2013;54(13):8181–90.
9. Zahid S, Jayasundera T, Rhoades W, Branham K, Khan N, Niziol LM, et al. Clinical phenotypes and prognostic full-field electroretinographic findings in Stargardt disease. Am J Ophthalmol. 2013;155(3):465–73 e463.
10. Lois N, Halfyard AS, Bird AC, Holder GE, Fitzke FW. Fundus autofluorescence in Stargardt macular dystrophy-fundus flavimaculatus. Am J Ophthalmol. 2004;138(1):55–63.
11. Cideciyan AV, Swider M, Aleman TS, Sumaroka A, Schwartz SB, Roman MI, et al. ABCA4-associated retinal degenerations spare structure and function of the human parapapillary retina. Invest Ophthalmol Vis Sci. 2005;46(12):4739–46.
12. Fujinami K, Zernant J, Chana RK, Wright GA, Tsunoda K, Ozawa Y, et al. Clinical and molecular characteristics of childhood-onset Stargardt disease. Ophthalmology. 2015;122(2):326–34.
13. Fishman GA, Farber M, Patel BS, Derlacki DJ. Visual acuity loss in patients with Stargardt's macular dystrophy. Ophthalmology. 1987;94(7):809–14.
14. Jayasundera T, Rhoades W, Branham K, Niziol LM, Musch DC, Heckenlively JR. Peripapillary dark choroid ring as a helpful diagnostic sign in advanced stargardt disease. Am J Ophthalmol. 2010;149(4):656–60 e652.
15. Kurz-Levin MM, Halfyard AS, Bunce C, Bird AC, Holder GE. Clinical variations in assessment of bull's-eye maculopathy. Arch Ophthalmol. 2002;120(5):567–75.
16. Maugeri A, Klevering BJ, Rohrschneider K, Blankenagel A, Brunner HG, Deutman AF, et al. Mutations in the ABCA4 (ABCR) gene are the major cause of autosomal recessive cone-rod dystrophy. Am J Hum Genet. 2000;67(4):960–6.
17. Birch DG, Peters AY, Locke KL, Spencer R, Megarity CF, Travis GH. Visual function in patients with cone-rod dystrophy (CRD) associated with mutations in the ABCA4(ABCR) gene. Exp Eye Res. 2001;73(6):877–86.
18. Souied EH1, Ducroq D, Rozet JM, Gerber S, Perrault I, Sterkers M, Benhamou N, Munnich A, Coscas G, Soubrane G, Kaplan J. A novel ABCR nonsense mutation responsible for late-onset fundus flavimaculatus. Invest Ophthalmol Vis Sci. 1999;40(11):2740–4.
19. Klevering BJ1, Deutman AF, Maugeri A, Cremers FP, Hoyng CB. The spectrum of retinal phenotypes caused by mutations in the ABCA4 gene. Graefes Arch Clin Exp Ophthalmol. 2005;243(2):90–100. Epub 2004 Dec 22.
20. Cremers FP, van de Pol DJ, van Driel M, den Hollander AI, van Haren FJ, Knoers NV, et al. Autosomal recessive retinitis pigmentosa and cone-rod dystrophy caused by splice site mutations in the Stargardt's disease gene ABCR. Hum Mol Genet. 1998;7(3):355–62.
21. Shroyer NF, Lewis RA, Yatsenko AN, Wensel TG, Lupski JR. Cosegregation and functional analysis of mutant ABCR (ABCA4) alleles in families that manifest both Stargardt disease and age-related macular degeneration. Hum Mol Genet. 2001;10(23):2671–8.
22. Zernant J, Schubert C, Im KM, Burke T, Brown CM, Fishman GA, et al. Analysis of the ABCA4 gene by next-generation sequencing. Invest Ophthalmol Vis Sci. 2011;52(11):8479–87.

2 AIPL1

AIPL1 encodes aryl-hydrocarbon interacting protein-like 1, which is a protein that may be important for protein folding and trafficking, expressed in the developing and adult photoreceptor layer. It has also been shown to affect photoreceptor function as well as signal transduction through its mediation of cone PDE6 and RetGC1, respectively [1]. Mutations in *AIPL1* cause recessive Leber congenital amaurosis (LCA) and juvenile-onset rod-cone dystrophy, dominant cone-rod dystrophy has also been reported.

AIPL1 mutations cause 4–8% of LCA [2]. Patients typically present within the first year of life. Patients may experience night blindness, photosensitivity, or photoattraction. Franceschetti's oculo-digital sign, pendular nystagmus, keratoconus (more common in patients with homozygous mutations), and cataracts are commonly observed. Visual acuities range from 20/400 to light perception (median of LP) [3]. The fundus may be normal at an early age, but later in disease it usually shows optic nerve pallor, bone-spicule pigmentary deposits in up to 84% of patients (ranging from mild mid-periphery deposits to severe, diffuse deposits and chorioretinal atrophy), and maculopathy in up to 80% of patients (ranging from mild foveal atrophy to macular stippling, aplasia, or atrophy within first decade) that worsens over time (Figs. 2.1, and 2.2) [4, 5]. Retinal white dots have also been reported in some patients by Tan et al. [6]. Maculopathy, keratoconus, and cataracts are more likely in patients with LCA caused by *AIPL1* mutations than in those with *RPE65* and *GUCY2D* mutations [4]. Electroretinogram (ERG) has been shown to be non-recordable in most patients at an early age, and Golmann visual field (GVF) reveals undetectable or very limited visual fields [7]. However, in three young patients with *AIPL1* mutations, Pennesi et al. reported some residual scotopic ERG function and more preserved visual fields [8]. Tan et al. have also reported residual rod function in a 2-year-old patient [6]. Optical coherence tomography (OCT) may reveal loss of foveal photoreceptors, loss of the outer nuclear layer, reduced foveal thickness, increased inner retinal thickness, or lamellar disorganization.

Juvenile-onset rod-cone dystrophy caused by recessively-inherited mutations in *AIPL1* has been reported in patients who presented with reduced acuity, decreased peripheral vision, and night blindness in the first decade of life. These patients gradually lose acuity and peripheral vision with time. Visual acuity may be as good as 20/60 in their 40s, but it declines steadily to worse than 20/400 within two decades [7]. Keratoconus has not been reported. Fundus findings may include preservation of RPE in the macula, with a bull's-eye lesion and pigmentary atrophy in the mid-periphery beyond the attenuated arcades (Fig. 2.3a–c). Optic nerve drusen have also been reported. Near-infrared imaging may reveal areas of depigmentation, and fundus autofluorescence may show areas of atrophy and hyperautofluorescent bone-spicule pigment deposits (using NIR-RAFI). OCT shows foveal atrophy, loss of photoreceptors and the ONL, and increased thickness in certain retinal areas [7]. GVF reveals a rod-cone pattern with peripheral constriction and loss, with a central functional island that is lost with age. ERG reveals residual but significantly reduced rod and cone parameters (90% reduction in one study) [7].

There has been a report by Sohocki et al. [2] of dominantly-inherited cone-rod dystrophy caused by a mutation in *AIPL1*.

S. Zahid et al., *Retinal Dystrophy Gene Atlas*, https://doi.org/10.1007/978-3-319-10867-4_2

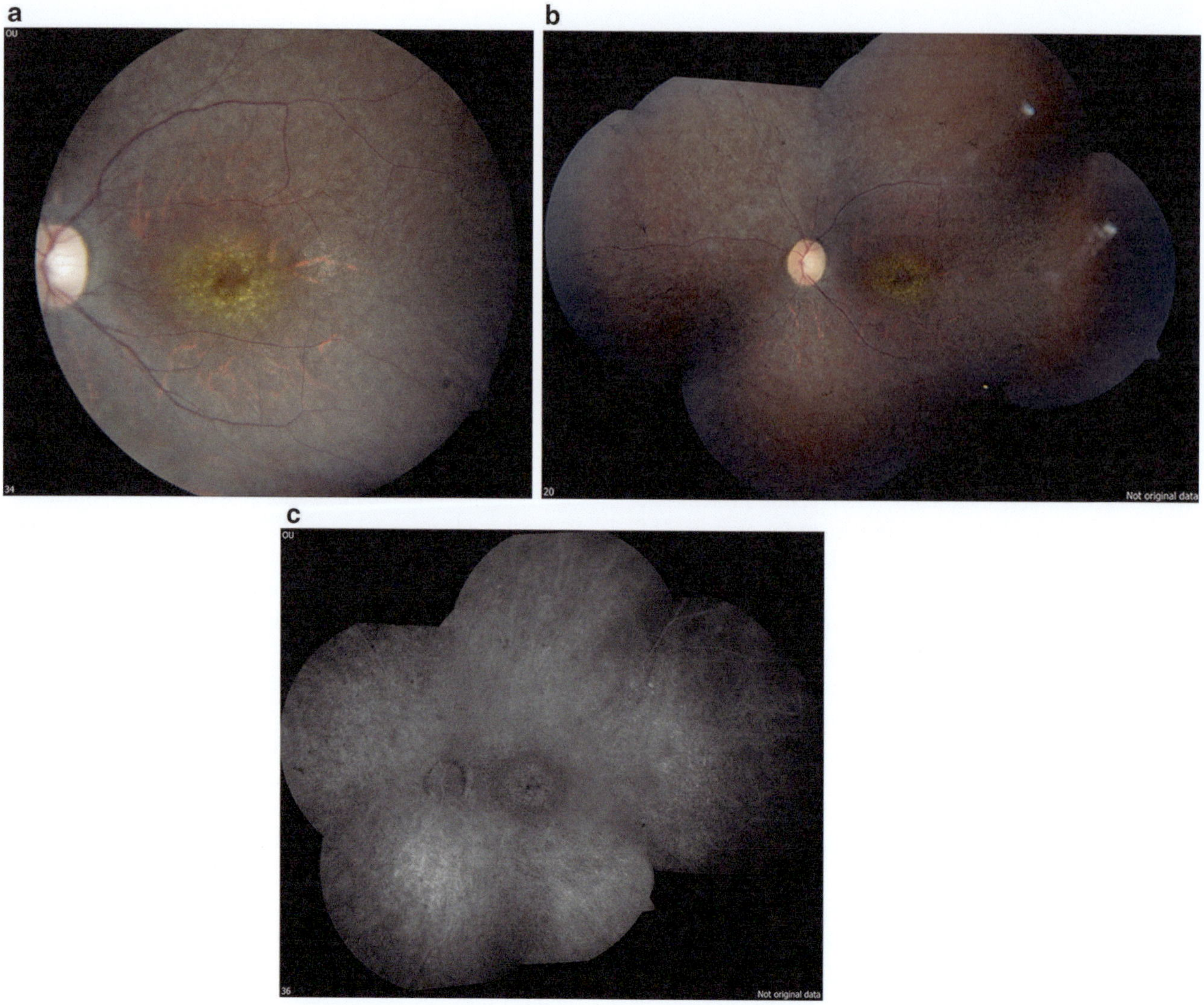

Fig. 2.1 Case summary: 24-year-old female with juvenile-onset rod-cone dystrophy. (**a**) Color fundus photographs of the right eye showing a bull's-eye lesion at the macula with atrophy at age 18. (**b**) Montage of color fundus photographs of the right eye showing a bull's-eye lesion at the macula with peripheral bone spicule pigmentation with atrophy at age 25. (**c**) Fluorescein angiography showing bull's eye lesion at the macula at age 18.

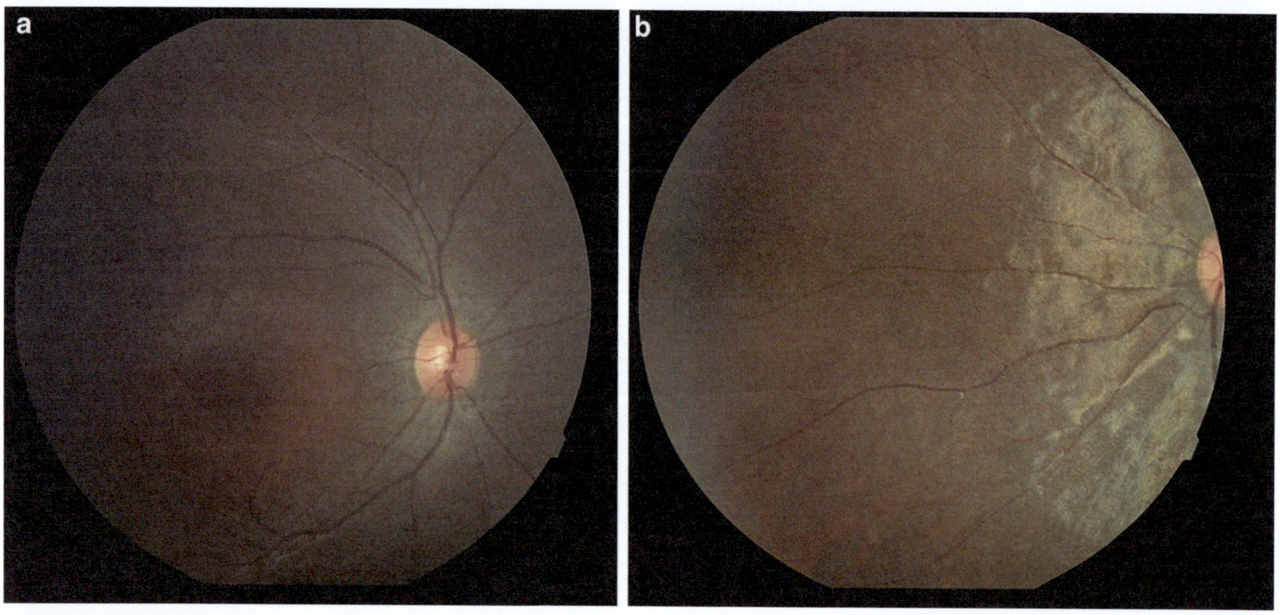

Fig. 2.2 Case summary: Color fundus photographs of the right and left eyes of a 6-year old (CEI24800) showing RPE mottling without obvious atrophy. (Courtesy of Richard G. Weleber).

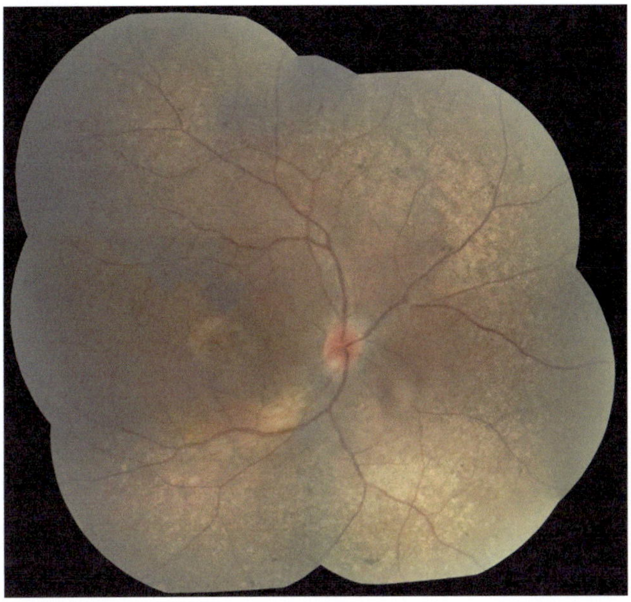

Fig. 2.3 Case summary: Color fundus photograph of the right eye of a 15-year-old male (CEI22551) showing extensive RPE atrophy including and outside the arcades with scant pigmentary deposits, as well as and macular atrophy. (Courtesy of Richard G. Weleber).

References

1. Kolandaivelu S, Singh RK, Ramamurthy V. AIPL1, A protein linked to blindness, is essential for the stability of enzymes mediating cGMP metabolism in cone photoreceptor cells. Hum Mol Genet. 2014;23(4):1002–12.
2. Sohocki MM, Perrault I, Leroy BP, Payne AM, Dharmaraj S, Bhattacharya SS, et al. Prevalence of AIPL1 mutations in inherited retinal degenerative disease. Mol Genet Metab. 2000;70(2):142–50.
3. Walia S, Fishman GA, Jacobson SG, Aleman TS, Koenekoop RK, Traboulsi EI, et al. Visual acuity in patients with Leber's congenital amaurosis and early childhood-onset retinitis pigmentosa. Ophthalmology. 2010;117(6):1190–8.
4. Dharmaraj S, Leroy BP, Sohocki MM, Koenekoop RK, Perrault I, Anwar K, et al. The phenotype of Leber congenital amaurosis in patients with AIPL1 mutations. Arch Ophthalmol. 2004; 122(7):1029–37.
5. Galvin JA, Fishman GA, Stone EM, Koenekoop RK. Evaluation of genotype-phenotype associations in leber congenital amaurosis. Retina. 2005;25(7):919–29.
6. Tan MH, Mackay DS, Cowing J, Tran HV, Smith AJ, Wright GA, et al. Leber congenital amaurosis associated with AIPL1: challenges in ascribing disease causation, clinical findings, and implications for gene therapy. PLoS One. 2012;7(3):e32330.
7. Jacobson SG, Cideciyan AV, Aleman TS, Sumaroka A, Roman AJ, Swider M, et al. Human retinal disease from AIPL1 gene mutations: foveal cone loss with minimal macular photoreceptors and rod function remaining. Invest Ophthalmol Vis Sci. 2011;52(1):70–9.
8. Pennesi ME, Stover NB, Stone EM, Chiang PW, Weleber RG. Residual electroretinograms in young Leber congenital amaurosis patients with mutations of AIPL1. Invest Ophthalmol Vis Sci. 2011;52(11):8166–73.

3 ALMS1

ALMS1 encodes a protein involved in ciliary function and/or ciliogenesis and is located at the ciliary basal body [1, 2]. Mutations are responsible for a progressive cone-rod dystrophy associated with systemic features—Alström syndrome (AS).

ALMS1 mutations are the only reported mutations responsible for AS [3], in the class of ciliopathies [4], and are inherited in an autosomal recessive pattern [5]. The prevalence of AS is about one per million [3]. Onset of the condition is in infancy, with photosensitivity and nystagmus as the commonly observed first symptoms [6–9]. Progressive cone-rod dystrophy is the hallmark of the disease [7]. The disease shows significant phenotypic interfamilial and intrafamilial variability with respect to age of onset and rate of progression [8]. In general, however, progression seems more rapid than is typical of other cone-rod dystrophies [8, 9]. In a cohort of three Swedish patients, all children showed 20/100–2/200 visual acuity at age 3 [8]. In another study of seven affected children from five unrelated non-consanguineous Chinese families, all patients observed (ages 5–14) exhibited best corrected visual acuity of 20/200 to light perception [3]. Bilateral subcapsular cataracts may also be observed in patients with AS [8, 10]. Fundus exam shows attenuation of retinal vessels [3, 10], optic disc pallor, retinal pigment epithelium (RPE) atrophy [8, 10], and may show the presence of drusen (Fig. 3.1a) [9]. Some individuals show narrowing of vessels and depigmentation early in life, but others may not show any abnormal features on fundus exam before the age of 8–10 years [8]. Asteroid hyalosis, optic disc drusen, and bone spicules may also be present [10]; one patient was reported to show a bull's-eye lesion in the macula [8]. Optical coherence tomography (OCT) shows thinning of the RPE and ellipsoid zone [3, 9] and early arrest of macular development in 5-year-old children [9, 10], with persistent inner retinal layers and absent connecting cilia in the outer retina (Fig. 3.1b) [9]. Electroretinography correlates with the degree of visual acuity loss, showing early cone involvement and subsequent rod degeneration. Cone response varies from undetectable at 4–6 months [8, 10] to slightly reduced at 10 years. Rod response is usually within normal limits in infancy and may show marked reduction or be nonresponsive by 5–6 years [8, 10], or may have only minor loss by age 10 [8]. Goldmann Visual Field (GVF) results vary widely between patients, with some showing fields as constricted as <5° on V:4e isopter by age 12 and others showing 50° of field on the I:4e isopter at age 10 [8]. Color vision also varies greatly, with some patients showing normal color vision at age 10 and others showing a complete loss of color vision at age 12 [8].

Other symptoms include bilateral sensorineural hearing loss, which often presents in childhood, but can present at any time from infancy to adulthood [10], type 2 diabetes mellitus, truncal obesity, dilated cardiomyopathy, craniofacial features, hypothyroidism, elevation of liver transaminases, renal insufficiency, gonadal dysfunction, menstrual irregularities [5, 11], and adolescent cessation of growth, leading to short stature and scoliosis [7]. Unlike Bardet-Biedl Syndrome, another ciliopathy, polydactyly is not generally seen (although there have been reports of polydactyly and syndactyly in up to 2% of patients with AS [8]), while sensorineural hearing loss is [4]. Morbidity and mortality are usually due to multiple organ failure from hepatic, cardiac, pulmonary, and renal fibrosis [7].

S. Zahid et al., *Retinal Dystrophy Gene Atlas*, https://doi.org/10.1007/978-3-319-10867-4_3

a

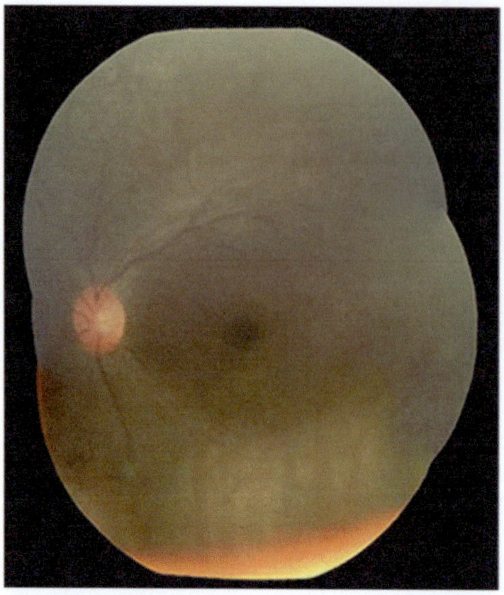

b

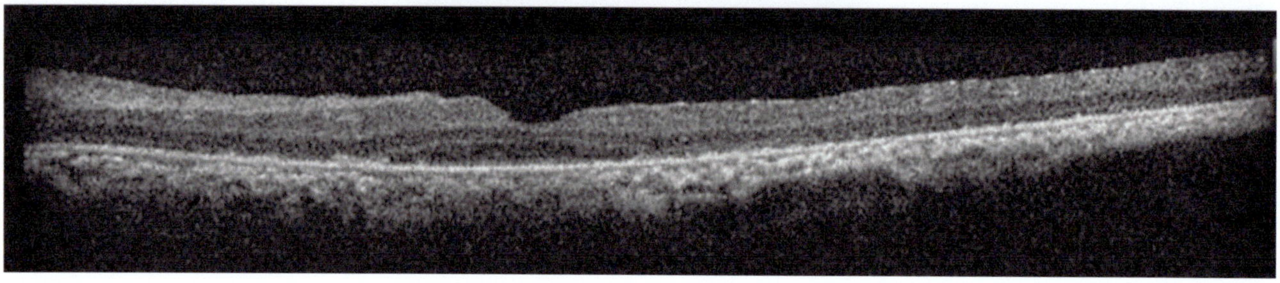

Fig. 3.1 Case summary: 11-year-old female (CEI24864) with homozygous *ALMS1* mutation c.6436C>T p.Arg2146X. Poor vision (LP OU). History of diabetes mellitus type 2, vitreous hemorrhage in both eyes, status-post pars plana vitrectomy in the left eye. (**a**) Color fundus photograph of the left eye showing peripheral retinal RPE changes. (**b**) Spectral domain-optical coherence tomography showing outer retinal atrophy with loss of the ellipsoid zone throughout the macula.

References

1. Jagger D, Collin G, Kelly J, Towers E, Nevill G, Longo-Guess C, et al. Alström syndrome protein ALMS1 localizes to basal bodies of cochlear hair cells and regulates ciulium-dependent planar cell polarity. Hum Mol Genet. 2011;20(3):466–81.
2. O'Neill MJF, McKusick VA. ALMS1 GENE; ALMS1. OMIM. 606844. 2012. Retrieved from http://www.omim.org/entry/606844.
3. Liang X, Hui L, Huajin L, Xu F, Dong F, Sui R, et al. Novel ALMS1 mutations in Chinese patients with Alström syndrome. Mol Vis. 2013;19:1885–91.
4. Piñeiro-Gallego T, Cortón M, Ayuso C, Baiget M, Valverde D. Molecular approach in the study of Alström syndrome: analysis of ten Spanish families. Mol Vis. 2012;18:1794–802.
5. Kaya A, Orbak Z, Çayir A, Döneray H, Taşdemir Ş, Ozantürk A, et al. Combined occurrence of Alström syndrome and bronchiectasis. Pediatrics. 2014;133(3):e780–3.
6. Casey J, McGettigan P, Brosnahan D, Curtis E, Treacy E, Ennis S, et al. Atypical Alstrom syndrome with novel ALMS1 mutations precluded by current diagnostic criteria. Eur J Med Genet. 2014;57(2–3):55–9.
7. Kuburovic V, Marshall JD, Collin GB, Nykamp K, Kuburović N, Milenković T, et al. Differences in the clinical spectrum of two adolescent male patients with Alström syndrome. Clin Dysmorphol. 2013;22(1):7–12.
8. Malm E, Ponjavic V, Nishina PM, Naggert JK, Hinman EG, Andréasson S, et al. Full-field electroretinography and marked variability in clinical phenotype of Alström syndrome. Arch Opthalmol. 2008;126(1):51–7.
9. Vingolo EM, Salvatore S, Grenga PL, Maffei P, Milan G, Marshall J. High-resolution spectral domain optical coherence tomography images of Alström syndrome. J Pediatr Ophthalmol Strabismus. 2010;47 Online:e1–3.
10. Marshall JD, Maffei P, Collin GB, Naggert JK. Alström syndrome: genetics and clinical overview. Curr Genomics. 2011;12(3):225–35.
11. Bahmad F Jr, Costa CS, Teixeira MS, Barros Filho JD, Viana LM, Marshall J. Familial Alström syndrome: a rare cause of bilateral progressive hearing loss. Braz J Otorhinolaryngol. 2014;80(2):99–104.

4 ARL6/BBS3

ARL6, or *BBS3*, encodes a protein that binds the ciliary membrane protein complex containing seven BBS (Bardet-Biedl syndrome) proteins [1]. Mutations are responsible for rod-cone (86.9%) and cone-rod (13.1%) dystrophies [2] and for syndromic features associated with Bardet-Biedl syndrome (BBS). *ARL6* mutations may also cause isolated retinitis pigmentosa (RP) [3, 4].

ARL6 mutations are responsible for a large percentage of cases of autosomal recessive Bardet-Biedl syndrome in Saudi patients, reported by Abu Safieh et al. [4] to have been seen in three out of seven families with BBS. Mutations in *ARL6* are rarely seen in other populations, however, with only two families affected with this mutation in a cohort of 163 families affected with BBS of North American, European, Newfoundlandian, Turkish, Iraqi, Pakistani, and Indian descent [5]. In a Danish study, mean age at diagnosis for BBS was 11.8 years [6]. In a study conducted in Brazil, only 21% of patients with BBS had a visual acuity above 20/40 in their better-seeing eye [2]. Night blindness may be observed in patients with *ARL6* mutations as early as age 5 [7]. Bilateral nystagmus has been observed in 26% of BBS patients, some of whom also demonstrated strabismus [2]. Central vision has been shown to decline 1 line per year on the logMAR chart, while peripheral vision declines at 0.19 log units per year in dark-adapted environments [2]; 73% of BBS patients are legally blind by their teens or twenties [8]. Some reports suggest that individuals with BBS caused by mutations in *BBS1* exhibit the mildest phenotype and best visual acuity [6, 9]. In contrast, Abu Safieh et al. [4] claim that mutations in *ARL6* tend to cause the mildest phenotypes. Patients with mutations in *ARL6* are also reportedly more likely to be myopic [8]. However, some researchers claim that there is no significant genotype-phenotype correlation for BBS [2]. On fundus exam, 42.8% of BBS patients show disc pallor, 67% show attenuated retinal vessels, 67% show widespread retinal pigment epithelium abnormalities, 42.8% show macular abnormalities, and 23.8% show peripheral pigmentation [2]. While the fundus findings include surface wrinkling or mild bone spicule-like pigmentation in some patients, most patients were sine pigmento (without pigment) [8]. Younger patients tend to show milder changes, such as peripapillary atrophy and mild patchy changes of the internal limiting membrane. Older patients with mutations in *ARL6* typically show more advanced retinal atrophy and macular atrophic changes. Some patients may exhibit posterior subcapsular cataracts [8]. Optical coherence tomography in patients with BBS shows thinning of the photoreceptor layer, with preservation of the inner retinal lamination [10]. On electroretinography, scotopic rod and maximal responses were non-detectable in 91.3%, while cone responses were non-detectable in 65.2%. All patients who could be assessed had elevated dark-adapted visual thresholds [2].

Syndromic features of those with Bardet-Biedl syndrome include hyperphagia-induced obesity, intellectual disability, renal anomalies, polydactyly, and hypogenitalism [11, 12]. Other features include developmental delay, speech delay, congenital heart disease, poor coordination, hypodontia, and increased incidence of diabetes mellitus and hypertension [11, 13]. It has been reported that individuals with mutations in *ARL6* more often have polydactyly of all four limbs [13].

There has been a reported case of an individual with a mutation in *ARL6* who had an isolated finding of retinitis pigmentosa [3, 4] without other systemic features.

References

1. Amberger JS, McKusick VA. ADP-ribosylation factor-like 6; ARL6. OMIM. 608845. 2004, updated 2015. http://omim.org/entry/608845. Accessed 1 Mar 2017.
2. Berezovsky A, Rocha DM, Sacai PY, Watanabe SS, Cavascan NN, Salomão SR. Visual acuity and retinal function in patients with Bardet-Biedl syndrome. Clinics (Sao Paulo). 2012;67(2):145–9.
3. Aldahmesh MA, Safieh LA, Alkuraya H, Al-Rajhi A, Shamseldin H, Hashem M, et al. Molecular characterization of retinitis pigmentosa in Saudi Arabia. Mol Vis. 2009;15:2464–9.

S. Zahid et al., *Retinal Dystrophy Gene Atlas*, https://doi.org/10.1007/978-3-319-10867-4_4

4. Abu Safieh L, Aldahmesh MA, Shamseldin H, Hashem M, Shaheen R, Alkuraya H, et al. Clinical and molecular characterization of Bardet-Biedl in consanguineous populations: the power of homozygosity mapping. J Med Genet. 2010;47(4):236–41.
5. Beales PL, Warner AM, Hitman GA, Thakker R, Flinter FA. Bardet-Biedl syndrome: a molecular and phenotypic study of 18 families. J Med Genet. 1997;34(2):92–8.
6. Hjortshøj TD, Grønskov K, Philp AR, Nishimura DY, Riise R, Sheffield VC, et al. Bardet-Biedl syndrome in Denmark—report of 13 novel sequence variations in six genes. Hum Mutat. 2010;31(4):429–36.
7. Khan S, Ullah I, Irfanullah TM, Basit S, Khan MN, et al. Novel homozygous mutations in the genes ARL6 and BBS10 underlying Bardet-Biedl syndrome. Gene. 2013;515(1):84–8.
8. Heon E, Westall C, Carmi R, Elbedour K, Panton C, Mackeen L, et al. Ocular phenotypes of three genetic variants of Bardet-Biedl syndrome. Am J Med Genet A. 2005;132A(3):283–7.
9. Daniels AB, Sandberg MA, Chen J, Weigel-DiFranco C, Fielding Hejtmancic J, Berson EL. Genotype-phenotype correlations in Bardet-Biedl syndrome. Arch Ophthalmol. 2012;130(7):901–7.
10. Billingsley G, Bin J, Fieggen KJ, Duncan JL, Gerth C, Ogata K, et al. Mutations in chaperonin-like BBS genes are a major contributor to disease development in a multiethnic Bardet-Biedl syndrome patient population. J Med Genet. 2010;47(7):453–63.
11. Xing DJ, Zhang HX, Huang N, KC W, Huang XF, Huang F, et al. Comprehensive molecular diagnosis of Bardet-Biedl syndrome by high-throughput targeted exome sequencing. PLoS One. 2014;9(3):e90599.
12. Zhang Q, Hu J, Ling K. Molecular views of Arf-like small GTPases in cilia and ciliopathies. Exp Cell Res. 2013;319(15):2316–22.
13. Pawlik B, Mir A, Iqbal H, Li Y, Nürnberg G, Becker C, et al. A novel familial BBS12 mutation associated with a mild phenotype: implications for clinical and molecular diagnostic strategies. Mol Syndromol. 2010;1(1):27–34.

5 BBS1

BBS1 encodes Bardet-Biedl syndrome 1 protein, which is part of the BBSome complex (*BBS1–9*) and is thought to be involved in ciliogenesis. Mutations in *BBS1* are associated with Bardet-Biedl syndrome (BBS) and non-syndromic retinitis pigmentosa [1, 2]. BBS is characterized by retinal degeneration and several systemic manifestations, including truncal obesity, muscular-skeletal abnormalities (such as polydactyly, syndactyly, brachydactyly, and/or clinodactyly), genitourinary tract abnormalities (renal cysts), impaired secondary sexual development (e.g., hypogonadism, virilism), deafness, and varying degrees of cognitive and behavioral abnormalities [3]. *BBS1*-related BBS follows an autosomal recessive pattern of inheritance. *BBS1* is the most commonly affected gene in BBS, accounting for approximately 23% of cases. Polydactyly is typically diagnosed in infancy and often the only residual evidence of this may be scars at the sites of removed digits. Patients with retinal manifestations may present with (syndromic) or without (non-syndromic) other extraocular manifestations of the spectrum of BBS [2].

Patients typically present with night blindness within their first two decades of life. Visual acuities may be good (20/40 to 20/50) initially, but progressively decrease over time. Visual acuities may be better in *BBS1*-related disease than in BBS caused by other genes, such as *BBS2*, *BBS3*, *BBS5*, *BBS7*, *BBS10*, and *BBS12* [4]. Cataracts are commonly observed in both the syndromic and non-syndromic RP populations with *BBS1* mutations. Fundus examination typically reveals bone spicules and arteriole attenuation [5]. There also may be atrophic maculopathy as the disease progresses, as well as bull's eye maculopathy (Figs. 5.1a, 5.2a, 5.3a, and 5.4a). Retinal pigment epithelium (RPE) atrophy may also be observed in the arcades. Goldmann visual fields typically reveal ring scotomas with field loss predominantly in the periphery. Electroretinogram (ERG) typically shows a rod-cone pattern of degeneration and often becomes nonrecordable at an early age [2, 6]. ERG parameters have been shown to be higher in retinopathy caused by *BBS1* than in RP caused by mutations in other genes [4]. Negative ERGs have also been reported in some patients [6, 7]. Optical coherence tomography (OCT) may reveal foveal, retinal, and outer nuclear layer thinning in the macula, including loss and disruption of the ellipsoid zone, but retinal lamination is usually maintained. Cystoid macular edema is common (Figs. 5.3c and 5.4c) [6–8]. Fundus autofluorescence may exhibit rings of foveal hyperfluorescence as well as hypofluorescent macular atrophy, sometimes in a bull's eye pattern (Figs. 5.1b, 5.2b, 5.3b, and 5.4b) [7]. There is significant phenotypic variability, even in patients harboring the same mutation, with manifestations ranging from a limited maculopathy to diffuse retinal dysfunction [6]. Some of the phenotypic variability is thought to be related to oligogenic epistatic interactions with mutations at other loci [9], but variability has also been demonstrated in the absence of such modifiers [6].

S. Zahid et al., *Retinal Dystrophy Gene Atlas*, https://doi.org/10.1007/978-3-319-10867-4_5

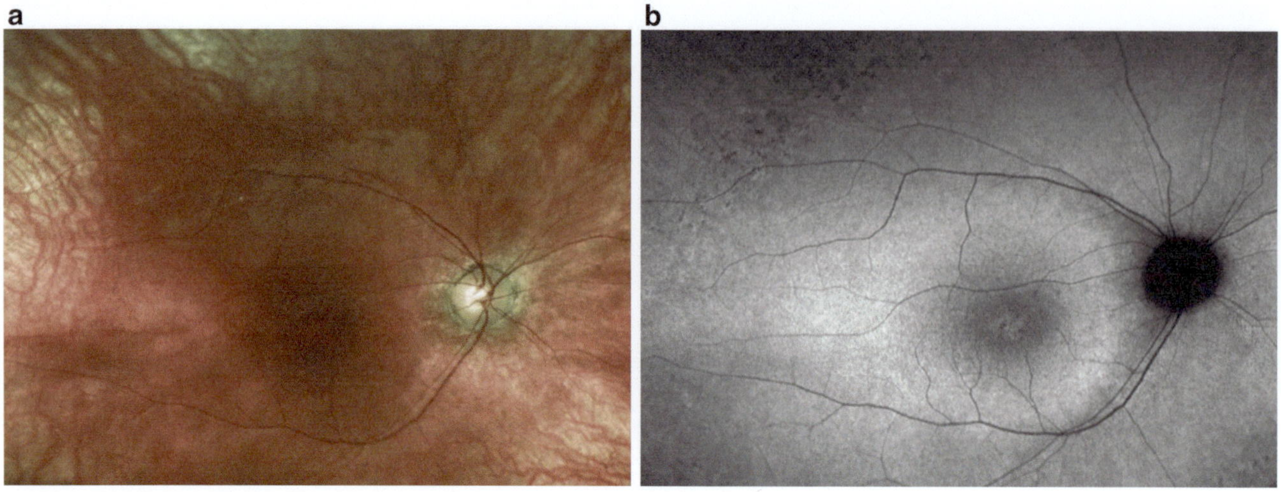

Fig. 5.1 Case summary: An 11-year-old boy with BBS. (**a**) Color fundus photograph of the right eye showing atrophic maculopathy with depigmentation at fovea. (**b**) Fundus autofluorescence showing abnormal macular hyperautofluorescence.

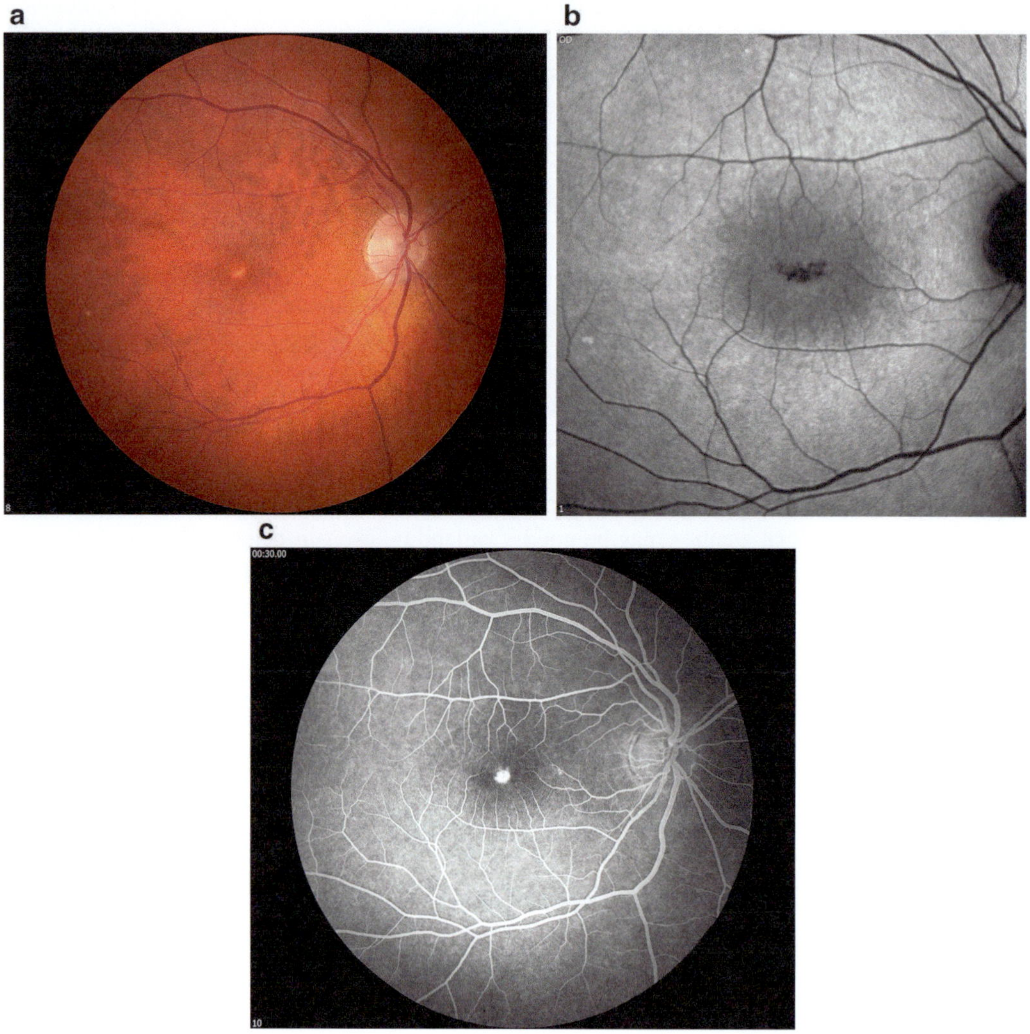

Fig. 5.2 Case summary: 35-year-old man with BBS. (**a**) Color fundus photograph of the right eye showing an atrophic maculopathy with foveal depigmentation. (**b**) Fundus autofluorescence showing foveal hypoautofluorescence. (**c**) Fluorescein angiography showing a window defect in the area of macular atrophy.

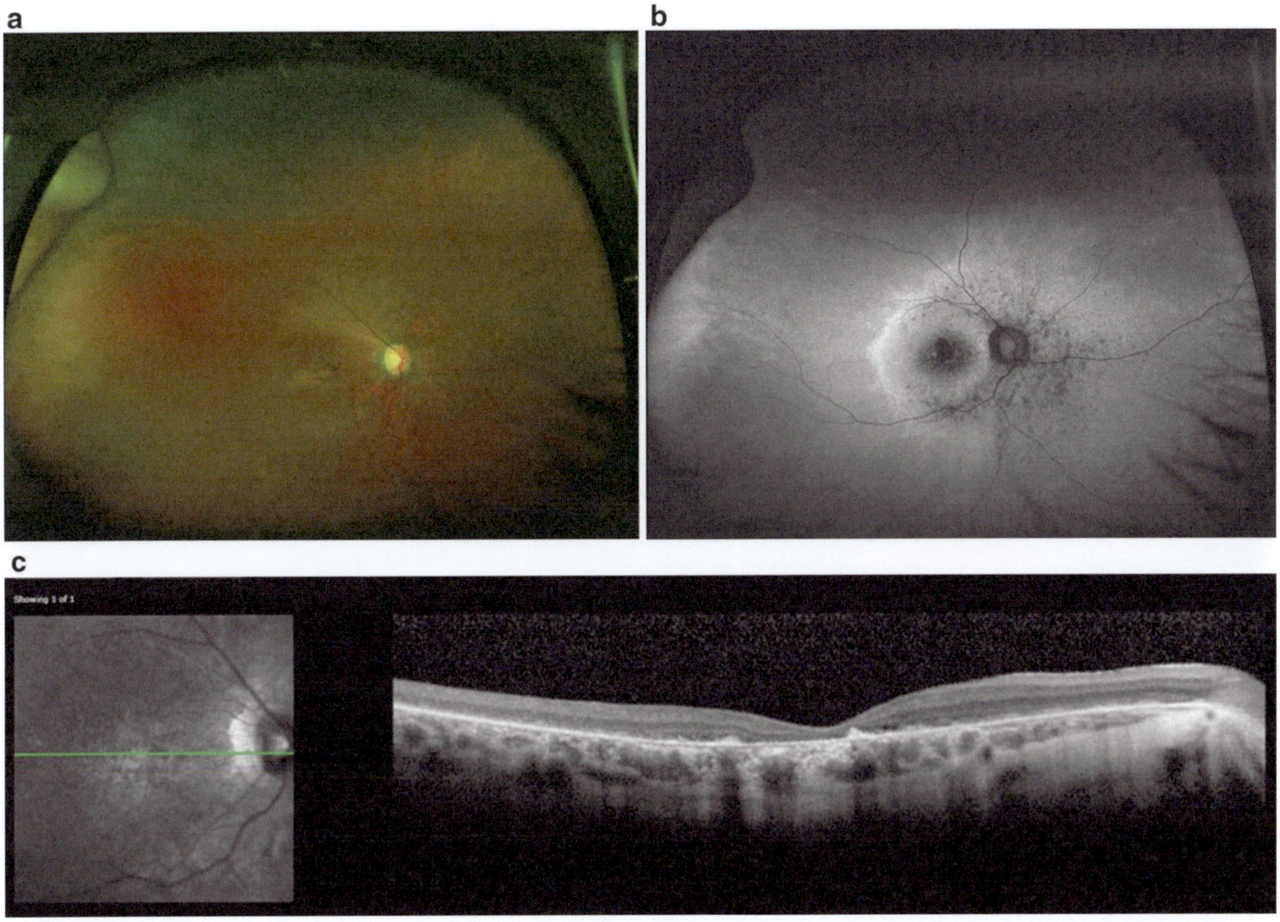

Fig. 5.3 Case summary: 35-year-old female (CEI28435) with retinitis pigmentosa with a history of polydactyly but without other syndromic features of BBS. Mutations: *BBS1* c.1169T>G:p.M390R; *BSS1* c.1169T>G:p.M390R. (**a**) Color fundus photograph of the right eye showing an atrophic maculopathy. (**b**) Fundus autofluorescence showing hypoautofluorescence at the fovea with a ring of hyperautofluorescence outside the arcades. (**c**) Spectral domain-optical coherence tomography showing outer retinal atrophy with loss of the ellipsoid zone.

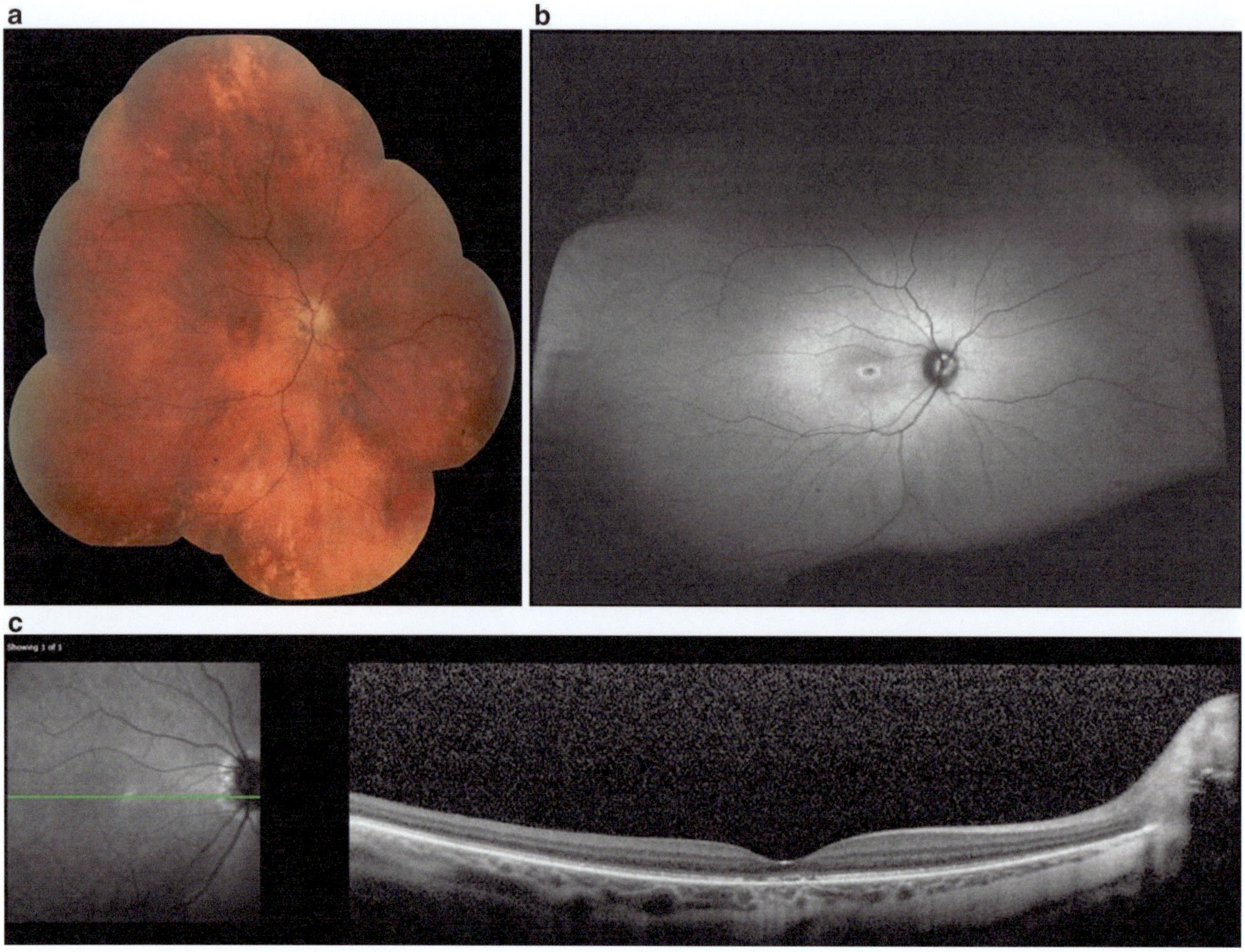

Fig. 5.4 Case summary: 26-year-old female (CEI28552) with syndromic retinitis pigmentosa with polydactyly. Mutations: *BBS1* c.T1169G:p.M390R; BBS1 c.T1169G:p.M390R. (**a**) Color fundus photograph of the right eye showing an atrophic maculopathy with peripheral pigment deposits and atrophy. (**b**) Fundus autofluorescence showing hypoautofluorescence at the fovea with a surrounding ring of hyperautofluorescence outside the fovea and a second more diffuse ring near the arcades. (**c**) Spectral domain-optical coherence tomography showing disruption of the ellipsoid zone (EZ) at the fovea, with maintenance of the EZ outside this region.

References

1. Mykytyn K, Nishimura DY, Searby CC, Shastri M, Yen HJ, Beck JS, et al. Identification of the gene (BBS1) most commonly involved in Bardet-Biedl syndrome, a complex human obesity syndrome. Nat Genet. 2002;31(4):435–8.
2. Estrada-Cuzcano A, Koenekoop RK, Senechal A, De Baere EB, de Ravel T, Banfi S, et al. BBS1 mutations in a wide spectrum of phenotypes ranging from nonsyndromic retinitis pigmentosa to Bardet-Biedl syndrome. Arch Ophthalmol. 2012;130(11):1425–32.
3. Green JS, Parfrey PS, Harnett JD, Farid NR, Cramer BC, Johnson G, et al. The cardinal manifestations of Bardet-Biedl syndrome, a form of Laurence-Moon-Biedl syndrome. N Engl J Med. 1989;321(15):1002–9.
4. Daniels AB, Sandberg MA, Chen J, Weigel-DiFranco C, Fielding Hejtmancic J, Berson EL. Genotype-phenotype correlations in Bardet-Biedl syndrome. Arch Ophthalmol. 2012;130(7):901–7.
5. Ajmal M, Khan MI, Neveling K, Tayyab A, Jaffar S, Sadeque A, et al. Exome sequencing identifies a novel and a recurrent BBS1 mutation in Pakistani families with Bardet-Biedl syndrome. Mol Vis. 2013;19:644–53.
6. Azari AA, Aleman TS, Cideciyan AV, Schwartz SB, Windsor EA, Sumaroka A, et al. Retinal disease expression in Bardet-Biedl syndrome-1 (BBS1) is a spectrum from maculopathy to retina-wide degeneration. Invest Ophthalmol Vis Sci. 2006;47(11):5004–10.
7. Cox KF, Kerr NC, Kedrov M, Nishimura D, Jennings BJ, Stone EM, et al. Phenotypic expression of Bardet-Biedl syndrome in patients homozygous for the common M390R mutation in the BBS1 gene. Vis Res. 2012;75:77–87.
8. Gerth C, Zawadzki RJ, Werner JS, Heon E. Retinal morphology in patients with BBS1 and BBS10 related Bardet-Biedl syndrome evaluated by Fourier-domain optical coherence tomography. Vis Res. 2008;48(3):392–9.
9. Badano JL, Leitch CC, Ansley SJ, May-Simera H, Lawson S, Lewis RA, et al. Dissection of epistasis in oligogenic Bardet-Biedl syndrome. Nature. 2006;439(7074):326–30.

6 BBS2

BBS2 encodes one of seven Bardet-Biedl Syndrome (BBS) proteins that form the stable core of a protein complex required for ciliogenesis and that have a likely function in membrane trafficking to the primary cilium [1]. Mutations are responsible for rod-cone (86.9%) and cone-rod (13.1%) dystrophies [2] and for syndromic features associated with Bardet-Biedl Syndrome.

BBS2 mutations are responsible for about 8–18% of autosomal recessive Bardet-Biedl syndrome [3–6]. Mutations in this gene are most common in the Bedouin population in the Negev Desert in Israel [4, 7]. They have also been seen at the increased frequency of 28.6% in a cohort of 14 Iranian families [8]. A recurring mutation in this gene is Y24X, which is most common in individuals with European ancestry [5]. Additionally, some researchers have reported digenic triallelic inheritance of BBS, also known as the triallelic hypothesis [3, 6, 9–11], but, statistically, this could just be due to the presence of rare polymorphisms or the recognized carrier frequency of mutations in these other BBS genes [6]. In a Danish study, mean age at diagnosis for individuals with mutations in *BBS2* was 7.8 years [6]. In a study conducted in Brazil, only 21% of patients with Bardet-Biedl had a visual acuity above 20/40 in their better-seeing eye [2]. Night blindness is typically observed in those with BBS by age 9, and bilateral nystagmus has been observed in 26% of BBS patients, some of whom also demonstrated strabismus [2]. Central vision has been shown to decline one line per year on the logMAR chart, while peripheral vision declines at 0.19 log units per year in dark-adapted environments [2]; 88% of BBS patients (from a cohort with mutations in *BBS6*, *BBS10*, or *BBS12*) are legally blind by age 18 [10]. It has been claimed that individuals with mutations in *BBS2* and *BBS10* have more severe phenotypes than those with mutations in *BBS1* [6], but obesity tends not to be as commonly observed in patients with mutations in *BBS2* [12]. Some investigators claim, however, that there is no significant genotype-phenotype correlation for BBS [2, 13]. In general, visual function has been seen to deteriorate with age in BBS, but the range of refractive errors has no significant trend [10]. There appears to be no statistically significant genotype-phenotype correlation for rod-cone vs. cone-rod dystrophy [10].

On fundus exam, 42.8% of BBS patients show disc pallor, 67% show attenuated retinal vessels, 67% show widespread retinal pigment epithelium abnormalities, 42.8% show macular abnormalities, and 23.8% show peripheral pigmentation (Fig. 6.1a, b) [2]. In an Israeli family with with individuals affected with mutations in *BBS2*, surface retinal wrinkling was seen mostly in childhood, primarily at the posterior pole, and was mostly observed around the vessels in older patients. There was no significant bone spicule-like pigmentation in the family [7]. OCT in individuals with BBS shows thinning of the photoreceptor layer, with preservation of the inner retinal lamination (Fig. 6.1c) [10]. On ERG, scotopic rod and maximal responses were non-detectable in 91.3% of those with BBS, and cone responses were non-detectable in 65.2%. In the Israeli family with *BBS2* mutations, the youngest child (age 4) had a mixed cone-rod response that was 11% of normal, while the 17-year-old demonstrated a nonrecordable ERG response. All patients with BBS who could be assessed had elevated dark-adapted visual thresholds [2].

Syndromic features of those with Bardet-Biedl Syndrome include hyperphagia-induced obesity, intellectual disability, renal anomalies, polydactyly, and hypogenitalism [14, 15]. Other features include developmental delay, speech delay, congenital heart disease, poor coordination, hypodontia, and increased incidence of diabetes mellitus and hypertension (Fig. 6.1) [12, 14].

S. Zahid et al., *Retinal Dystrophy Gene Atlas*, https://doi.org/10.1007/978-3-319-10867-4_6

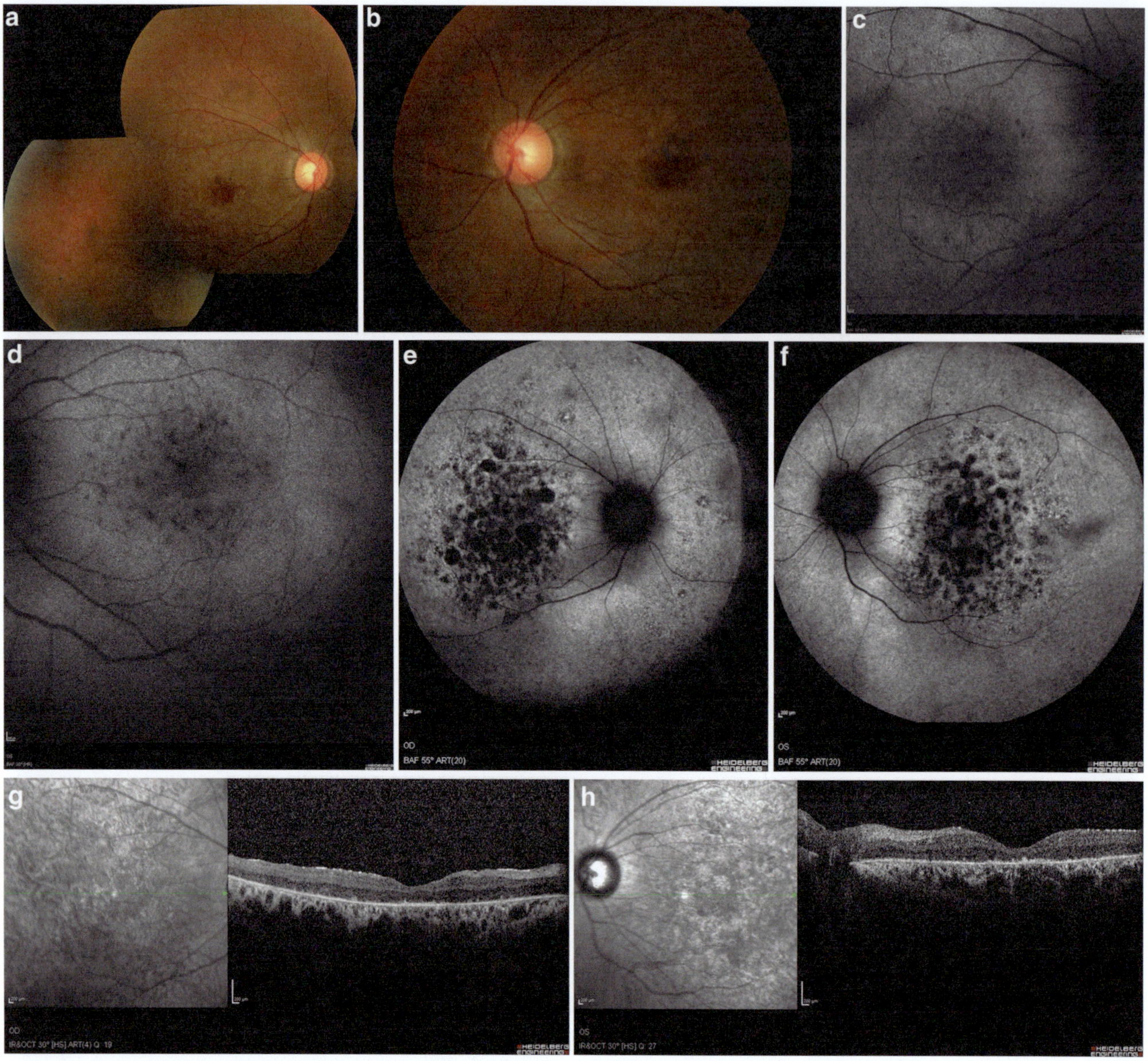

Fig. 6.1 Case Summary: 27-year-old female with Bardet–Biedl syndrome (BBS) with homozygous mutations in *BBS2* (c.1237C > T) with best-corrected visual acuity 3/36 in both eyes. (**a**, **b**) Color fundus photos of the right (montage) and left eyes showing patchy RPE atrophy throughout the macula, macular atrophy, and sparse peripheral pigment deposits. The macular atrophy in the left fundus is associated with dense pigmentary changes. (**c**, **d**) Fundus autofluorescence of the right and left eyes showing small areas of hypoautofluorescence (corresponding to RPE atrophy) early in the disease state, followed by (**e**, **f**) larger areas of hypoautofluorescence in a background of relative hyperautofluorescence, showing disease progression over the course of years. (**g**, **h**) Spectral domain optical coherence tomography of the right and left eyes showing extensive macular ellipsoid zone loss, deposits above the RPE, and trace epiretinal membranes in both eyes.

References

1. Hamosh A, Tiller GE. BBS2 gene; BBS2. In:OMIM–online mendelian inheritance in man; 2013. http://omim.org/entry/606151. Accessed 10 Jan 2017.
2. Berezovsky A, Rocha DM, Sacai PY, Watanabe SS, Cavascan NN, Salomão SR. Visual acuity and retinal function in patients with Bardet-Biedl syndrome. Clinics (Sao Paulo). 2012;67(2):145–9.
3. Beales PL, Badano JL, Ross AJ, Ansley SJ, Hoskins BE, Kirsten B. Genetic interaction of BBS1 mutations with alleles at other BBS loci can result in non-Mendelian Bardet-Biedl syndrome. Am J Hum Genet. 2003;72(5):1187–99.
4. Daniels AB, Sandberg MA, Chen J, Weigel-DiFranco C, Fielding Hejtmancic J, Berson EL. Genotype-phenotype correlations in Bardet-Biedl syndrome. Arch Ophthalmol. 2012;130(7):901–7.
5. Deveault C, Billingsley G, Duncan JL, Bin J, Theal R, Vincent A, et al. BBS genotype-phenotype assessment of a multiethnic patient cohort calls for a revision of the disease definition. Hum Mutat. 2011;32(6):610–9.
6. Hjortshøj TD, Grønskov K, Philp AR, Nishimura DY, Riise R, Sheffield VC, et al. Bardet-Biedl syndrome in Denmark –

report of 13 novel sequence variations in six genes. Hum Mutat. 2010;31(4):429–36.
7. Héon E, Westall C, Carmi R, Elbedour K, Panton C, Mackeen L, et al. Ocular phenotypes of three genetic variants of Bardet-Biedl syndrome. Am J Med Genet A. 2005;132A(3):283–7.
8. Fattahi Z, Rostami P, Najmabadi A, Mohseni M, Kahrizi K, Akbari MR, et al. Mutation profile of BBS genes in Iranian patients with Bardet-Biedl syndrome: genetic characterization and report of nine novel mutations in five BBS genes. J Hum Genet. 2014;59(7):368–75.
9. Badano JL, Kim JC, Hoskins BE, Lewis RA, Ansley SJ, Cutler DJ, et al. Heterozygous mutations in BBS1, BBS2 and BBS6 have a potential epistatic effect on Bardet-Biedl patients with two mutations at a second BBS locus. Hum Mol Genet. 2003;12(14):1651–9.
10. Billingsley G, Bin J, Fieggen KJ, Duncan JL, Gerth C, Ogata K, et al. Mutations in chaperonin-like BBS genes are a major contributor to disease development in a multiethnic Bardet-Biedl syndrome patient population. J Med Genet. 2010;47(7):453–63.
11. Katsanis N, Ansley SJ, Badano JL, Eichers ER, Lewis RA, Hoskins BE, et al. Triallelic inheritance in Bardet-Biedl syndrome, a Mendelian recessive disorder. Science. 2001;293(5538):2256–9.
12. Pawlik B, Mir A, Iqbal H, Li Y, Nürnberg G, Becker C, et al. A novel familial BBS12 mutation associated with a mild phenotype: implications for clinical and molecular diagnostic strategies. Mol Syndromol. 2010;1(1):27–34.
13. Stoetzel C, Muller J, Laurier V, Davis EE, Zaghloul NA, Vicaire S, et al. Identification of a novel BBS gene (BBS12) highlights the major role of a vertebrate-specific branch of chaperonin-related proteins in Bardet-Biedl syndrome. Am J Hum Genet. 2007;80(1):1–11.
14. Xing DJ, Zhang HX, Huang N, KC W, Huang XF, Huang F, et al. Comprehensive molecular diagnosis of Bardet-Biedl syndrome by high-throughput targeted exome sequencing. PLoS One. 2014;9(3):e90599.
15. Zhang Q, Hu J, Ling K. Molecular views of Arf-like small GTPases in cilia and ciliopathies. Exp Cell Res. 2013;319(15):2316–22.

7 BBS4

BBS4 encodes one of seven Bardet-Biedl Syndrome (BBS) proteins that form the stable core of a protein complex required for ciliogenesis and that have a likely function in membrane trafficking to the primary cilium [1, 2]. Mutations are responsible for rod-cone (86.9%) and cone-rod (13.1%) dystrophies [3] and for syndromic features associated with Bardet-Biedl Syndrome.

BBS4 mutations were responsible for about 14% of autosomal recessive Bardet-Biedl syndrome cases in a study of 14 Iranian families [4] and for about 1.2% of cases seen at the Berman-Gund laboratory in Massachusetts [5]. *BBS4* mutations are more frequently found in populations in the Middle East [6]. It is the most commonly mutated gene in cases of Bardet-Biedl in Turkish and Pakistani populations [4, 7] and is also one of the more commonly mutated genes in cases of BBS in the Bedouin population in the Negev Desert in Israel [5].

Additionally, some researchers have reported digenic triallelic inheritance of BBS, also known as the triallelic hypothesis [8–12], but, statistically, this could just be due to the presence of rare polymorphisms or the recognized carrier frequency of mutations in these other BBS genes [11].

In a study of three pairs of siblings with BBS due to mutations in *BBS4*, the mean age of onset of retinal dystrophy was 4 years, with a range of 2–7 years [13]. In a study conducted in Brazil, only 21% of patients with Bardet-Biedl had a visual acuity above 20/40 in their better-seeing eye [3]. Night blindness is typically observed in those with BBS by age 9, and bilateral nystagmus has been observed in 26% of BBS patients, some of whom also demonstrated strabismus [3]. Central vision for those with BBS is expected to decline one line per year on the logMAR chart, while peripheral vision declines at 0.19 log units per year in dark-adapted environments [3]; 88% of BBS patients (from a cohort with mutations in *BBS6*, *BBS10*, or *BBS12*) are legally blind by age 18 [10].

It has been claimed that individuals with mutations in *BBS4* are more likely to have high myopia than other patients with BBS [5, 14], that they tend to have more significant and earlier-onset obesity [6, 15], and that they more frequently have polydactyly only of the upper limbs [6, 16]. Some researchers claim, however, that there is no significant genotype-phenotype correlation for BBS [3, 17]. In general, visual function has been seen to deteriorate with age in BBS, but the range of refractive errors has no significant trend [10]. There appears to be no statistically significant genotype-phenotype correlation for rod-cone vs. cone-rod dystrophy [10].

On fundus exam, 42.8% of BBS patients show disc pallor, 67% show attenuated retinal vessels, 67% show widespread retinal epithelium abnormalities, 42.8% show macular abnormalities, and 23.8% show peripheral pigmentation [3]. In a study with three pairs of siblings with *BBS4* mutations, all six patients had "amorphous" pigment deposits rather than bone spicules [13]. Fundus autofluorescence may show hyperautofluorescence at the fovea and peripheral patchy hypoautofluorescence in areas of retinal pigment epithelium atrophy and pigment deposition (Fig. 7.1a). Optical coherence tomography in individuals with BBS shows thinning of the photoreceptor layer, with preservation of the inner retinal lamination (Fig. 7.1b) [10]. On electroretinography, scotopic rod and maximal responses were non-detectable in 91.3% of those with BBS, and cone responses were non-detectable in 65.2% [3]. In a study of three pairs of siblings with *BBS4* mutations, all had non-recordable rod and cone responses on ERG, and the youngest was 13 years old at the age of evaluation [17]. In a study of 23 patients with BBS, all patients who could be assessed had elevated dark-adapted visual thresholds [3].

Syndromic features of those with Bardet-Biedl Syndrome include hyperphagia-induced obesity, intellectual disability, renal anomalies, polydactyly, and hypogenitalism [18, 19]. Other features include developmental delay, speech delay, congenital heart disease, poor coordination, hypodontia, and increased incidence of diabetes mellitus and hypertension [16, 18] (Fig. 7.1).

S. Zahid et al., *Retinal Dystrophy Gene Atlas*, https://doi.org/10.1007/978-3-319-10867-4_7

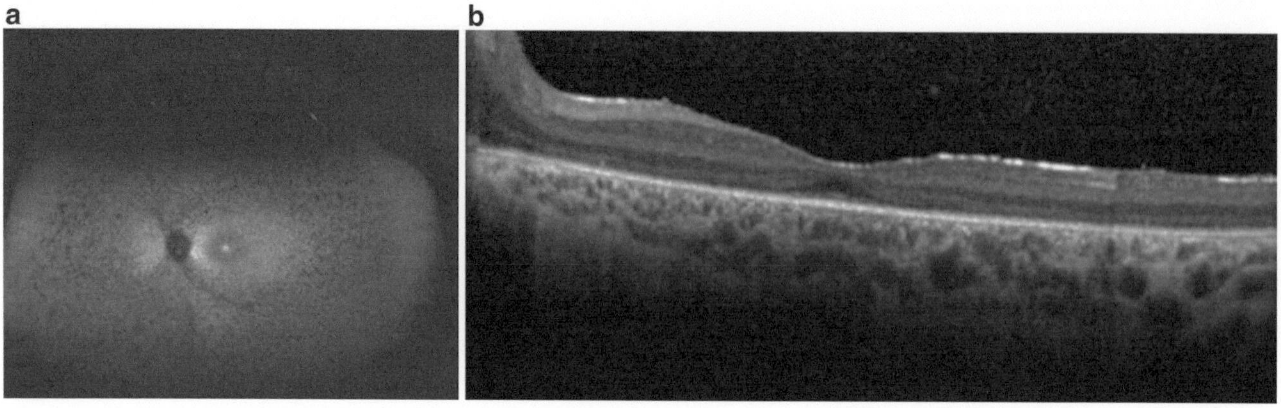

Fig. 7.1 Case Summary: 13-year-old female (CEI25963) with rod-cone dystrophy as a manifestation of Bardet-Biedl Syndrome with a homozygous splicing donor site mutation (IVS10 + 1G > A. CEI 2011) in *BBS4*. (**a**) Fundus autofluorescence of the left eye showing hyperautofluorescence at the fovea and peripheral patchy retinal pigment epithelium atrophy. (**b**) Spectral domain optical coherence tomography showing a faint epiretinal membrane and extensive loss of the ellipsoid zone.

References

1. Hamosh A, Tiller GE. BBS2 gene; BBS2. In:OMIM–online mendelian inheritance in man; 2013. http://omim.org/entry/606151. Accessed 10 Jan 2017.
2. Hartz PA, McKusick VA. BBS4 gene; BBS4. In:OMIM–online mendelian inheritance in man; 2014. http://www.omim.org/entry/600374. Accessed 10 Jan 2017.
3. Berezovsky A, Rocha DM, Sacai PY, Watanabe SS, Cavascan NN, Salomão SR. Visual acuity and retinal function in patients with Bardet-Biedl syndrome. Clinics (Sao Paulo). 2012;67(2):145–9.
4. Fattahi Z, Rostami P, Najmabadi A, Mohseni M, Kahrizi K, Akbari MR, et al. Mutation profile of BBS genes in Iranian patients with Bardet-Biedl syndrome: genetic characterization and report of nine novel mutations in five BBS genes. J Hum Genet. 2014;59(7):368–75.
5. Daniels AB, Sandberg MA, Chen J, Weigel-DiFranco C, Fielding Hejtmancic J, Berson EL. Genotype-phenotype correlations in Bardet-Biedl syndrome. Arch Ophthalmol. 2012;130(7):901–7.
6. Ghadami M, Tomita HA, Najafi MT, Damavandi E, Farahvash MS, Yamada K, et al. Bardet-Biedl syndrome type 3 in an Iranian family: clinical study and confirmation of disease location. Am J Med Genet. 2000;94(5):433–7.
7. Beales PL, Katsanis N, Lewis RA, Ansley SJ, Elcioglu N, Raza J, et al. Genetic and mutational analyses of a large multiethnic Bardet-Biedl cohort reveal a minor involvement of BBS6 and delineate the critical intervals of other loci. Am J Hum Genet. 2001;68(3):606–16.
8. Badano JL, Kim JC, Hoskins BE, Lewis RA, Ansley SJ, Cutler DJ, et al. Heterozygous mutations in BBS1, BBS2 and BBS6 have a potential epistatic effect on Bardet-Biedl patients with two mutations at a second BBS locus. Hum Mol Genet. 2003;12(14):1651–9.
9. Beales PL, Badano JL, Ross AJ, Ansley SJ, Hoskins BE, Kirsten B. Genetic interaction of BBS1 mutations with alleles at other BBS loci can result in non-Mendelian Bardet-Biedl syndrome. Am J Hum Genet. 2003;72(5):1187–99.
10. Billingsley G, Bin J, Fieggen KJ, Duncan JL, Gerth C, Ogata K, et al. Mutations in chaperonin-like BBS genes are a major contributor to disease development in a multiethnic Bardet-Biedl syndrome patient population. J Med Genet. 2010;47(7):453–63.
11. Hjortshøj TD, Grønskov K, Philp AR, Nishimura DY, Riise R, Sheffield VC, et al. Bardet-Biedl syndrome in Denmark – report of 13 novel sequence variations in six genes. Hum Mutat. 2010;31(4):429–36.
12. Katsanis N, Ansley SJ, Badano JL, Eichers ER, Lewis RA, Hoskins BE, et al. Triallelic inheritance in Bardet-Biedl syndrome, a Mendelian recessive disorder. Science. 2001;293(5538):2256–9.
13. Riise R, Tornqvist K, Wright AF, Mykytyn K, Sheffield VC. The phenotype in Norwegian patients with Bardet-Biedl syndrome with mutations in the BBS4 gene. Arch Ophthalmol. 2002;120(10):1364–7.
14. Héon E, Westall C, Carmi R, Elbedour K, Panton C, Mackeen L, et al. Ocular phenotypes of three genetic variants of Bardet-Biedl syndrome. Am J Med Genet A. 2005;132A(3):283–7.
15. Beales PL, Warner AM, Hitman GA, Thakker R, Flinter FA. Bardet-Biedl syndrome: a molecular and phenotypic study of 18 families. J Med Genet. 1997;34(2):92–8.
16. Pawlik B, Mir A, Iqbal H, Li Y, Nürnberg G, Becker C, et al. A novel familial BBS12 mutation associated with a mild phenotype: implications for clinical and molecular diagnostic strategies. Mol Syndromol. 2010;1(1):27–34.
17. Stoetzel C, Muller J, Laurier V, Davis EE, Zaghloul NA, Vicaire S, et al. Identification of a novel BBS gene (BBS12) highlights the major role of a vertebrate-specific branch of chaperonin-related proteins in Bardet-Biedl syndrome. Am J Hum Genet. 2007;80(1):1–11.
18. Xing DJ, Zhang HX, Huang N, Wu KC, Huang XF, Huang F, et al. Comprehensive molecular diagnosis of Bardet-Biedl syndrome by high-throughput targeted exome sequencing. PLoS One. 2014;9(3):e90599.
19. Zhang Q, Hu J, Ling K. Molecular views of Arf-like small GTPases in cilia and ciliopathies. Exp Cell Res. 2013;319(15):2316–22.

8 BBS5

BBS5 encodes one of seven Bardet-Biedl Syndrome (BBS) proteins that form the stable core of a protein complex required for ciliogenesis and that have a likely function in membrane trafficking to the primary cilium [1]. *BBS5* in particular has a possible role in regulating light-dependent translocation of arrestin1, which moves between photoreceptor inner and outer segments according to light conditions [2]. Mutations are responsible for rod-cone (86.9%) and cone-rod (13.1%) dystrophies [3] and for syndromic features associated with BBS.

BBS5 mutations are responsible for about 2–3% of autosomal recessive BBS [4–6], mostly from non-European ethnic backgrounds [7]. Mutations in *BBS5*, along with mutations in *BBS4* and *BBS8*, are particularly common in patients with BBS from the Middle East and Africa [8]. Additionally, some researchers have reported digenic triallelic inheritance of BBS, also known as the triallelic hypothesis [9–13], but, statistically, this could be simply due to the presence of rare polymorphisms or the recognized carrier frequency of mutations in these other BBS genes [12].

In a Danish study, mean age at diagnosis for BBS was 11.8 years [12]. In a study conducted in Brazil, only 21% of patients with BBS had a visual acuity above 20/40 in their better-seeing eye [3]. Night blindness is typically observed in those with BBS by age 9, and bilateral nystagmus has been observed in 26% of BBS patients, some of whom also demonstrated strabismus [3]. Central vision for those with BBS is expected to decline 1 line per year on the logMAR chart, while peripheral vision declines at 0.19 log units per year in dark-adapted environments [3]; 88% of BBS patients (from a cohort with mutations in *BBS6*, *BBS10*, or *BBS12*) are legally blind by age 18 [11]. Visual function has been seen to deteriorate with age in BBS, but the range of refractive errors has no significant trend [11]. There appears to be no statistically significant genotype-phenotype correlation for rod-cone versus cone-rod dystrophy [11].

On fundus examination, 42.8% of BBS patients show disc pallor, 67% show attenuated retinal vessels, 67% show widespread retinal epithelium abnormalities, 42.8% show macular abnormalities, and 23.8% show peripheral pigmentation [3]. Optical coherence tomography shows thinning of the photoreceptor layer, with preservation of the inner retinal lamination [11]. On ERG, scotopic rod and maximal responses were non-detectable in 91.3% of those with BBS, and cone responses were non-detectable in 65.2%. All patients who could be assessed had elevated dark-adapted visual thresholds [3].

Syndromic features of those with BBS include hyperphagia-induced obesity, intellectual disability, renal anomalies, polydactyly, and hypogenitalism [14, 15]. Other features include developmental delay, speech delay, congenital heart disease, poor coordination, hypodontia, and increased incidence of diabetes mellitus and hypertension [14, 16].

S. Zahid et al., *Retinal Dystrophy Gene Atlas*, https://doi.org/10.1007/978-3-319-10867-4_8

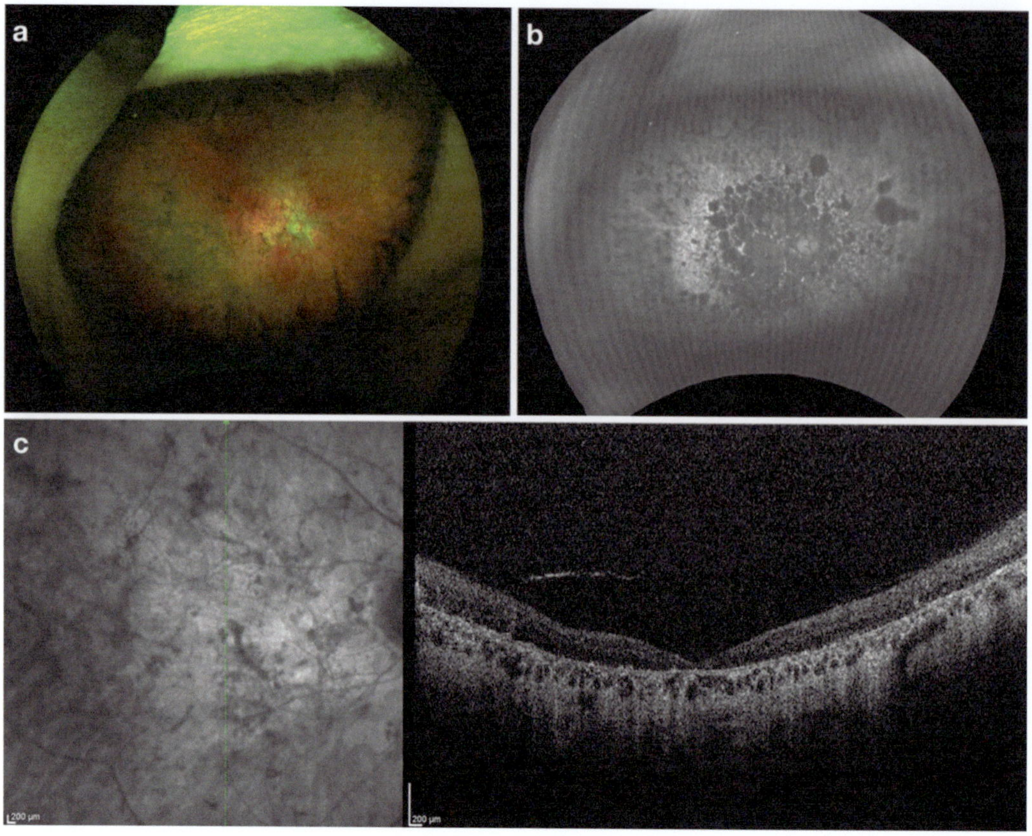

Fig. 8.1 Case summary: 42 year old man with Bardet-Biedl Syndrome. (**a**) Widefield color fundus photo of the right eye, showing diffuse retinal atrophy and pigment clumping. (**b**) Widefield fundus autofluorescence of the right eye, demonstrating patches of hypoautofluorescence in the posterior pole, with widespread mottled hypoautofluorescence throughout the retina. (**c**) Spectral Domain Optical Coherence Tomography of the right eye, showing diffuse retinal thinning, loss of the ellipsoid zone, and foveal atrophy.

References

1. Hamosh A, Tiller GE. BBS2 gene; BBS2. OMIM. 606151. 2013. http://omim.org/entry/606151. Accessed 6 Mar 2017.
2. Smith TS, Spitzbarth B, Li J, Dugger DR, Stern-Schneider G, Sehn E, et al. Light-dependent phosphorylation of Bardet-Biedl syndrome 5 in photoreceptor cells modulates its interaction with arrestin1. Cell Mol Life Sci. 2013;70(23):4603–16.
3. Berezovsky A, Rocha DM, Sacai PY, Watanabe SS, Cavascan NN, Salomão SR. Visual acuity and retinal function in patients with Bardet-Biedl syndrome. Clinics (Sao Paulo). 2012;67(2):145–9.
4. Daniels AB, Sandberg MA, Chen J, Weigel-DiFranco C, Fielding Hejtmancic J, Berson EL. Genotype-phenotype correlations in Bardet-Biedl syndrome. Arch Ophthalmol. 2012;130(7):901–7.
5. Deveault C, Billingsley G, Duncan JL, Bin J, Theal R, Vincent A, et al. BBS genotype-phenotype assessment of a multiethnic patient cohort calls for a revision of the disease definition. Hum Mutat. 2011;32(6):610–9.
6. Li JB, Gerdes JM, Haycraft CJ, Fan Y, Teslovich TM, May-Simera H, et al. Comparative genomics identifies a flagellar and basal body proteome that includes the BBS5 human disease gene. Cell. 2004;117(4):541–52.
7. Hjortshøj TD, Grønskov K, Philp AR, Nishimura DY, Adeyemo A, Rotimi CN, et al. Novel mutations in BBS5 highlight the importance of this gene in non-Caucasian Bardet-Biedl syndrome patients. Am J Med Genet A. 2008;146A(4):517–20.
8. Fattahi Z, Rostami P, Najmabadi A, Mohseni M, Kahrizi K, Akbari MR, et al. Mutation profile of BBS genes in Iranian patients with Bardet-Biedl syndrome: genetic characterization and report of nine novel mutations in five BBS genes. J Hum Genet. 2014;59(7):368–75.
9. Badano JL, Kim JC, Hoskins BE, Lewis RA, Ansley SJ, Cutler DJ, et al. Heterozygous mutations in BBS1, BBS2 and BBS6 have a potential epistatic effect on Bardet-Biedl patients with two mutations at a second BBS locus. Hum Mol Genet. 2003;12(14):1651–9.
10. Beales PL, Badano JL, Ross AJ, Ansley SJ, Hoskins BE, Kirsten B, et al. Genetic interaction of BBS1 mutations with alleles at other BBS loci can result in non-Mendelian Bardet-Biedl syndrome. Am J Hum Genet. 2003;72(5):1187–99.
11. Billingsley G, Bin J, Fieggen KJ, Duncan JL, Gerth C, Ogata K, et al. Mutations in chaperonin-like BBS genes are a major contributor to disease development in a multiethnic Bardet-Biedl syndrome patient population. J Med Genet. 2010;47(7):453–63.
12. Hjortshøj TD, Grønskov K, Philp AR, Nishimura DY, Riise R, Sheffield VC, et al. Bardet-Biedl syndrome in Denmark – report of 13 novel sequence variations in six genes. Hum Mutat. 2010;31(4):429–36.
13. Katsanis N, Ansley SJ, Badano JL, Eichers ER, Lewis RA, Hoskins BE, et al. Triallelic inheritance in Bardet-Biedl syndrome, a Mendelian recessive disorder. Science. 2001;293(5538):2256–9.
14. Xing DJ, Zhang HX, Huang N, Wu KC, Huang XF, Huang F, et al. Comprehensive molecular diagnosis of Bardet-Biedl syndrome by high-throughput targeted exome sequencing. PLoS One. 2014;9(3):e90599.
15. Zhang Q, Hu J, Ling K. Molecular views of Arf-like small GTPases in cilia and ciliopathies. Exp Cell Res. 2013;319(15):2316–22.
16. Pawlik B, Mir A, Iqbal H, Li Y, Nürnberg G, Becker C, et al. A novel familial BBS12 mutation associated with a mild phenotype: implications for clinical and molecular diagnostic strategies. Mol Syndromol. 2010;1(1):27–34.

9 BBS7

BBS7 encodes one of seven Bardet-Biedl Syndrome (BBS) proteins that form the stable core of a protein complex required for ciliogenesis and that have a likely function in membrane trafficking to the primary cilium [1]. Mutations are responsible for rod-cone (86.9%) and cone-rod (13.1%) dystrophies [2] and for syndromic features associated with BBS. Ocular features vary widely, however. In a Chinese family with *BBS7* mutations, patients were found to have macular dystrophy rather than typical retinitis pigmentosa (RP) findings [3].

BBS7 mutations are usually described as being responsible for about 2–9% of autosomal recessive Bardet-Biedl syndrome [4–8]. Additionally, some researchers have reported digenic triallelic inheritance of BBS, also known as the triallelic hypothesis [9–13], but, statistically, this could be due simply to the presence of rare polymorphisms or the recognized carrier frequency of mutations in these other BBS genes [12].

In a Danish study, mean age at diagnosis for BBS was 11.8 years [12]. In a study conducted in Brazil, only 21% of patients with Bardet-Biedl had a visual acuity above 20/40 in their better eye [2]. Night blindness is typically observed in those with BBS by age 9, and bilateral nystagmus has been observed in 26% of BBS patients, some of whom also demonstrated strabismus [2]. Central vision for those with BBS is expected to decline 1 line per year on the logMAR chart, while peripheral vision declines at 0.19 log units per year in dark-adapted environments [2]; 88% of BBS patients (from a cohort with mutations in *BBS6*, *BBS10*, or *BBS12*) are legally blind by age 18 [11]. In general, visual function has been seen to deteriorate with age in BBS, but the range of refractive errors has no significant trend. There appears to be no statistically significant genotype-phenotype correlation for rod-cone vs. cone-rod dystrophy [11].

On fundus exam, 42.8% of BBS patients show disc pallor, 67% show attenuated retinal vessels, 67% show widespread retinal epithelium abnormalities, 42.8% show macular abnormalities, and 23.8% show peripheral pigmentation [2]. In a Chinese family with BBS due to *BBS7* mutations, patients had attenuated vessels, chorioretinal atrophy and scarring, as well as optic disc pallor [3]. OCT in individuals with BBS shows thinning of the photoreceptor layer, with preservation of the inner retinal lamination [11]. It was observed that five patients from Toronto with *BBS7* mutations had reduced retinal thickness, with less preservation of retinal layers across similar age groups than patients with mutations in *BBS1* and *BBS10*, who had previously been reported [4]. On ERG, scotopic rod and maximal responses were non-detectable in 91.3% of those with BBS, and cone responses were non-detectable in 65.2%. All patients with BBS who could be assessed had elevated dark-adapted visual thresholds [2].

Syndromic features of those with Bardet-Biedl Syndrome include hyperphagia-induced obesity, intellectual disability, renal anomalies, polydactyly, and hypogenitalism [14, 15]. Other features include developmental delay, speech delay, congenital heart disease, poor coordination, hypodontia, and increased incidence of diabetes mellitus and hypertension [14, 16].

S. Zahid et al., *Retinal Dystrophy Gene Atlas*, https://doi.org/10.1007/978-3-319-10867-4_9

References

1. Hamosh A, Tiller GE. BBS2 gene; BBS2. OMIM. 606151. 2013. http://omim.org/entry/606151. Accessed 6 Mar 2017.
2. Berezovsky A, Rocha DM, Sacai PY, Watanabe SS, Cavascan NN, Salomão SR. Visual acuity and retinal function in patients with Bardet-Biedl syndrome. Clinics (Sao Paulo). 2012;67(2):145–9.
3. Yang Z, Yang Y, Zhao P, Chen K, Chen B, Lin Y, et al. A novel mutation in BBS7 gene causes Bardet-Biedl syndrome in a Chinese family. Mol Vis. 2008;14:2304–8.
4. Bin J, Madhavan J, Ferrini W, Mok CA, Billingsley G, Héon E. BBS7 and TTC8 (BBS8) mutations play a minor role in the mutational load of Bardet-Biedl syndrome in a multiethnic population. Hum Mutat. 2009;30(7):E737–46.
5. Daniels AB, Sandberg MA, Chen J, Weigel-DiFranco C, Fielding Hejtmancic J, Berson EL. Genotype-phenotype correlations in Bardet-Biedl syndrome. Arch Ophthalmol. 2012;130(7):901–7.
6. Badano JL, Ansley SJ, Leitch CC, Lewis RA, Lupski JR, Katsanis N. Identification of a novel Bardet-Biedl syndrome protein, BBS7, that shares structural features with BBS1 and BBS2. Am J Hum Genet. 2003;72(3):650–8.
7. Deveault C, Billingsley G, Duncan JL, Bin J, Theal R, Vincent A, et al. BBS genotype-phenotype assessment of a multiethnic patient cohort calls for a revision of the disease definition. Hum Mutat. 2011;32(6):610–9.
8. Fattahi Z, Rostami P, Najmabadi A, Mohseni M, Kahrizi K, Akbari MR, et al. Mutation profile of BBS genes in Iranian patients with Bardet-Biedl syndrome: genetic characterization and report of nine novel mutations in five BBS genes. J Hum Genet. 2014;59(7):368–75.
9. Badano JL, Kim JC, Hoskins BE, Lewis RA, Ansley SJ, Cutler DJ, et al. Heterozygous mutations in BBS1, BBS2 and BBS6 have a potential epistatic effect on Bardet-Biedl patients with two mutations at a second BBS locus. Hum Mol Genet. 2003;12(14):1651–9.
10. Beales PL, Badano JL, Ross AJ, Ansley SJ, Hoskins BE, Kirsten B, et al. Genetic interaction of BBS1 mutations with alleles at other BBS loci can result in non-Mendelian Bardet-Biedl syndrome. Am J Hum Genet. 2003;72(5):1187–99.
11. Billingsley G, Bin J, Fieggen KJ, Duncan JL, Gerth C, Ogata K, et al. Mutations in chaperonin-like BBS genes are a major contributor to disease development in a multiethnic Bardet-Biedl syndrome patient population. J Med Genet. 2010;47(7):453–63.
12. Hjortshøj TD, Grønskov K, Philp AR, Nishimura DY, Riise R, Sheffield VC, et al. Bardet-Biedl syndrome in Denmark – report of 13 novel sequence variations in six genes. Hum Mutat. 2010;31(4):429–36.
13. Katsanis N, Ansley SJ, Badano JL, Eichers ER, Lewis RA, Hoskins BE, et al. Triallelic inheritance in Bardet-Biedl syndrome, a Mendelian recessive disorder. Science. 2001;293(5538):2256–9.
14. Xing DJ, Zhang HX, Huang N, Wu KC, Huang XF, Huang F, et al. Comprehensive molecular diagnosis of Bardet-Biedl syndrome by high-throughput targeted exome sequencing. PLoS One. 2014;9(3):e90599.
15. Zhang Q, Hu J, Ling K. Molecular views of Arf-like small GTPases in cilia and ciliopathies. Exp Cell Res. 2013;319(15):2316–22.
16. Pawlik B, Mir A, Iqbal H, Li Y, Nürnberg G, Becker C, et al. A novel familial BBS12 mutation associated with a mild phenotype: implications for clinical and molecular diagnostic strategies. Mol Syndromol. 2010;1(1):27–34.

10 BBS9

BBS9 encodes one of seven Bardet-Biedl Syndrome (BBS) proteins that form the stable core of a protein complex required for ciliogenesis and that have a likely function in membrane trafficking to the primary cilium [1]. Mutations are responsible for rod-cone (86.9%) and cone-rod (13.1%) dystrophies [2] and for syndromic features associated with BBS.

BBS9 mutations are generally reported to be responsible for about 1–4% of autosomal recessive BBS [3, 4]. In a cohort of 14 patients with BBS in Iran, however, 14% of the patients had mutations in *BBS9* [4]. Additionally, some researchers have reported digenic triallelic inheritance of BBS, also known as the triallelic hypothesis [5–9], but, statistically, this could be due simply to the presence of rare polymorphisms or the recognized carrier frequency of mutations in these other BBS genes [8].

In a Danish study, mean age at diagnosis for BBS was 11.8 years [8]. In a study conducted in Brazil, only 21% of patients with Bardet-Biedl had a visual acuity above 20/40 in their better eye [2]. Night blindness is typically observed in those with BBS by age 9, and bilateral nystagmus has been observed in 26% of BBS patients, some of whom also demonstrated strabismus [2]. Central vision for those with BBS is expected to decline 1 line per year on the logMAR chart, while peripheral vision declines at 0.19 log units per year in dark-adapted environments [2]; about 88% of BBS patients (from a cohort with mutations in *BBS6*, *BBS10*, or *BBS12*) are legally blind by age 18 [7]. In general, visual function has been seen to deteriorate with age in BBS, but the range of refractive errors has no significant trend [7]. There appears to be no statistically significant genotype-phenotype correlation for rod-cone vs. cone-rod dystrophy [7].

On fundus exam, 42.8% of BBS patients show disc pallor, 67% show attenuated retinal vessels, 67% show widespread retinal epithelium abnormalities, 42.8% show macular abnormalities, and 23.8% show peripheral pigmentation [2]. OCT in individuals with BBS shows thinning of the photoreceptor layer, with preservation of the inner retinal lamination [7]. On ERG, scotopic rod and maximal responses were non-detectable in 91.3% of those with BBS, and cone responses were non-detectable in 65.2%. All patients with BBS who could be assessed had elevated dark-adapted visual thresholds [2].

Syndromic features of those with BBS include hyperphagia-induced obesity, intellectual disability, renal anomalies, polydactyly, and hypogenitalism [10, 11]. Other features include developmental delay, speech delay, congenital heart disease, poor coordination, hypodontia, and increased incidence of diabetes mellitus and hypertension [10, 12].

S. Zahid et al., *Retinal Dystrophy Gene Atlas*, https://doi.org/10.1007/978-3-319-10867-4_10

References

1. Hamosh A, Tiller GE. BBS2 gene; BBS2. OMIM. 606151. 2013. http://omim.org/entry/606151. Accessed 6 Mar 2017.
2. Berezovsky A, Rocha DM, Sacai PY, Watanabe SS, Cavascan NN, Salomão SR. Visual acuity and retinal function in patients with Bardet-Biedl syndrome. Clinics (Sao Paulo). 2012;67(2):145–9.
3. Deveault C, Billingsley G, Duncan JL, Bin J, Theal R, Vincent A, et al. BBS genotype-phenotype assessment of a multiethnic patient cohort calls for a revision of the disease definition. Hum Mutat. 2011;32(6):610–9.
4. Fattahi Z, Rostami P, Najmabadi A, Mohseni M, Kahrizi K, Akbari MR, et al. Mutation profile of BBS genes in Iranian patients with Bardet-Biedl syndrome: genetic characterization and report of nine novel mutations in five BBS genes. J Hum Genet. 2014;59(7):368–75.
5. Badano JL, Kim JC, Hoskins BE, Lewis RA, Ansley SJ, Cutler DJ, et al. Heterozygous mutations in BBS1, BBS2 and BBS6 have a potential epistatic effect on Bardet-Biedl patients with two mutations at a second BBS locus. Hum Mol Genet. 2003;12(14):1651–9.
6. Beales PL, Badano JL, Ross AJ, Ansley SJ, Hoskins BE, Kirsten B, et al. Genetic interaction of BBS1 mutations with alleles at other BBS loci can result in non-Mendelian Bardet-Biedl syndrome. Am J Hum Genet. 2003;72(5):1187–99.
7. Billingsley G, Bin J, Fieggen KJ, Duncan JL, Gerth C, Ogata K, et al. Mutations in chaperonin-like BBS genes are a major contributor to disease development in a multiethnic Bardet-Biedl syndrome patient population. J Med Genet. 2010;47(7):453–63.
8. Hjortshøj TD, Grønskov K, Philp AR, Nishimura DY, Riise R, Sheffield VC, et al. Bardet-Biedl syndrome in Denmark – report of 13 novel sequence variations in six genes. Hum Mutat. 2010;31(4):429–36.
9. Katsanis N, Ansley SJ, Badano JL, Eichers ER, Lewis RA, Hoskins BE, et al. Triallelic inheritance in Bardet-Biedl syndrome, a Mendelian recessive disorder. Science. 2001;293(5538):2256–9.
10. Xing DJ, Zhang HX, Huang N, Wu KC, Huang XF, Huang F, et al. Comprehensive molecular diagnosis of Bardet-Biedl syndrome by high-throughput targeted exome sequencing. PLoS One. 2014;9(3):e90599.
11. Zhang Q, Hu J, Ling K. Molecular views of Arf-like small GTPases in cilia and ciliopathies. Exp Cell Res. 2013;319(15):2316–22.
12. Pawlik B, Mir A, Iqbal H, Li Y, Nürnberg G, Becker C, et al. A novel familial BBS12 mutation associated with a mild phenotype: implications for clinical and molecular diagnostic strategies. Mol Syndromol. 2010;1(1):27–34.

11 BBS10

BBS10 encodes a protein that is part of the type II chaperonin family and that, along with *BBS12*, localizes to the basal body of primary cilia and is responsible for ciliogenesis and adipogenesis [1, 2]. Mutations are responsible for rod-cone (86.9%) and cone-rod (13.1%) dystrophies [3] and for syndromic features associated with Bardet-Biedl syndrome (BBS).

BBS10 mutations are responsible for around 20% [1, 4, 5] to 43% [6] of autosomal recessive Bardet-Biedl syndrome, which appears to have a similar frequency in families of European and Middle Eastern ancestry [4]. However, this frequency was found to be as low as 7.6% in a Spanish cohort [7]. The most common mutation in *BBS10* is a 1-bp insertion (271dupT), causing premature termination 4 codons later (C91LfsX5). This mutation accounts for about 26% [1] to 46% [4] of *BBS10* mutant alleles and is most frequent in those of European descent [4, 8], but it is also seen in Turkish and Afghan families [4]. Additionally, some researchers have reported digenic triallelic inheritance of BBS, also known as the triallelic hypothesis [1, 6, 9, 10], but, statistically, this could just be due to the presence of rare polymorphisms or the recognized carrier frequency of mutations in these other BBS genes [6]. There has also been a reported case of an individual with four mutations in *BBS10* who was shown to have a more severe phenotype overall [1]. In a Danish study, mean age at diagnosis for individuals with mutations in *BBS10* was 8.7 years [6]. In a study conducted in Brazil, only 21% of patients with Bardet-Biedl had a visual acuity above 20/40 in their better eye [3]. Night blindness is typically observed in those with BBS by age 9, and bilateral nystagmus has been observed in 26% of BBS patients, some of whom also demonstrated strabismus [3]. Central vision for those with BBS is expected to decline one line per year on the logMAR chart, while peripheral vision declines at 0.19 log units per year in dark-adapted environments [3]; about 88% of BBS patients (from a cohort with mutations in *BBS6*, *BBS10*, or *BBS12*) are legally blind by age 18 [1]. It has been claimed that the phenotype of individuals with mutations in *BBS10* is more severe and has a lower visual acuity and smaller visual field areas [11] than those with mutations in *BBS1* [1, 5, 8, 11]. Some researchers claim, however, that there is no significant genotype-phenotype correlation for BBS [3]. In general, visual function has been seen to deteriorate with age, but the range of refractive errors has no significant trend [1]. There appears to be no statistically significant genotype-phenotype correlation for rod-cone vs. cone-rod dystrophy [1]. For patients with mutations in *BBS10*, nystagmus was observed in 16 of 23 patients, and cataract (including "mild" cataract) was noted in 9 of 20 [1].

On fundus exam, 42.8% of BBS patients show disc pallor, 67% show attenuated retinal vessels, 67% show widespread retinal pigment epithelium abnormalities, 42.8% show macular abnormalities, and 23.8% show peripheral pigmentation (Fig. 11.1a–d) [3]. On OCT, those with mutations in *BBS10* and *BBS1* show preserved inner retinal layers and outer nuclear layer, disrupted IS/OS layer, thinned RPE, and reduced (but present) photoreceptor inner or outer segment layer in the foveal area (Fig. 11.1e–f) [11]. Deposits adjacent and anterior to Bruch's membrane, which could be related to retinal reorganization, are more evident in those with *BBS10* than with *BBS1* mutations [11]. Internal limiting membrane wrinkling was seen in 3 of 8 patients with *BBS10* or *BBS1* mutations [11]. On ERG, scotopic rod and maximal responses were non-detectable in 91.3% of those with BBS, and cone responses were non-detectable in 65.2%. All patients who could be assessed had elevated dark-adapted visual thresholds [3].

Syndromic features of those with Bardet-Biedl syndrome include hyperphagia-induced obesity, intellectual disability, renal anomalies, polydactyly, and hypogenitalism [12, 13]. Other features include developmental delay, speech delay, congenital heart disease, poor coordination, hypodontia, and increased incidence of diabetes mellitus and hypertension [12, 14].

S. Zahid et al., *Retinal Dystrophy Gene Atlas*, https://doi.org/10.1007/978-3-319-10867-4_11

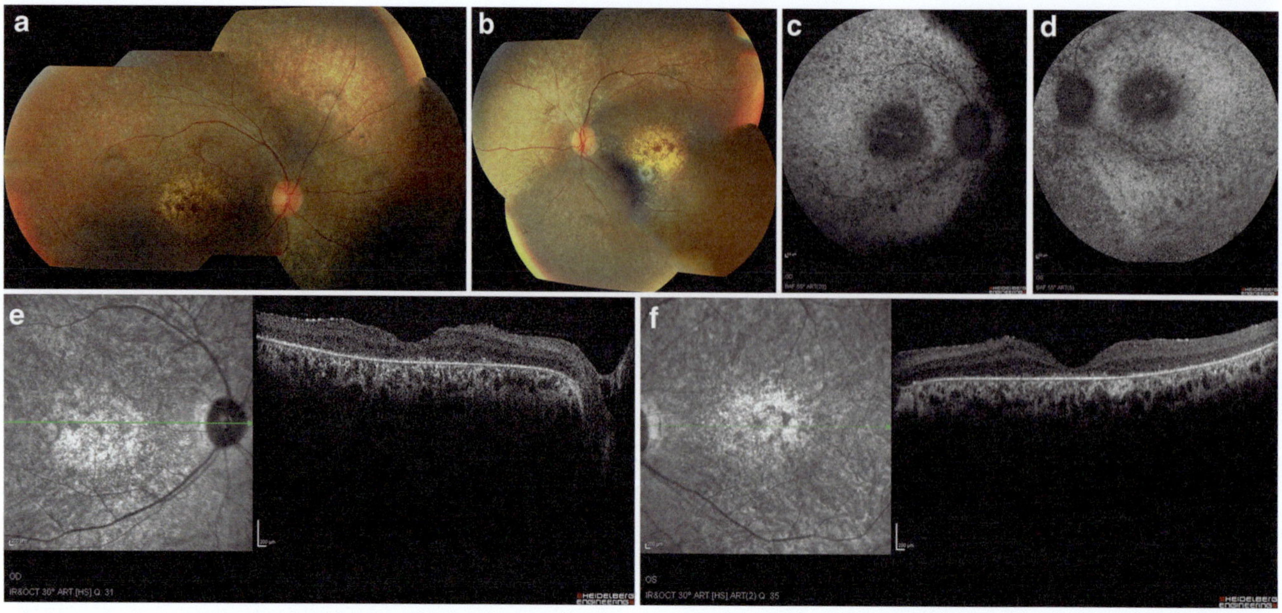

Fig. 11.1 Case Summary: 26-year-old female with Bardet-Biedl syndrome with heterozygous mutations in *BBS10* (c.899A > C; c.306delCAGA) with best-corrected visual acuity of 1/60 in both eyes. (**a**, **b**) Color fundus photos of the right and left eyes showing extensive macular atrophy with pigmentary changes and diffuse RPE dropout along the arcades and midperipheral retina with pigmentary changes. (**c**, **d**) Fundus autofluorescence of the right and left eyes showing macular and diffuse patchy areas of hypoautofluorescence corresponding to areas of atrophy. (**e**, **f**) Spectral domain optical coherence tomography of the right and left eyes showing extensive macular ellipsoid zone loss and subretinal deposits above the RPE.

References

1. Billingsley G, Bin J, Fieggen KJ, Duncan JL, Gerth C, Ogata K, et al. Mutations in chaperonin-like BBS genes are a major contributor to disease development in a multiethnic Bardet-Biedl syndrome patient population. J Med Genet. 2010;47(7):453–63.
2. Kniffin CL, VA MK. BBS10 GENE; BBS10. In:OMIM–online Mendelian inheritance in man; 2011. http://www.omim.org/entry/610148. Accessed 11 Jan 2017.
3. Berezovsky A, Rocha DM, Sacai PY, Watanabe SS, Cavascan NN, Salomão SR. Visual acuity and retinal function in patients with Bardet-Biedl syndrome. Clinics (Sao Paulo). 2012;67(2):145–9.
4. Stoetzel C, Laurier V, Davis EE, Muller J, Rix S, Badano JL, et al. BBS10 encodes a vertebrate-specific chaperonin-like protein and is a major BBS locus. Nat Genet. 2006;38(5):521–4.
5. Daniels AB, Sandberg MA, Chen J, Weigel-DiFranco C, Fielding Hejtmancic J, Berson EL. Genotype-phenotype correlations in Bardet-Biedl syndrome. Arch Ophthalmol. 2012;130(7):901–7.
6. Hjortshøj TD, Grønskov K, Philp AR, Nishimura DY, Riise R, Sheffield VC, et al. Bardet-Biedl syndrome in Denmark – report of 13 novel sequence variations in six genes. Hum Mutat. 2010;31(4):429–36.
7. Alvarez-Satta M, Castro-Sánchez S, Pereiro I, Piñeiro-Gallego T, Baiget M, Ayuso C, et al. Overview of Bardet-Biedl syndrome in Spain: identification of novel mutations in BBS1, BBS10 and BBS12 genes. Clin Genet. 2014;89(6):601–2.
8. Deveault C, Billingsley G, Duncan JL, Bin J, Theal R, Vincent A, et al. BBS genotype-phenotype assessment of a multiethnic patient cohort calls for a revision of the disease definition. Hum Mutat. 2011;32(6):610–9.
9. Badano JL, Kim JC, Hoskins BE, Lewis RA, Ansley SJ, Cutler DJ, et al. Heterozygous mutations in BBS1, BBS2 and BBS6 have a potential epistatic effect on Bardet-Biedl patients with two mutations at a second BBS locus. Hum Mol Genet. 2003;12(14):1651–9.
10. Beales PL, Badano JL, Ross AJ, Ansley SJ, Hoskins BE, Kirsten B. Genetic interaction of BBS1 mutations with alleles at other BBS loci can result in non-Mendelian Bardet-Biedl syndrome. Am J Hum Genet. 2003;72(5):1187–99.
11. Gerth C, Zawadzki RJ, Werner JS, Héon E. Retinal morphology in patients with BBS1 and BBS10 related Bardet-Biedl syndrome evaluated by Fourier-domain optical coherence tomography. Vis Res. 2008;48(3):392–9.
12. Xing DJ, Zhang HX, Huang N, KC W, Huang XF, Huang F, et al. Comprehensive molecular diagnosis of Bardet-Biedl syndrome by high-throughput targeted exome sequencing. PLoS One. 2014;9(3):e90599.
13. Zhang Q, Hu J, Ling K. Molecular views of Arf-like small GTPases in cilia and ciliopathies. Exp Cell Res. 2013;319(15):2316–22.
14. Pawlik B, Mir A, Iqbal H, Li Y, Nürnberg G, Becker C, et al. A novel familial BBS12 mutation associated with a mild phenotype: implications for clinical and molecular diagnostic strategies. Mol Syndromol. 2010;1(1):27–34.

12 BBS12

BBS12 encodes a protein that is part of the chaperonin family and that, along with BBS10, localizes to the basal body of primary cilia and is responsible for ciliogenesis and adipogenesis [1, 2]. Mutations are responsible for rod-cone (86.9%) and cone-rod (13.1%) dystrophies [3] and for syndromic features associated with Bardet-Biedl syndrome (BBS).

BBS12 mutations are responsible for about 3–11% [1, 4–7] of autosomal recessive Bardet-Biedl syndrome. A study conducted in France and the US showed most of these families to be Caucasian [7], while a study conducted in Canada showed most of them to be of non-European ancestry [1]. A study of 14 Iranian families with BBS reported the prevalence of mutations in *BBS12* to be as high as 21.4% [8]. Additionally, some researchers have reported digenic triallelic inheritance of BBS, also known as the triallelic hypothesis [1, 6, 9, 10], although statistically, this could just be due to the presence of rare polymorphisms or the recognized carrier frequency of mutations in these other BBS genes [6]. It also appears that *BBS12* is rarely a partner in digenic inheritance [11]. In a Danish study, mean age at diagnosis for BBS was 11.8 years [6]. In a study conducted in Brazil, only 21% of patients with Bardet-Biedl had a visual acuity above 20/40 in their better eye [3]. Night blindness (nyctalopia) is generally observed in those with BBS by age 9, and bilateral nystagmus has been observed in 26% of BBS patients, some of whom also demonstrated strabismus [3]. Central vision for those with BBS is expected to decline one line per year on the logMAR chart, while peripheral vision declines at 0.19 log units per year in dark-adapted environments [3]; about 88% of BBS patients (from a cohort with mutations in *BBS6*, *BBS10*, or *BBS12*) are legally blind by age 18 [1]. It has been claimed that the phenotype of individuals with mutations in *BBS12* and *BBS10* have a more rapid progression of visual loss than those with mutations in *BBS6* [1], but it has also been claimed those with mutations in *BBS12* and *BBS1* have a milder phenotype than those with *BBS10* mutations [12]. Some researchers claim, however, that there are no significant genotype-phenotype correlations for BBS [3, 7]. In general, visual function has been seen to deteriorate with age in BBS, but the range of refractive errors has no significant trend [1]. There appears to be no statistically significant genotype-phenotype correlation for rod-cone vs. cone-rod dystrophy [1].

On fundus exam, 42.8% of BBS patients show disc pallor, 67% show attenuated retinal vessels, 67% show widespread retinal pigment epithelium abnormalities, 42.8% show macular abnormalities, and 23.8% show peripheral pigmentation [3] (Fig. 12.1a–d). OCT shows thinning of the photoreceptor layer, with preservation of the inner retinal lamination [1] (Fig. 12.1e–f). On ERG, scotopic rod and maximal responses were non-detectable in 91.3% of those with BBS, and cone responses were non-detectable in 65.2%. All patients who could be assessed had elevated dark-adapted visual thresholds [3].

Syndromic features of those with Bardet-Biedl syndrome include hyperphagia-induced obesity, intellectual disability, renal anomalies, polydactyly, and hypogenitalism [13, 14]. Other features include developmental delay, speech delay, congenital heart disease, poor coordination, hypodontia, and increased incidence of diabetes mellitus and hypertension [13, 15].

There has been a report of three individuals who carried the homozygous mutation p.S701X in the *BBS12* gene, which is closer to the C-terminal end of the encoded protein than any other reported pathogenic mutations in *BBS12* [15]. These patients were siblings from a consanguineous Pakistani family who exhibited a milder phenotype for BBS, showing only postaxial polydactyly, hypodontia, and late-onset retinal dysfunction; with no renal or genital anomalies, obesity, learning disability, or other symptoms of BBS. Night blindness for these patients began at age 13–15, while daytime vision was only mildly impaired by the ages of 30, 27, and 19. All three exhibited rod-cone dystrophy, myopia, and astigmatism, and none of them met clinical diagnostic criteria for BBS [15].

S. Zahid et al., *Retinal Dystrophy Gene Atlas*, https://doi.org/10.1007/978-3-319-10867-4_12

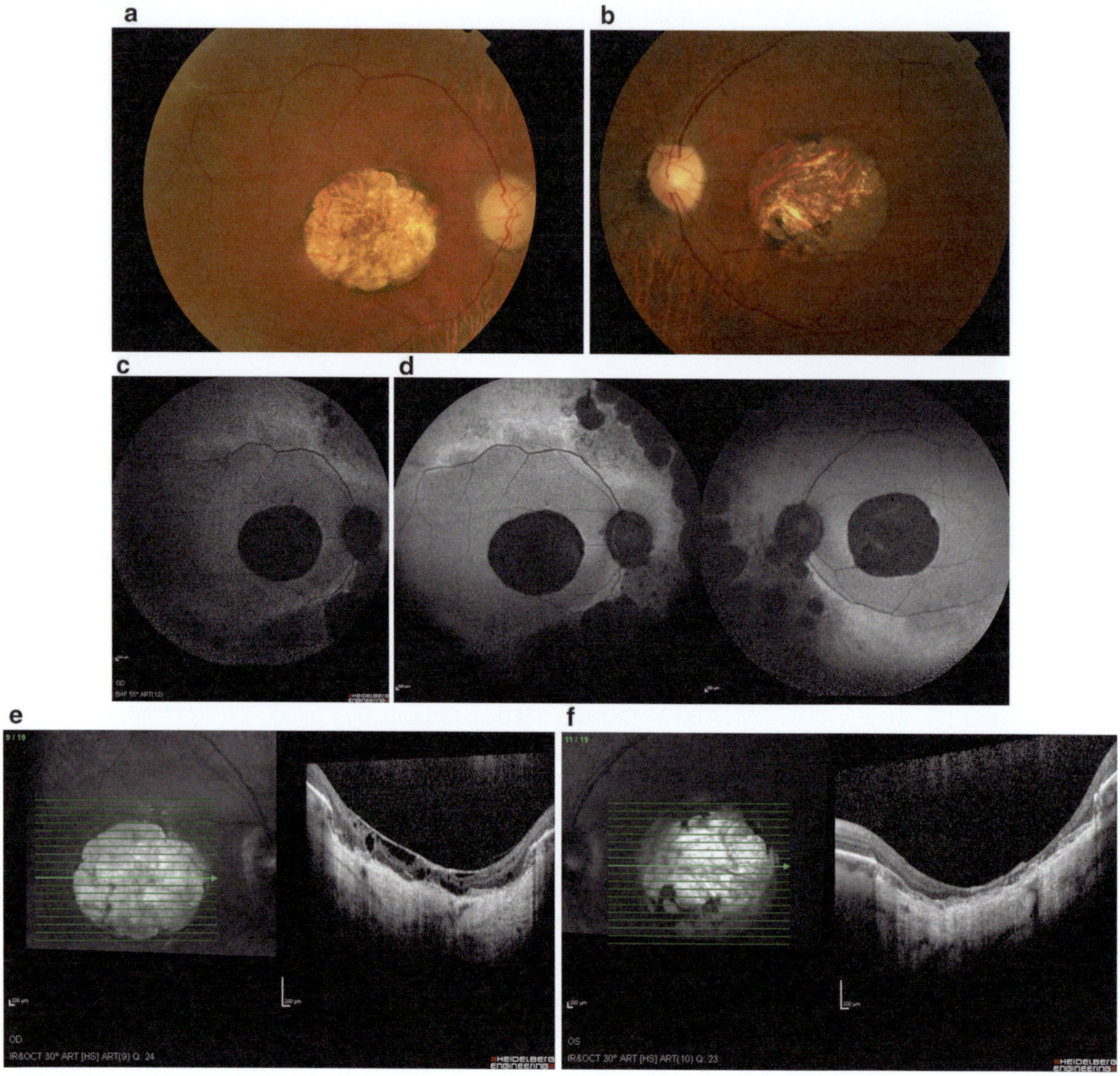

Fig. 12.1 Case summary: 51-year-old male with Bardet-Biedl syndrome with homozygous mutations in *BBS12* (c.1418_1420del) with best-corrected visual acuity of 2/60 in the right eye and 3/20 in the left eye. (**a**, **b**) Color fundus photographs of the right and left eyes showing large circular areas of chorioretinal atrophy limited to the central maculae in both eyes. Retinal pigment epithelium atrophy is also apparent in areas along the arcades in both eyes. (**c**, **d**) Fundus autofluorescence of the right and left eyes showing circular areas of hypoautofluorescence in the macula and outside the arcades in both eyes, corresponding to areas of RPE/photoreceptor atrophy. There are also areas of hyperautofluorescence along the arcades in both eyes in areas without atrophy. In the right eye, there is progression of atrophy demonstrated along the superior arcades, with the areas of hypoautofluorescence extending to areas that were previously hyperautofluorescent. (**e**, **f**) Spectral domain optical coherence tomography of the right and left eyes showing profound RPE and ellipsoid zone atrophy with areas of scarring in both eyes, and showing inner retinal cystic cavities and an epiretinal membrane in the right eye.

References

1. Billingsley G, Bin J, Fieggen KJ, Duncan JL, Gerth C, Ogata K, et al. Mutations in chaperonin-like BBS genes are a major contributor to disease development in a multiethnic Bardet-Biedl syndrome patient population. J Med Genet. 2010;47(7):453–63.
2. Kniffin CL, VA MK. BBS10 GENE; BBS10. In:OMIM–online Mendelian inheritance in man; 2011. http://www.omim.org/entry/610148. Accessed 11 Jan 2017.
3. Berezovsky A, Rocha DM, Sacai PY, Watanabe SS, Cavascan NN, Salomão SR. Visual acuity and retinal function in patients with Bardet-Biedl syndrome. Clinics (Sao Paulo). 2012;67(2):145–9.
4. Alvarez-Satta M, Castro-Sánchez S, Pereiro I, Piñeiro-Gallego T, Baiget M, Ayuso C, et al. Overview of Bardet-Biedl syndrome

in Spain: identification of novel mutations in BBS1, BBS10 and BBS12 genes. Clin Genet. 2014;89(6):601–2.
5. Daniels AB, Sandberg MA, Chen J, Weigel-DiFranco. C, Fielding Hejtmancic J, Berson EL. Genotype-phenotype correlations in Bardet-Biedl syndrome. Arch Ophthalmol. 2012;130(7):901–7.
6. Hjortshøj TD, Grønskov K, Philp AR, Nishimura DY, Riise R, Sheffield VC, et al. Bardet-Biedl syndrome in Denmark – report of 13 novel sequence variations in six genes. Hum Mutat. 2010;31(4):429–36.
7. Stoetzel C, Muller J, Laurier V, Davis EE, Zaghloul NA, Vicaire S, et al. Identification of a novel BBS gene (BBS12) highlights the major role of a vertebrate-specific branch of chaperonin-related proteins in Bardet-Biedl syndrome. Am J Hum Genet. 2007;80(1):1–11.
8. Fattahi Z, Rostami P, Najmabadi A, Mohseni M, Kahrizi K, Akbari MR, et al. Mutation profile of BBS genes in Iranian patients with Bardet-Biedl syndrome: genetic characterization and report of nine novel mutations in five BBS genes. J Hum Genet. 2014;59(7):368–75.
9. Badano JL, Kim JC, Hoskins BE, Lewis RA, Ansley SJ, Cutler DJ, et al. Heterozygous mutations in BBS1, BBS2 and BBS6 have a potential epistatic effect on Bardet-Biedl patients with two mutations at a second BBS locus. Hum Mol Genet. 2003;12(14):1651–9.
10. Beales PL, Badano JL, Ross AJ, Ansley SJ, Hoskins BE, Kirsten B. Genetic interaction of BBS1 mutations with alleles at other BBS loci can result in non-Mendelian Bardet-Biedl syndrome. Am J Hum Genet. 2003;72(5):1187–99.
11. Dulfer E, Hoefsloot LH, Timmer A, Mom C, van Essen AJ. Two sibs with Bardet-Biedl syndrome due to mutations in BBS12: no clues for modulation by a third mutation in BBS10. Am J Med Genet A. 2010;152A(10):2666–9.
12. Deveault C, Billingsley G, Duncan JL, Bin J, Theal R, Vincent A, et al. BBS genotype-phenotype assessment of a multiethnic patient cohort calls for a revision of the disease definition. Hum Mutat. 2011;32(6):610–9.
13. Xing DJ, Zhang HX, Huang N, Wu KC, Huang XF, Huang F, et al. Comprehensive molecular diagnosis of Bardet-Biedl syndrome by high-throughput targeted exome sequencing. PLoS One. 2014;9(3):e90599.
14. Zhang Q, Hu J, Ling K. Molecular views of Arf-like small GTPases in cilia and ciliopathies. Exp Cell Res. 2013;319(15):2316–22.
15. Pawlik B, Mir A, Iqbal H, Li Y, Nürnberg G, Becker C, et al. A novel familial BBS12 mutation associated with a mild phenotype: implications for clinical and molecular diagnostic strategies. Mol Syndromol. 2010;1(1):27–34.

13 *BEST1*

BEST1 encodes bestrophin-1, a Ca^{2+}-dependent protein in the RPE. Mutations in *BEST1* cause dominant Best vitelliform macular dystrophy (BVMD), adult-onset foveomacular vitelliform dystrophy (AOFVD), autosomal dominant vitreoretinochoroidopathy (ADVRC), microcornea, rod-cone dystrophy, cataract, posterior staphyloma (MRCS) syndrome, and autosomal recessive bestrophinopathy (ARB) [1].

BVMD is an autosomal-dominant macular dystrophy that presents with reduced visual acuity, metamorphopsia, photophobia, or night blindness, with an age of onset ranging from early childhood to the sixties (mean 33 years) [1]. Hyperopia is very common. Visual acuity gradually declines with age, especially during the vitelliform disease stages, but may remain stable in some patients for many years. Choroidal neovascularization (CNV), which may result in a more rapid reduction of visual acuity, has been reported to occur in up to 9% of patients with BVMD and usually occurs in the context of scarring (Fig. 13.1a–b). CNV typically responds to conventional anti-VEGF treatments.

The fundus exhibits classical stages as depicted, beginning with normal to slightly altered macular RPE changes (pre-vitelliform stage), and then progressing to a characteristic "egg-yolk" macular lesion (Fig. 13.2a), which then becomes "scrambled" in the subsequent stage (Figs. 13.3 and 13.4a). Thereafter, there is a "pseudohypopyon" stage that exhibits a fluid level containing yellow material inferiorly, which is followed by atrophy and scarring of the choroid and retina. There was previously thought to be a linear progression between these stages, but there is evidence that patients can progress and regress between stages, and they often exhibit two different stages in each eye; there may even be variable stages represented within a single lesion. There have been reports of patients in the final scarred stage who maintain good visual acuity [2].

In early stages of disease, fluorescein angiography reveals hypofluorescence due to the vitelliform lesion obstructing the choroidal signal, while later stages of disease are characterized by hyperfluorescence in areas of atrophy, which manifest as window defects. Fundus autofluorescence (FAF) reveals a high intensity signal in the areas where yellowish fundoscopic lesions are located (Figs. 13.2b and 13.4b); the inferior yellow material-filled region of the pseudohypopyon lesion is usually hyperautofluorescent on FAF. As with AMD, this progresses to well-defined hypofluorescence in the atrophic stages.

The earliest OCT finding is thickening of the photoreceptor outer segments, which can be observed to elongate during light adaption. Later OCT findings, including scars and CNV, are characterized by hyperreflective sub-retinal material and occasional sub-RPE deposits (Fig. 13.2c) [3]. As the disease progresses, the subretinal material often partially liquefies and becomes hyporeflective on OCT. In the final stages, OCT demonstrates central retinal atrophy.

The electro-oculogram (EOG), a measure of the ocular standing potential, is abnormal, with an Arden ratio less than 1.5. This can be abnormal even before patients exhibit any fundoscopic signs of disease. The reduction in the light peak of the EOG is due to the mutant Bestrophin (expressed in both and macular and peripheral RPE) having an abnormal large scale voltage-gated chloride channel conductance in the RPE [4]. However, there have also been reports of several patients with BVMD with normal EOGs. Full-field ERG and dark adaptation are usually normal, while multifocal ERG is usually abnormal. One study, which used multifocal ERG in the context of subretinal fluid, has shown that the extent of structural abnormalities correlates with the extent of functional abnormalities [5].

Of note, some mutations have been reported to exhibit a more rapid decline in visual acuity than others [1]. Genotype-phenotype correlations have been challenging, given extensive intra- and interfamilial phenotypic variability [1, 6–10]. There has also been a report of a patient with a homozygous dominant mutation and a more severe phenotype, with early reduction of rod ERG parameters and a multifocal vitelliform retinopathy [11].

Null *BEST1* mutations carried in the homozygous or compound heterozygous states cause autosomal recessive

S. Zahid et al., *Retinal Dystrophy Gene Atlas*, https://doi.org/10.1007/978-3-319-10867-4_13

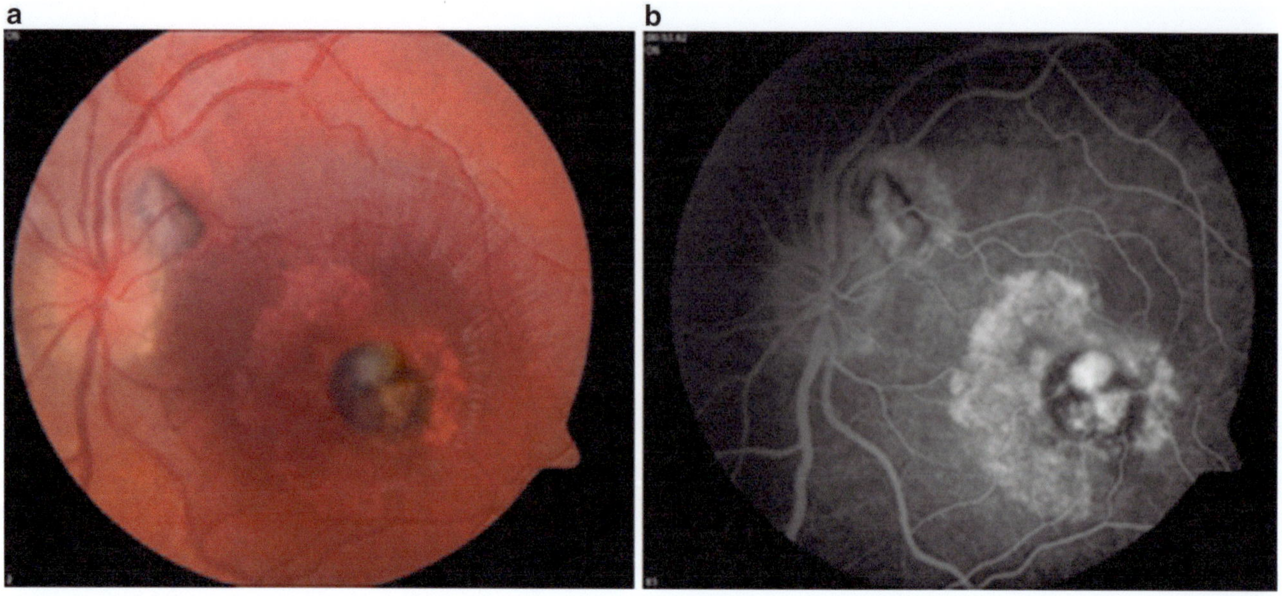

Fig. 13.1 Case summary: 8-year-old with Best disease. (**a**) Color fundus photograph of the left eye showing two pigmented lesions, one near the fovea and another superotemporal to the optic nerve. The central lesion represents choroidal neovascularization, is surrounded by RPE depigmentation, and appears to be elevated. (**b**) Late-phase fluorescein angiography of the left eye showing leakage at the neovascular membrane in the central macula, and window defects with staining surrounding the lesion.

bestrophinopathy (ARB), in which patients present at an average age of 23 years (range 4–40 years) with central vision deficits, hyperopia, and shallow anterior chambers [12]. These patients are at elevated risk of developing angle-closure glaucoma due to their shallow anterior chamber anatomy. Fundus findings include central RPE changes with vitelliform deposits, edema, and subretinal fluid. EOG, pattern ERG, multifocal ERG, and full-field ERG are all usually abnormal. FFA reveals patchy areas of hyper- and hypofluorescence corresponding to areas of atrophy and edema, while FAF shows areas of increased signal, with lipofuscin accumulation and decreased signal in areas of atrophy. Carriers of mutations associated with autosomal recessive bestrophinopathy are completely normal. There have been reports of some patients with biallelic mutations in *BEST1* who exhibit a BVMD phenotype rather than recessive bestrophinopathy [13].

BEST1 mutations may also cause a proportion of AOFVD, a subtype of pattern dystrophy, with an average age of onset of reduced visual acuity and metamorphopsia in the fifties. Visual acuity may remain stable or progressively deteriorate with time, depending on foveal atrophy or CNV (up to 15%). The characteristic fundoscopic lesion is round and yellow/white with a pigmented spot in the fovea bilaterally; the size of the lesion is variable, but it is usually smaller than the optic disc. The lesion may appear similar to the lesions seen in the spectrum of BVMD (vitelliform "egg-yolk" lesion >1DD), and there may be multiple lesions in the same eye. EOG and full-field ERG are typically normal or mildly reduced, whereas multifocal ERG reveals central dysfunction. Color vision may be abnormal, and central scotoma may be present in up to half of patients [16]. Fluorescein angiography usually reveals blockage of fluorescence at the lesion, but, some may exhibit areas of patchy increased signal. FAF patterns seen in AFVD are variable. One study has shown that reduced foveal OCT cross-sectional thickness correlates with worse visual acuity [14]. Some studies have suggested that AOFVD caused by *BEST1* mutations may actually just be a milder form of BVMD, given the later average age of onset and better visual acuity early in the disease course [15, 16].

BEST1 mutations also cause ADVIRC. This disease can present with rotary nystagmus, cataracts (usually at a young age and often posterior subcapsular), hyperopia, shallow anterior chamber, and nanophthalmos, and many patients develop angle-closure glaucoma. Fundus findings are characterized by circumferential dark pigmentary deposits that start in the peripheral retina and progress inwards, chorioretinal atrophy surrounding the disc and in the mid-periphery, white punctate deposits, and fibrillar degenerative vitreous strands; retinal vascular attenuation and disc pallor may also be observed [17, 18].

Visual acuity is generally stable throughout life, given the macular sparing, but it may deteriorate in patients who develop macular edema, central macular atrophy, retinal detachment, or vitreous hemorrhage. EOG and full-field ERG are usually abnormal, displaying loss of rod and cone function, although both of these modalities have been

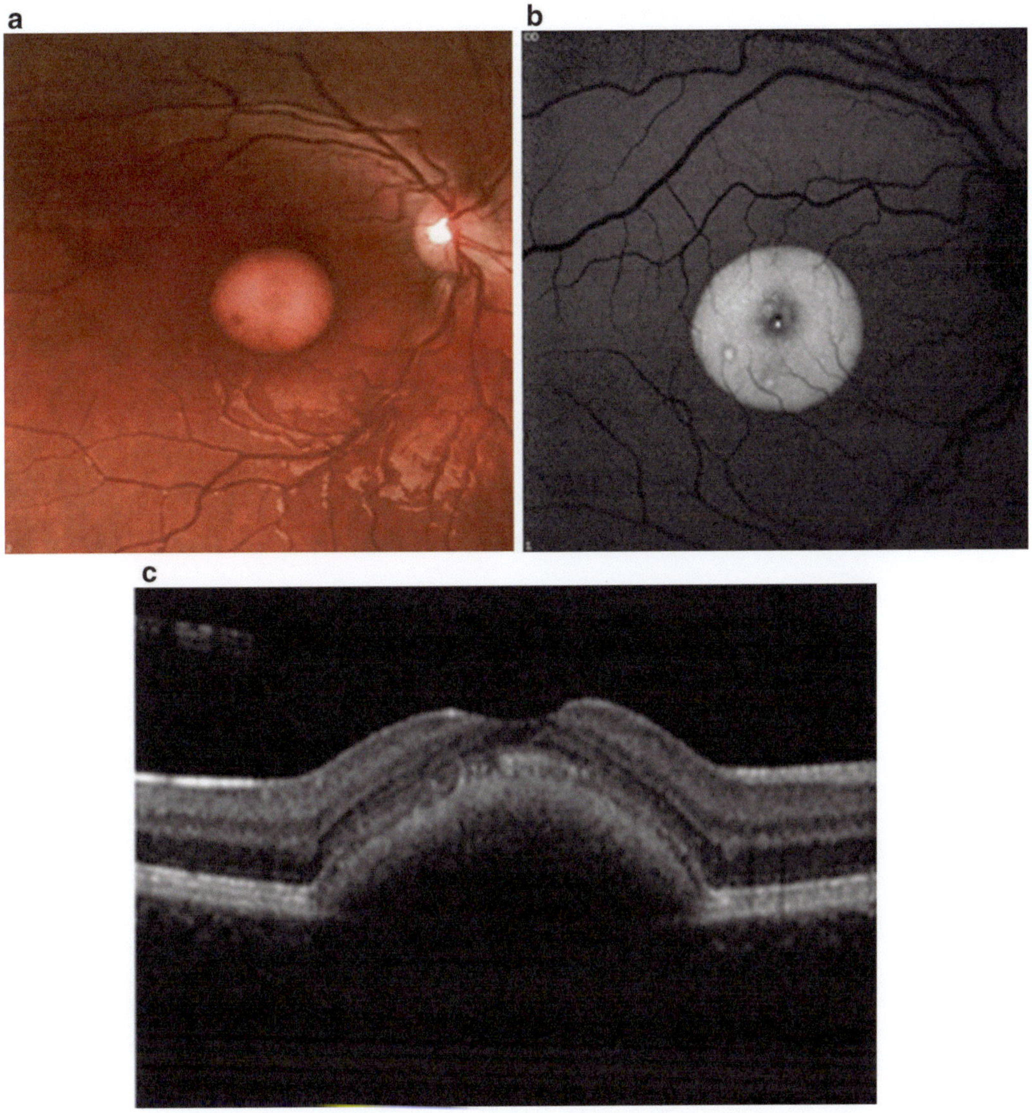

Fig. 13.2 Case summary: 7-year-old girl with Best disease. (**a**) Color fundus photograph of the right eye showing a classic egg yolk vitelliform lesion in the macula. (**b**) Fundus autofluorescence of the right eye showing hyperautofluorescence within the classic egg yolk vitelliform lesion. (**c**) Spectral domain optical coherence tomography of the right eye showing the extent of the vitelliform lesion in the subretinal space with disruption of the ellipsoid zone and shadowing posteriorly to the lesion.

reported to be within normal limits in some patients. As in rod-cone dystrophy, the GVF reveals a gradually constricting peripheral field.

MRCS syndrome is caused by mutations in *BEST1* and is characterized by microcornea, rod-cone dystrophy, cataract, and staphyloma [19]. Some patients experience night blindness as the initial symptom, and visual acuity usually declines after the third decade due to a combination of cataracts and photoreceptor dysfunction. Posterior staphyloma with normal ocular axial lengths and pulverulent cataracts at a young age are both very common. Fundus features include peripheral atrophy and pigment deposits that progress centrally with age. Full-field ERG reveals a rod-cone pattern of degeneration, and the EOG is invariably abnormal. Some studies have suggested that MRCS syndrome is on a spectrum of disease with ADVIRC, given reports of some patients in a family carrying an MRCS-associated mutation exhibiting nanophthalmos without posterior staphyloma. Mutations affecting splicing are associated with ADVIRC and MRCS.

Of note, there has also been a case series showing an association between *BEST1* mutations and retinoschisis in two siblings [20]. In these cases, patients presented with blurry vision and reduced visual acuity during childhood. Fundoscopy and OCT revealed retinoschisis, serous retinal detachments, and increased retinal thickness, while FFA demonstrated hyperfluorescent spots in the retina, and full-field ERG parameters were within normal limits.

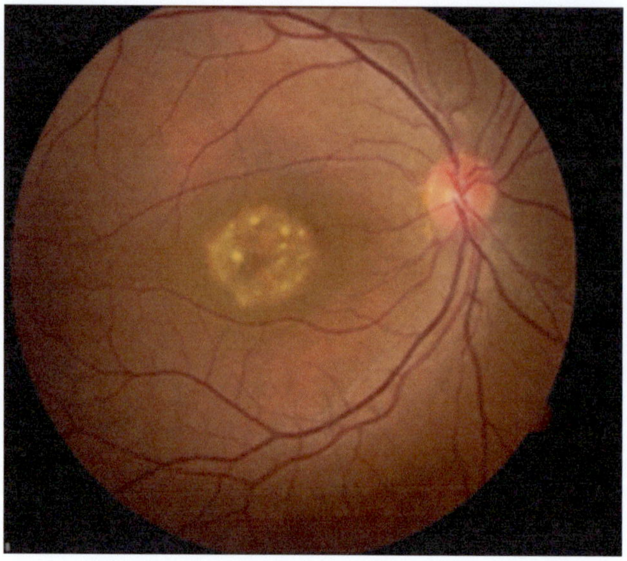

Fig. 13.3 Color fundus photograph of the right eye from a 34-year-old women with Best disease showing the vitelleruptive (scrambled egg appearance) phase.

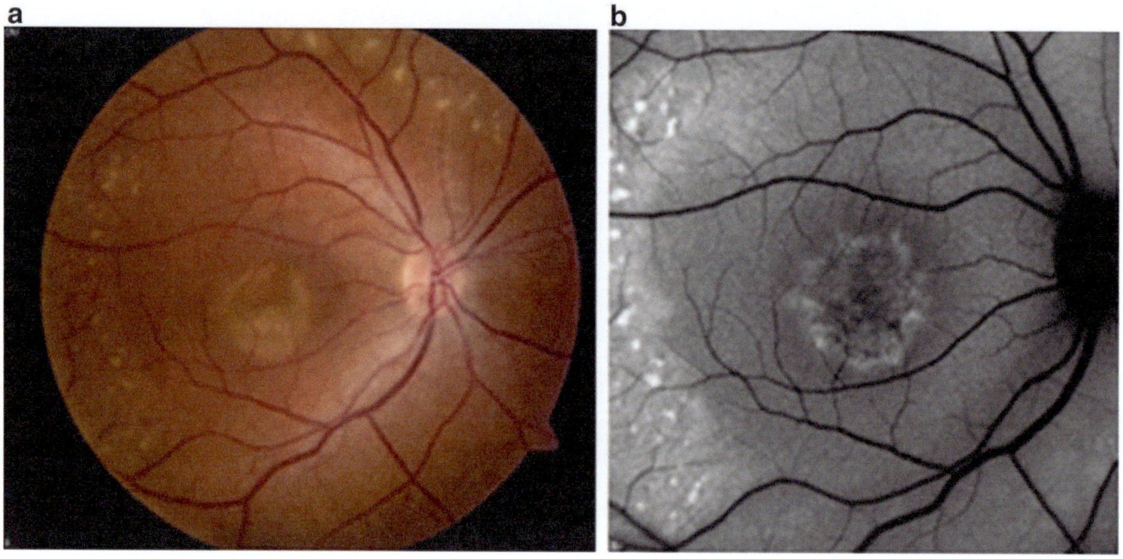

Fig. 13.4 Case summary: 37-year-old woman with homozygous null alleles in *BEST1*. (**a**) Color fundus photograph of the right eye showing macular atrophy and patchy RPE atrophy associated with a vitelliform lesion with fleck-like deposits in the temporal macula and outside the vascular arcades (superiorly). (**b**) Fundus autofluorescence of the right eye showing a ring of hyperautofluorescence surrounding patchy hypofluorescent patches. The fleck-like deposits shown in (a) are also hyperautofluorescent.

References

1. Boon CJF, Klevering BJ, Leroy BP, Hoyng CB, Keunen JEE, den Hollander AI. The spectrum of ocular phenotypes caused by mutations in the BEST1 gene. Prog Retin Eye Res. 2009;28(3):187–205.
2. Mohler CW, Fine SL. Long-term evaluation of patients with Best's vitelliform dystrophy. Ophthalmology. 1981;88(7):688–92.
3. Kay CN, Abramoff MD, Mullins RF, Kinnick TR, Lee K, Eyestone ME, et al. Three-dimensional distribution of the vitelliform lesion, photoreceptors, and retinal pigment epithelium in the macula of patients with best vitelliform macular dystrophy. Arch Ophthalmol. 2012;130(3):357–64.
4. Abramoff MD, Mullins RF, Lee K, Hoffmann JM, Sonka M, Critser DB, et al. Human photoreceptor outer segments shorten during light adaptation. Invest Ophthalmol Vis Sci. 2013;54(5):3721–8.
5. Bitner H, Schatz P, Mizrahi-Meissonnier L, Sharon D, Rosenberg T. Frequency, Genotype, and Clinical Spectrum of Best Vitelliform Macular Dystrophy: Data From a National Center in Denmark. Am J Ophthalmol. 2012;154(2):403–12.e404.

6. Querques G, Zerbib J, Santacroce R, Margaglione M, Delphin N, Rozet JM, et al. Functional and clinical data of Best vitelliform macular dystrophy patients with mutations in the BEST1 gene. Mol Vis. 2009;15:2960–72.
7. Cohn AC, Turnbull C, Ruddle JB, Guymer RH, Kearns LS, Staffieri S, et al. Best's macular dystrophy in Australia: phenotypic profile and identification of novel BEST1 mutations. Eye (Lond). 2010;25(2):208–17.
8. Lacassagne E, Dhuez A, Rigaudiere F, Dansault A, Vêtu C, Bigot K, et al. Phenotypic variability in a French family with a novel mutation in the BEST1 gene causing multifocal best vitelliform macular dystrophy. Mol Vis. 2011;17:309–22.
9. Pineiro-Gallego T, Alvarez M, Pereiro I, Campos S, Sharon D, Schatz P, et al. Clinical evaluation of two consanguineous families with homozygous mutations in BEST1. Mol Vis. 2011;17:1607–17.
10. Sohn EH, Francis PJ, Duncan JL, Weleber RG, Saperstein DA, Farrell DF, et al. Phenotypic variability due to a novel Glu292Lys variation in exon 8 of the BEST1 gene causing best macular dystrophy. Arch Ophthalmol. 2009;127(7):913–20.
11. Schatz P, Bitner H, Sander B, Holfort S, Andreasson S, Larsen M, et al. Evaluation of macular structure and function by OCT and electrophysiology in patients with vitelliform macular dystrophy due to mutations in BEST1. Invest Ophthalmol Vis Sci. 2010;51(9):4754–65.
12. Burgess R, Millar ID, Leroy BP, Urquhart JE, Fearon IM, De Baere E, et al. Biallelic mutation of BEST1 causes a distinct retinopathy in humans. Am J Hum Genet. 2008;82(1):19–31.
13. Sodi A, Menchini F, Manitto MP, Passerini I, Murro V, Torricelli F, et al. Ocular phenotypes associated with biallelic mutations in BEST1 in Italian patients. Mol Vis. 2011;17:3078–87.
14. Querques G, Bux AV, Prato R, Iaculli C, Souied EH, Delle Noci N. Correlation of visual function impairment and optical coherence tomography findings in patients with adult-onset foveomacular vitelliform macular dystrophy. Am J Ophthalmol. 2008;146(1):135–42.
15. Glacet-Bernard A, Soubrane G, Coscas G. Macular vitelliform degeneration in adults. Retrospective study of a series of 85 patients. J Fr Ophtalmol. 1990;13(8–9):407–20.
16. Renner AB, Tillack H, Kraus H, Kohl S, Wissinger B, Mohr N, et al. Morphology and functional characteristics in adult vitelliform macular dystrophy. Retina. 2004;24(6):929–39.
17. Lafaut BA, Loeys B, Leroy BP, Spileers W, De Laey JJ, Kestelyn P. Clinical and electrophysiological findings in autosomal dominant vitreoretinochoroidopathy: report of a new pedigree. Graefes Arch Clin Exp Ophthalmol. 2001;239(8):575–82.
18. Yardley J, Leroy BP, Hart-Holden N, Lafaut BA, Loeys B, Messiaen LM, et al. Mutations of VMD2 splicing regulators cause nanophthalmos and autosomal dominant vitreoretinochoroidopathy (ADVIRC). Invest Ophthalmol Vis Sci. 2004;45(10):3683–9.
19. Reddy MA, Francis PJ, Berry V, Bradshaw K, Patel RJ, Maher ER, et al. A clinical and molecular genetic study of a rare dominantly inherited syndrome (MRCS) comprising of microcornea, rod-cone dystrophy, cataract, and posterior staphyloma. Br J Ophthalmol. 2003;87(2):197–202.
20. Silva RA, Berrocal AM, Lam BL, Albini TA. Novel Mutation in BEST1 Associated With Retinoschisis. JAMA Ophthalmol. 2013;9:1–5.

CACNA1F

14

CACNA1F encodes a voltage-dependent calcium channel involved in signal transmission from rod and cone photoreceptors to the inner retina [1]. Mutations are X-linked and have been reported to cause 55% of congenital stationary night blindness (CSNB). They have also been associated with cone-rod dystrophy, Aland Eye Disease, and retinal and optic disc atrophy [2–7].

Patients with CSNB present in the first decade with nystagmus (52%) or at a later age with reduced visual acuity (range 20/30–20/200), night blindness (observed in only 39% of patients), low-to-moderate myopia, abnormal color vision (normal, tritan, or non-specific), and strabismus (24%) [8]. The fundus is usually normal, but myopic degeneration can be seen in patients with high myopia (Figs. 14.1 and 14.2a). ERG reveals a characteristic negative ERG, in which the b-wave to a-wave ratio is less than 1 for the bright flash scotopic b-wave (Fig. 14.2b). Unlike patients with mutations in *NYX,* patients with *CACNA1F* mutations often demonstrate some preservation of the dim scotopic b-wave (giving rise to the term "incomplete CSNB"), and not all patients with *CACNA1F* mutations exhibit a negative ERG (75% in some studies) [8]. The flicker amplitude is often reduced, although not extinguished, and it can exhibit a double-peaked wave [2].

Cone-rod dystrophy caused by mutations in *CACNA1F* may present in childhood or adulthood [9, 10]. Patients present with reduced visual acuity (20/40–20/300), central scotomata, and color vision defects (protan defects or normal color vision is also possible). Myopia is commonly observed; nystagmus is uncommon. ERG reveals reduced flicker amplitudes and may exhibit a negative ERG. The fundus is often normal, but there may be myopic degeneration in patients with high myopia.

Mutations in *CACNA1F* can also cause Aland Eye Disease, which is characterized by a hypopigmented fundus, reduced visual acuity secondary to foveal hypoplasia, nystagmus, and color vision deficits (often protan) [5]. It has been described as a stationary disease except for the progressive myopia. ERG reveals defects in both rods and cones.

Nakamura et al. have also reported a unique phenotype caused by mutations in *CACNA1F* [6]. These patients experience progressively deteriorating visual acuity and visual fields that correspond to funduscopic evidence of retinal and optic disc atrophy with attenuated retinal vessels. GVF may show central scotomata and visual field constriction. ERG has been reported to reveal a negative waveform, but it generally shows more severe and diffuse retinal dysfunction than is typically patients with CSNB as described above. The same mutations that cause this unique phenotype may also cause CSNB, illustrating the phenotypic variability associated with *CACNA1F* mutations.

S. Zahid et al., *Retinal Dystrophy Gene Atlas*, https://doi.org/10.1007/978-3-319-10867-4_14

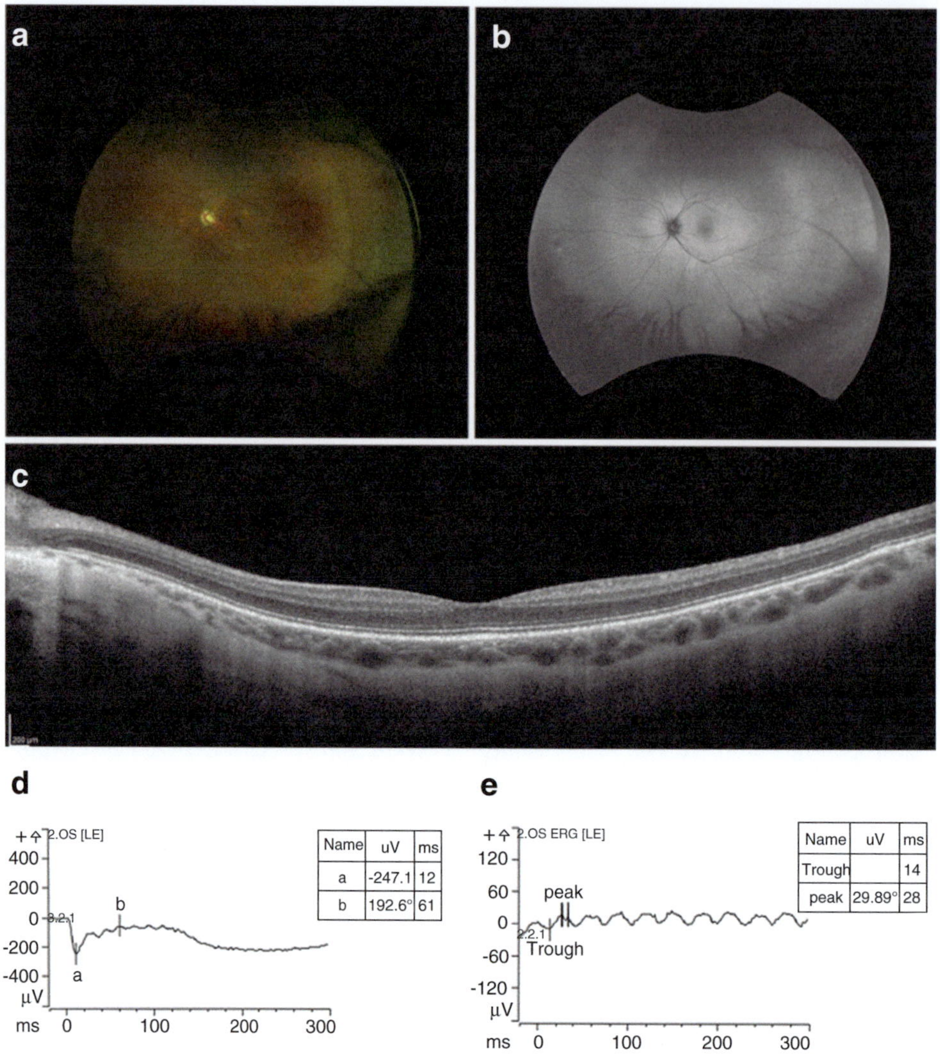

Fig. 14.1 Case summary: 28-year-old male with CSNB. Color fundus photograph showing a myopic-appearing fundus.

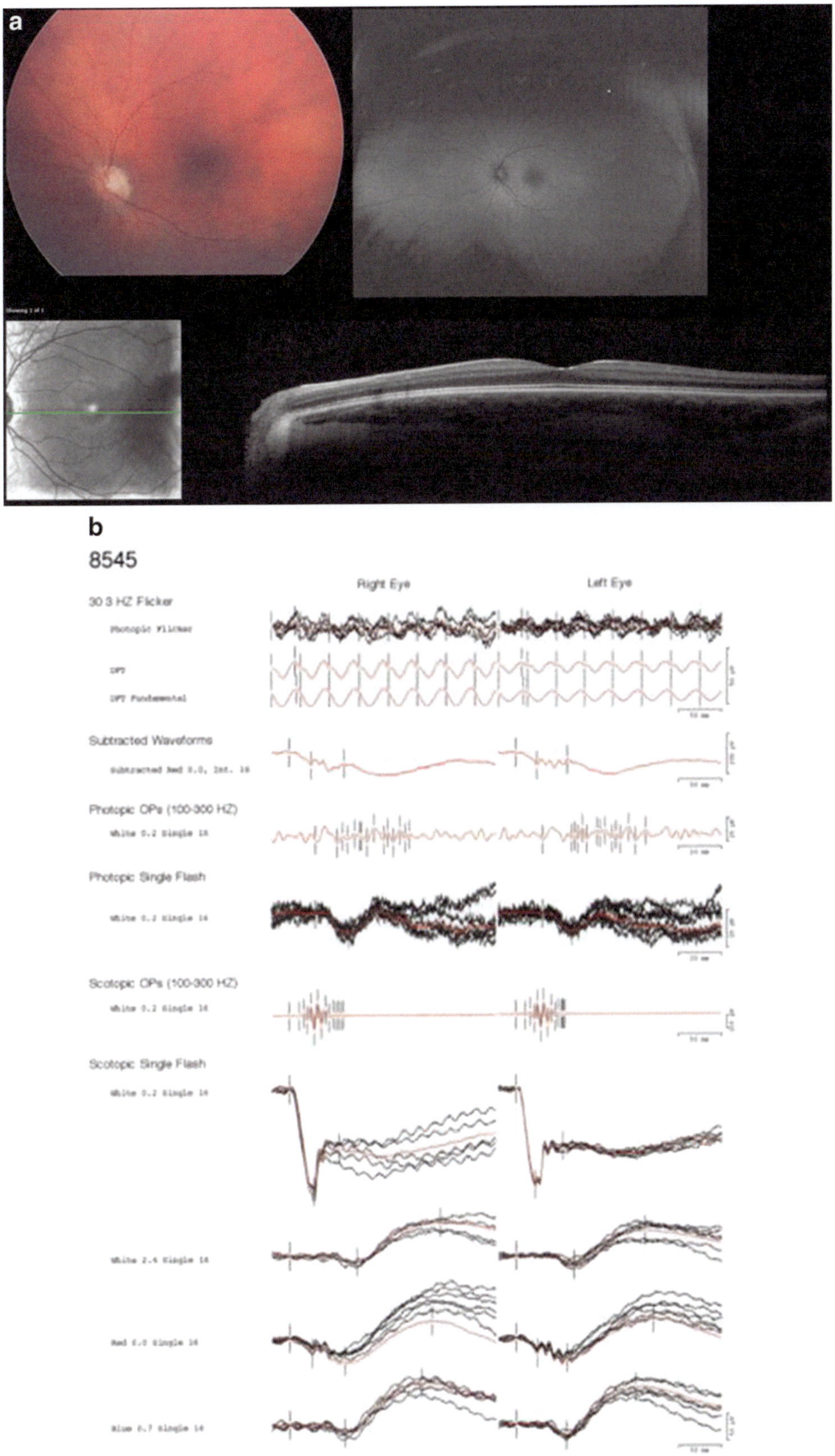

Fig. 14.2 Case summary: 19-year-old male (CEI26323) with CSNB. (**a**) Color fundus photograph, fundus autofluorescence and spectral domain-optical coherence tomography showing an essentially unremarkable left eye. (**b**) Full-field electroretinogram of both eyes, showing an electronegative b-wave on dark-adapted bright flash and a double-peaked wave on flicker.

References

1. Hemara-Wahanui A, Berjukow S, Hope CI, Dearden PK, SB W, Wilson-Wheeler J, et al. A CACNA1F mutation identified in an X-linked retinal disorder shifts the voltage dependence of Cav1.4 channel activation. Proc Natl Acad Sci U S A. 2005;102(21):7553–8.
2. Boycott KM, Sauve Y, MacDonald IM. X-linked congenital stationary night blindness. In: Pagon RA, Adam MP, Ardinger HH, Wallace SE, Amemiya A, Bean LJH, et al., editors. GeneReviews® [Internet]. Seattle WA: University of Washington, Seattle; 1993–2016. 2008. [updated 2012 Apr 26].
3. Strom TM, Nyakatura G, Apfelstedt-Sylla E, Hellebrand H, Lorenz B, Weber BH, et al. An L-type calcium-channel gene mutated in incomplete X-linked congenital stationary night blindness. Nat Genet. 1998;19(3):260–3.
4. Boycott KM, Maybaum TA, Naylor MJ, Weleber RG, Robitaille J, Miyake Y, et al. A summary of 20 CACNA1F mutations identified in 36 families with incomplete X-linked congenital stationary night blindness, and characterization of splice variants. Hum Genet. 2001;108(2):91–7.
5. Jalkanen R, Bech-Hansen NT, Tobias R, Sankila EM, Mäntyjärvi M, Forsius H, et al. A novel CACNA1F gene mutation causes Aland Island eye disease. Invest Ophthalmol Vis Sci. 2007;48(6):2498–502.
6. Nakamura M, Ito S, Piao CH, Terasaki H, Miyake Y. Retinal and optic disc atrophy associated with a CACNA1F mutation in a Japanese family. Arch Ophthalmol. 2003;121(7):1028–33.
7. Wutz K, Sauer C, Zrenner E, Lorenz B, Alitalo T, Broghammer M, et al. Thirty distinct CACNA1F mutations in 33 families with incomplete type of XLCSNB and Cacna1f expression profiling in mouse retina. Eur J Hum Genet. 2002;10(8):449–56.
8. Lodha N, Loucks CM, Beaulieu C, Parboosingh JS, Bech-Hansen NT. Congenital stationary night blindness: mutation update and clinical variability. Adv Exp Med Biol. 2012;723:371–9.
9. Jalkanen R, Mantyjarvi M, Tobias R, Isosomppi J, Sankila EM, Alitalo T, et al. X linked cone-rod dystrophy, CORDX3, is caused by a mutation in the CACNA1F gene. J Med Genet. 2006;43(8):699–704.
10. Jalkanen R, Demirci FY, Tyynismaa H, Bech-Hansen T, Meindl A, Peippo M, et al. A new genetic locus for X linked progressive cone-rod dystrophy. J Med Genet. 2003;40(6):418–23.

15 CEP290

CEP290 encodes a centrosomal protein involved in ciliary assembly and ciliary trafficking. Mutations are responsible for autosomal recessive Leber's congenital amaurosis (LCA), Joubert syndrome, and Bardet-Biedl Syndrome [1–3].

Recessive *CEP290* mutations are responsible for 15–20% of LCA. Patients typically have profound vision loss that manifests at birth or within the first few months of life, with one study showing that 64% of patients exhibit CF acuity in the better eye at presentation [4]. However, there have been reports of intrafamilial variability in visual acuity in affected families, and some patients may have acuities better than 20/200 [1]. In some patients, visual acuity may even be as good as 20/25 [4]. This same study suggests that vision may remain relatively stable over time in this disease. Symptomatology includes pendular nystagmus, high hypermetropia, photodysphoria, oculodigital sign, keratoconus, and cataracts [5]. Some patients may have associated systemic findings, such as abnormal proprioception, infertility, and mental retardation. Funduscopic appearance is variable and may include peripapillary atrophy, arteriolar narrowing, foveal dysgenesis, RPE atrophy with nummular or bone spicule pigmentation, and optic disc pallor (Figs. 15.1a and 15.2a). Fundus autofluorescence may show a hyperautofluorescent ring around the fovea (Figs. 15.1b and 15.2b). Coloboma and Coats-like vasculopathy are also observed. Electroretinography (ERG) exhibits globally reduced rod and cone function.

Joubert syndrome is a genetic disease resulting from cerebellar vermis hypo/a-plasia that manifests with hypotonia; ataxia; mental retardation; hyperpnea; oculomotor apraxia; polydactyly; cleft lip/palate; tongue, kidney, and liver defects; and seizures. Patients with recessive *CEP290* mutations may also exhibit retinopathy as part of Joubert syndrome and associated disorders, manifesting vision loss within the first few months to years of life [2]. Clinical findings may include chorioretinal colobomas and classical findings of retinitis pigmentosa (RP) (e.g., bone-spicule pigment deposits, retinal vascular attenuation, etc).

Recessively-inherited mutations in *CEP290* are also associated with Bardet-Biedl Syndrome, a pleiotropic genetic disorder that includes a diverse array of manifestations, most commonly including obesity, polydactyly, hypogonadism, renal dysfunction, and retinitis pigmentosa [5–7]. The ophthalmic manifestations occur early in life and usually begin with night blindness in the first decade, progressing to peripheral visual loss and a maculopathy later in life, accompanied by the classical RP findings of bone-spicule pigmentary deposits and progressive retinal atrophy and concomitant loss of visual fields. However, patients may also present with central visual deficits and progress to subsequent peripheral vision loss. By the second to third decade, almost 75% of patients are legally blind.

S. Zahid et al., *Retinal Dystrophy Gene Atlas*, https://doi.org/10.1007/978-3-319-10867-4_15

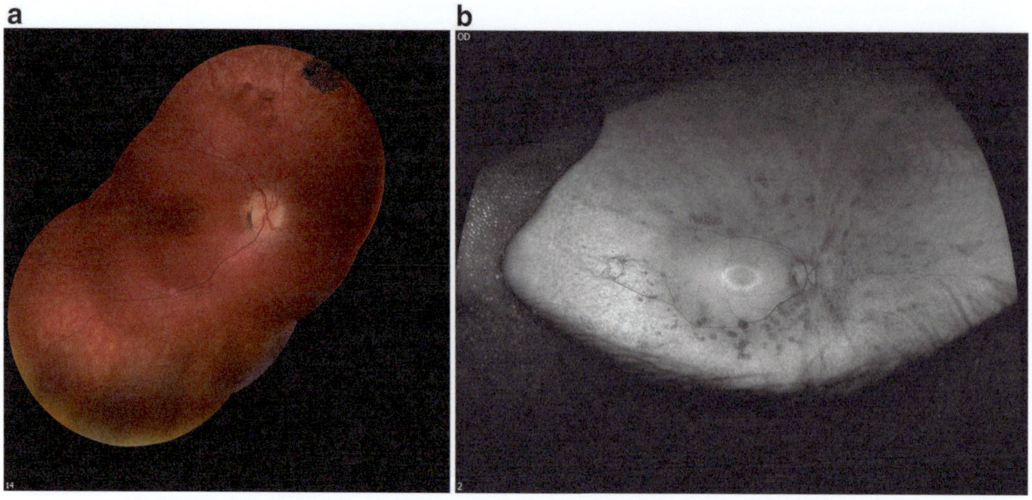

Fig. 15.1 Case summary: 14-year-old girl with LCA. (**a**) Color fundus photo of a 14-year-old girl showing peripheral RPE atrophy and a CHRPE superonasally. (**b**) Wide-field fundus autofluorescence image of the same patient's eye at age 20 showing parafoveal hyperfluorescent ring and hypopigmented areas around the fundus.

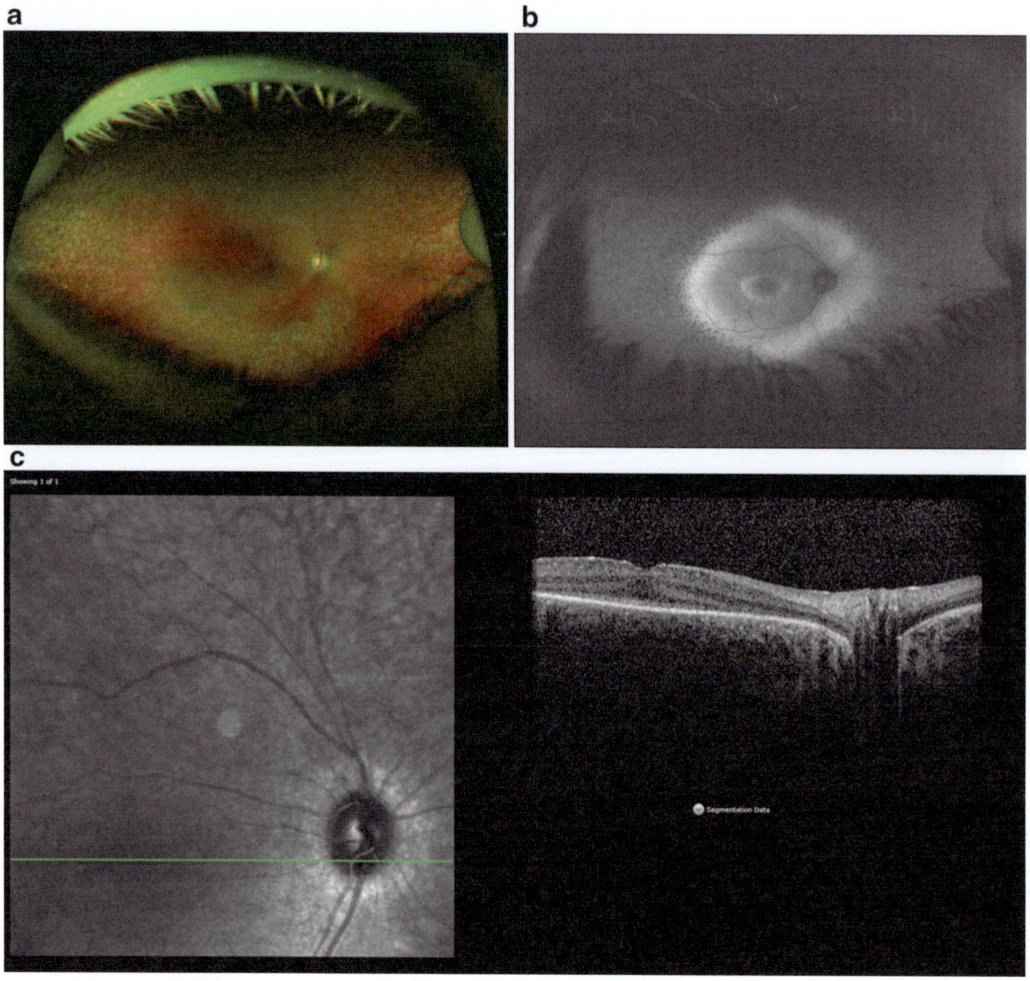

Fig. 15.2 Case summary: 9-year-old male (CEI25602) (*Image courtesy of* Richard Weleber). (**a**) Wide-field color fundus photo showing diffuse RPE atrophy with peripheral retinal deposits. (**b**) Wide-field fundus autofluorescence image showing a hyperautofluorescent ring around the fovea with hyperautofluorescence around the arcades. (**c**) Spectral domain-OCT showing diffuse outer retinal atrophy and an epiretinal membrane.

References

1. den Hollander AI, Koenekoop RK, Yzer S, Lopez I, Arends ML, Voesenek KE, et al. Mutations in the CEP290 (NPHP6) gene are a frequent cause of Leber congenital amaurosis. Am J Hum Genet. 2006;79(3):556–61.
2. Brancati F, Barrano G, Silhavy JL, Marsh SE, Travaglini L, Bielas SL, et al. CEP290 mutations are frequently identified in the oculo-renal form of Joubert syndrome-related disorders. Am J Hum Genet. 2007;81(1):104–13.
3. Coppieters F, Lefever S, Leroy BP, De Baere E. CEP290, a gene with many faces: mutation overview and presentation of CEP290base. Hum Mutat. 2010;31(10):1097–108.
4. McAnany JJ, Genead MA, Walia S, Drack AV, Stone EM, Koenekoop RK, et al. Visual acuity changes in patients with leber congenital amaurosis and mutations in CEP290. JAMA Ophthalmol. 2013;131(2):178–82.
5. Chung DC, Traboulsi EI. Leber congenital amaurosis: clinical correlations with genotypes, gene therapy trials update, and future directions. J AAPOS. 2009;13(6):587–92.
6. Waters AM, Beales PL. Bardet-Biedl syndrome. In: Pagon RA, Adam MP, Bird TD, Dolan CR, Fong CT, Stephens K, editors. GeneReviews. Seattle: University of Washington; 1993.
7. Leitch CC, Zaghloul NA, Davis EE, Stoetzel C, Diaz-Font A, Rix S, et al. Hypomorphic mutations in syndromic encephalocele genes are associated with Bardet-Biedl syndrome. Nat Genet. 2008;40(4):443–8.

16 CERKL

CERKL encodes ceramide kinase-like protein, and mutations in this gene are associated with autosomal recessive cone-rod dystrophy [1–7]. Biallelic *CERKL* mutations cause up to 5% of recessive retinitis pigmentosa in Spain and are also common in the Yemenite Jewish population [2, 3, 5].

Patients with *CERKL*-related cone-rod dystrophy typically present in their teens or twenties (median of 23 years) with night blindness and central visual deficits, but symptoms may occur as early as the first decade [3, 5, 8]. Photophobia is very common. Some patients may exhibit early-onset posterior subcapsular cataracts [2, 5]. Visual acuity is usually maintained into early adulthood but then rapidly declines with macular atrophy (range from 20/50 to LP in older patients) [2]. Fundus findings feature macular abnormalities, ranging from mild pigmentary changes to macular atrophy, attenuated retinal vessels, and variable degrees of peripheral changes (ranging from mid-peripheral bone spicule deposits to a "salt and pepper" appearance) [3, 8]. Macular and peripheral atrophy worsen with time and are clinically manifested as a progressive loss of visual fields and acuity. Some patients may exhibit pigment accumulation in areas of well-defined macular atrophy (Figs. 16.1a and 16.2a); atrophic areas may become confluent and resemble gyrate atrophy [2, 5]. Macular changes may be evident as early as 15 years of age, and in some patients with maculopathy, the periphery is initially normal [3]. Many patients exhibit normal coloration of the optic disc [1, 2]. Full-field ERGs demonstrate severe abnormalities of both rod- and cone-driven function, and these recordings may demonstrate a cone-rod pattern in some patients [3, 4]. ERGs are non-recordable in many older patients [2]. GVF often reveals constriction of peripheral fields with a central scotoma in the context of macular atrophy or annular loss of fields surrounding a residual central island. Late in the disease process, some patients exhibit absolute scotoma [2–4]. FAF reveals hypoautofluorescence in areas of macular atrophy and a broad ring of hyperfluorescence around the perifovea (Figs. 16.1b and 16.2b). OCT may show thinning of the fovea with loss of the outer nuclear layer (ONL) or abnormal lamination. Some patients may exhibit areas of OCT hyperreflectivity in the ONL and inner segment-outer segment line (Fig. 16.1c); these areas exhibit heterogenous FAF signals, characterized by both hyper- and hypoautofluorescence [4]. The ONL and ellipsoid zone are reduced in and around the fovea, especially in the areas of highest cone and rod densities [4]. Given the early macular involvement, many patients receive a diagnosis of cone-rod dystrophy.

S. Zahid et al., *Retinal Dystrophy Gene Atlas*, https://doi.org/10.1007/978-3-319-10867-4_16

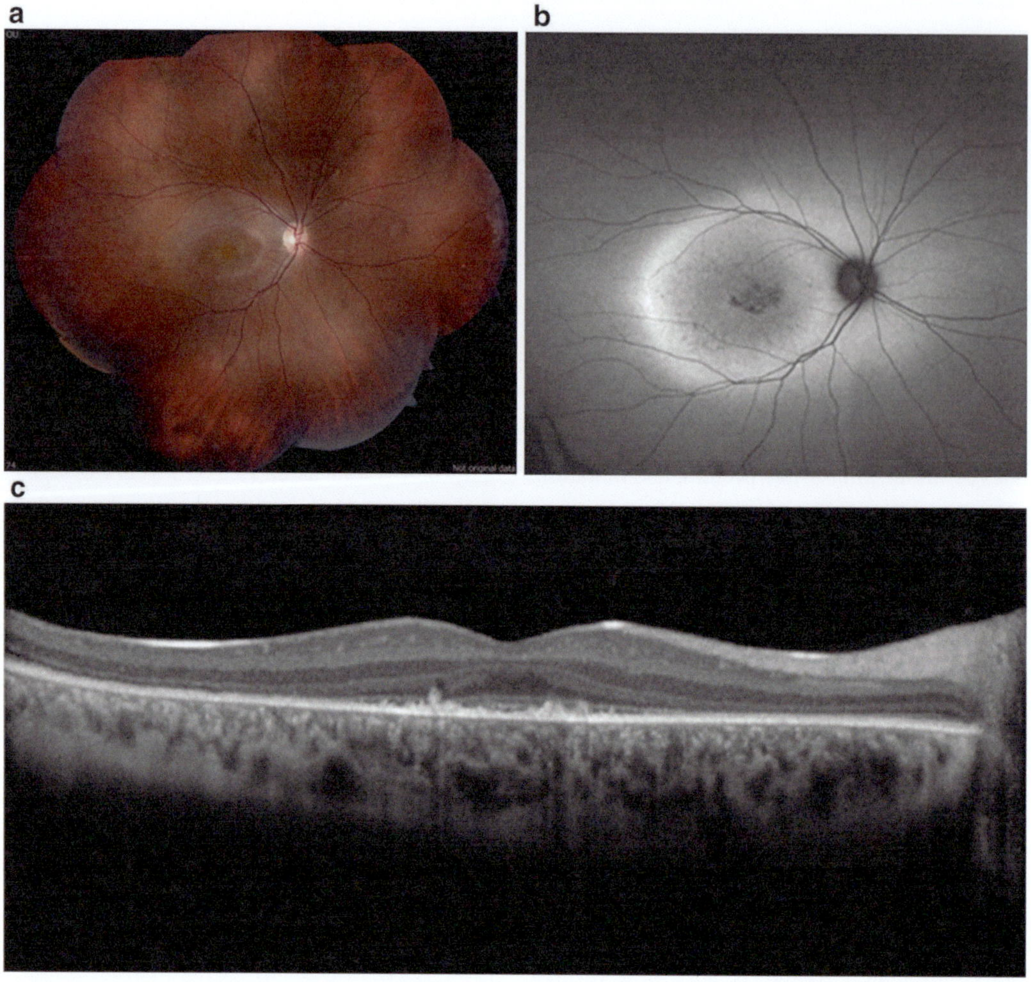

Fig. 16.1 Case summary: 20 year-old-man with a cone-rod dystrophy with mutations in *CERKL*. (**a**) Montage color fundus photograph of the right eye showing macular atrophy with subretinal deposits. (**b**) Fundus autofluorescence of the right eye showing macular hypoautofluorescence in areas of atrophy with a hyperautofluorescent ring near the vascular arcades. (**c**) Spectral domain optical coherence tomography of the right eye showing extrafoveal ellipsoid zone and outer nuclear layer loss with subretinal deposits in areas of residual photoreceptors.

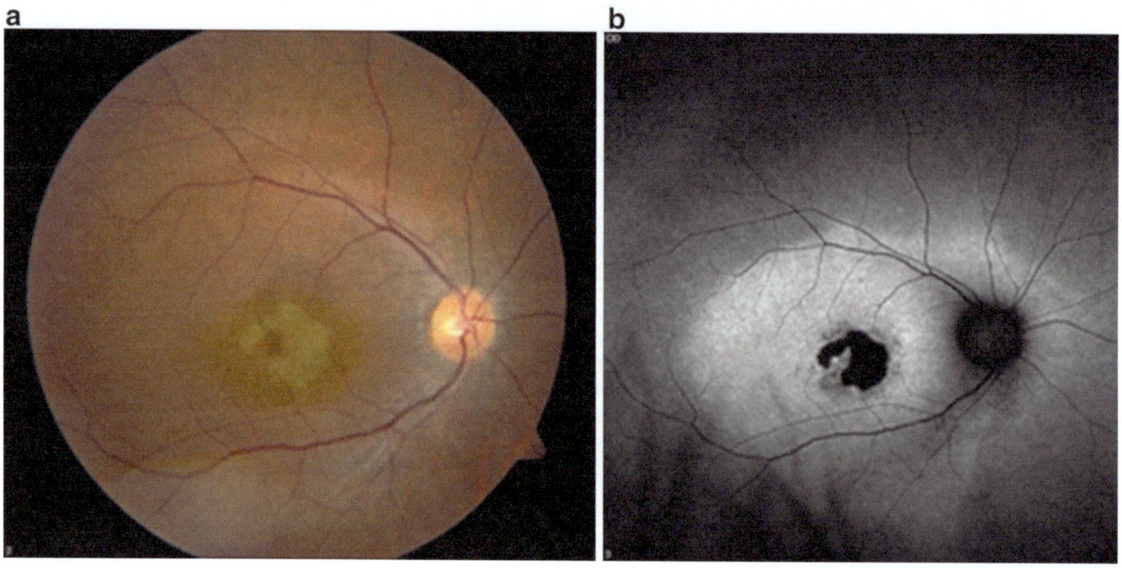

Fig. 16.2 Case summary: 37-year-old male with macular atrophy. (**a**) Color fundus photograph of the right eye showing macular atrophy. (**b**) Fundus autofluorescence of the right eye showing a dense hypoautofluorescent area corresponding to the area of atrophy within a background of macular hyperautofluorescence.

References

1. Tang Z, Wang Z, Wang Z, Ke T, Wang QK, Liu M. Novel compound heterozygous mutations in CERKL cause autosomal recessive retinitis pigmentosa in a nonconsanguineous Chinese family. Arch Ophthalmol. 2009;127(8):1077–8.
2. Avila-Fernandez A, Cantalapiedra D, Aller E, Vallespín E, Aguirre-Lambán J, Blanco-Kelly F, et al. Mutation analysis of 272 Spanish families affected by autosomal recessive retinitis pigmentosa using a genotyping microarray. Mol Vis. 2010;16:2550–8.
3. Auslender N, Sharon D, Abbasi AH, Garzozi HJ, Banin E, Ben-Yosef T. A common founder mutation of CERKL underlies autosomal recessive retinal degeneration with early macular involvement among Yemenite Jews. Invest Ophthalmol Vis Sci. 2007;48(12):5431–8.
4. Aleman TS, Soumittra N, Cideciyan AV, Sumaroka AM, Ramprasad VL, Herrera W, et al. CERKL mutations cause an autosomal recessive cone-rod dystrophy with inner retinopathy. Invest Ophthalmol Vis Sci. 2009;50(12):5944–54.
5. Avila-Fernandez A, Riveiro-Alvarez R, Vallespin E, Wilke R, Tapias I, Cantalapiedra D, et al. CERKL mutations and associated phenotypes in seven Spanish families with autosomal recessive retinitis pigmentosa. Invest Ophthalmol Vis Sci. 2008;49(6):2709–13.
6. Tuson M, Marfany G, Gonzalez-Duarte R. Mutation of CERKL, a novel human ceramide kinase gene, causes autosomal recessive retinitis pigmentosa (RP26). Am J Hum Genet. 2004;74(1):128–38.
7. Ali M, Ramprasad VL, Soumittra N, Mohamed MD, Jafri H, Rashid Y, et al. A missense mutation in the nuclear localization signal sequence of CERKL (p.R106S) causes autosomal recessive retinal degeneration. Mol Vis. 2008;14:1960–4.
8. Bayes M, Goldaracena B, Martinez-Mir A, Iragui-Madoz MI, Solans T, Chivelet P, et al. A new autosomal recessive retinitis pigmentosa locus maps on chromosome 2q31-q33. J Med Genet. 1998;35(2):141–5.

CHM

17

CHM encodes Rab Escort Protein, or REP1, which binds unprenylated Rab proteins involved in vesicle transport. Mutations in *CHM* are associated with choroideremia [1, 2].

Choroideremia is an X-linked progressive chorioretinal dystrophy. Affected male patients typically experience night blindness in the first or second decade of life, followed by progressive visual field constriction [1]. Visual acuities are usually 20/40 or better in the first-to-fourth decades but subsequently deteriorate to 20/200 or less and in some cases to no light perception in the elderly [1, 3–5]. Visual fields show mid-peripheral isolated scotomata with progressive constriction over time [3, 5, 6]. Fundus examination typically shows lobular choroidal and retinal/RPE atrophy, which starts in the periphery and later coalesces into widespread chorioretinal atrophy down to bare sclera, with progressive constriction over time and macular sparing until the fifth to sixth decades (Figs. 17.1a, 17.2, and 17.4) [1, 3, 5]. Unlike retinitis pigmentosa, retinal vascular caliber and optic nerve appearance remain relatively normal. Fundus autofluorescence (FAF) demonstrates isolated peripheral areas of reduced autofluorescence (AF) early in the disease, which progress to large lobular areas of reduced AF in advanced disease (Fig. 17.3a) [8]. Optical coherence tomography (OCT) shows outer retinal atrophy with foveal sparing until later stages and outer choroidal thinning with increased reflectance due to RPE loss (Figs. 17.1b and 17.3b) [5, 9]. Cystoid macular edema may be seen. Full-field electroretinograms (ERG) show significantly reduced rod and cone responses, which may be non-recordable in later stages of disease [5, 6]. Rarely, there may be a negative electroretinogram [8].

Female carriers are typically asymptomatic, but, due to skewed X-inactivation, may show areas of peripheral retinal and RPE pigmentary disturbance with variable increasing chorioretinal involvement with age (Fig. 17.4). OCT of female carriers may vary, but when abnormal it may demonstrate remodeling over time, including focal thickening of the outer retina and drusen-like deposits corresponding with areas of increased AF [9]. ERGs may be normal or show mild reduction of amplitudes [1, 6, 7].

S. Zahid et al., *Retinal Dystrophy Gene Atlas*, https://doi.org/10.1007/978-3-319-10867-4_17

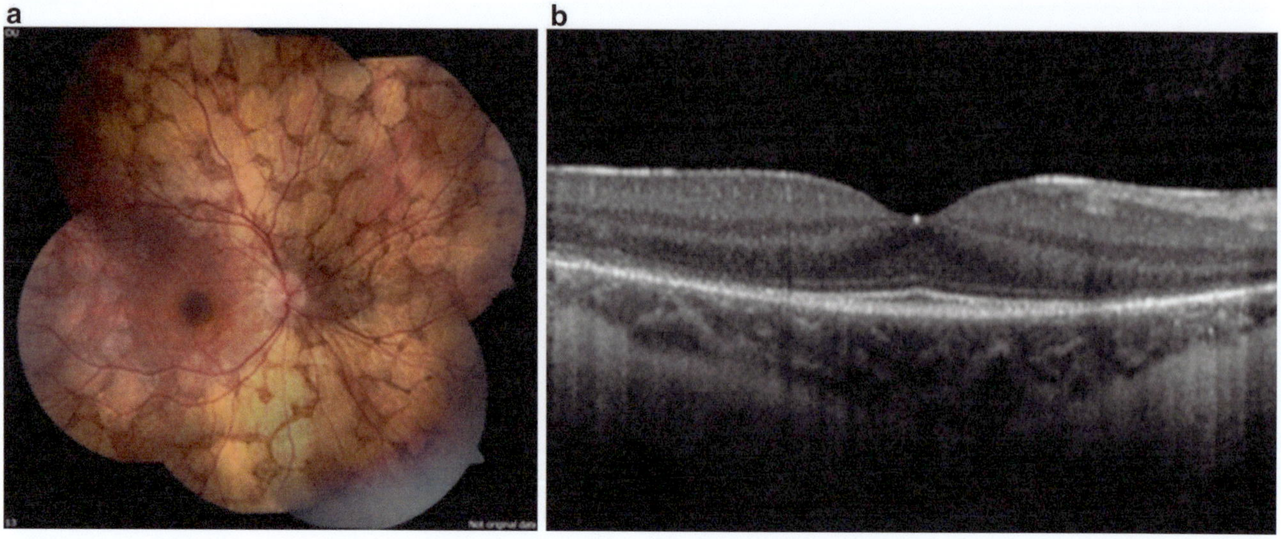

Fig. 17.1 Case summary: 8-year-old boy with choroideremia. (**a**) Montage color fundus photograph of the right eye showing lobular choroidal and retinal/RPE atrophy starting in the periphery and extending to the vascular arcades. (**b**) Spectral domain optical coherence tomography of the right eye showing extrafoveal loss of the ellipsoid zone and a trace epiretinal membrane.

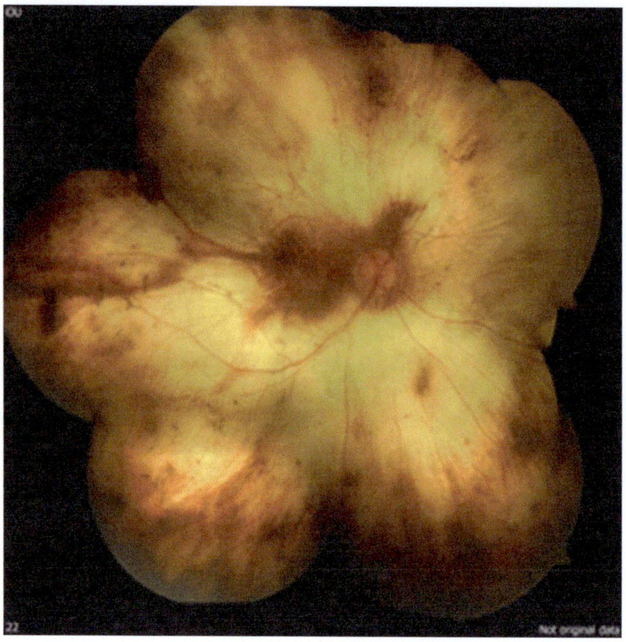

Fig. 17.2 Montage color fundus photograph of the right eye from a 62-year-old male with choroideremia, showing extensive chorioretinal atrophy, associated with scant pigment deposits, which start in the periphery and extend to the vascular arcades.

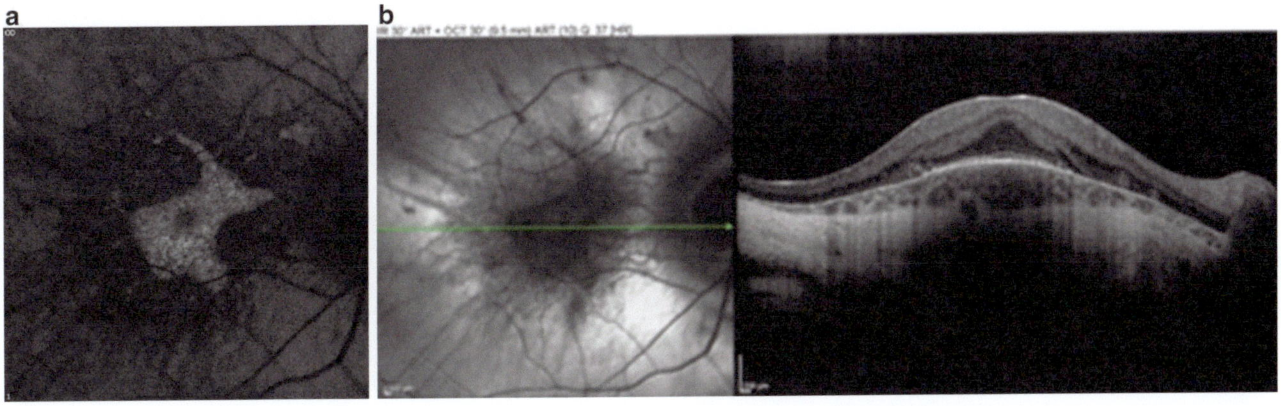

Fig. 17.3 26-year-old man with choroideremia. (**a**) Fundus autofluorescence of the right eye showing loss of macular autofluorescence with residual abnormal hyperautofluorescence in the central macula. (**b**) Spectral domain optical coherence tomography showing extrafoveal loss of the ellipsoid zone and outer nuclear layer as well as choroidal and RPE atrophy.

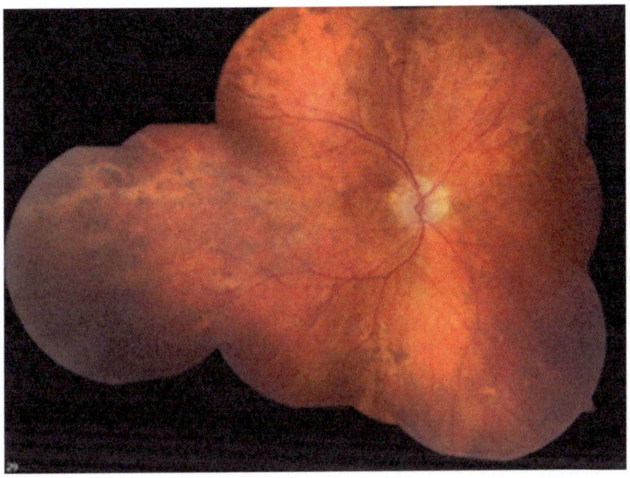

Fig. 17.4 48-year-old female carrier of choroideremia. Montage color fundus photograph of the right eye, showing scattered patchy areas of peripheral retinal and RPE pigmentary changes.

References

1. MacDonald IM, Hume S, Chan S, Seabra MC. Choroideremia. 2003 [Updated 2015]. In: Pagon RA, Adam MP, Ardinger HH, et al., editors. GeneReviews [Internet]. Seattle: University of Washington; .1993–2017. Available from: https://www.ncbi.nlm.nih.gov/books/NBK1337. Accessed 20 Jan 2017.
2. Cremers FP, Sankila EM, Brunsmann F, Jay M, Jay B, Wright A, et al. Deletions in patients with classical choroideremia vary in size from 45 kb to several megabases. Am J Hum Genet. 1990;47(4):622–8.
3. Esposito G, De Falco F, Tinto N, Testa F, Vitagliano L, Tandurella IC, et al. Comprehensive mutation analysis (20 families) of the choroideremia gene reveals a missense variant that prevents the binding of REP1 with Rab geranylgeranyl transferase. Hum Mutat. 2011;32(12):1460–9.
4. Roberts MF, Fishman GA, Roberts DK, Heckenlively JR, Weleber RG, Anderson RJ, et al. Retrospective, longitudinal, and cross sectional study of visual acuity impairment in choroideraemia. Br J Ophthalmol. 2002;86(6):658–62.
5. Lin Y, Liu X, Luo L, Qu B, Jiang S, Yang H, et al. Molecular analysis of the choroideremia gene related clinical findings in two families with choroideremia. Mol Vis. 2011;17:2564–9.
6. Zhou Q, Liu L, Xu F, Li H, Sergeev Y, Dong F, et al. Genetic and phenotypic characteristics of three Mainland Chinese families with choroideremia. Mol Vis. 2012;18:309–16.
7. Mura M, Sereda C, Jablonski MM, MacDonald IM, Iannaccone A. Clinical and functional findings in choroideremia due to complete deletion of the CHM gene. Arch Ophthalmol. 2007;125(8):1107–13.
8. Renner AB, Kellner U, Cropp E, Preising MN, MacDonald IM, van den Hurk JA, et al. Choroideremia: variability of clinical and electrophysiological characteristics and first report of a negative electroretinogram. Ophthalmology. 2006;113(11):2066 e1–10.
9. Huang AS, Kim LA, Fawzi AA. Clinical characteristics of a large choroideremia pedigree carrying a novel CHM mutation. Arch Ophthalmol. 2012;130(9):1184–9.

18 CLN3

CLN3 encodes battenin, a protein involved in lysosomal function and neuronal transport. Mutations in this gene are associated with a syndromic retinal degeneration, Batten disease, or juvenile neuronal ceroid lipofuscinosis (JNCL), as well as non-syndromic retinal degeneration [1].

CLN3-related JNCL follows an autosomal recessive pattern of inheritance. Although over 50 mutations in this gene have been reported, 80–90% of patients with JNCL have a 1.02 kB deletion, resulting in a frameshift and prematurely truncated protein [2].

Children with JNCL usually present with vision impairment as the first reported symptom. The average age of onset ranges from 4–10 years [2]. Patients typically exhibit a rapidly progressive deterioration in vision, leading to legal blindness within 3 years, which is atypical when compared with other juvenile-onset maculopathies [3]. Other visual symptoms include esotropia, photophobia, nyctalopia, nystagmus, and dyschromatopsia [4]. Systemic features include seizures, behavioral abnormalities, motor dysfunction, impaired cognition, dementia, and premature death [3].

Fundoscopy may reveal a bull's-eye maculopathy, macular or peripheral pigmentary retinopathy, optic atrophy or optic disc pallor, bone-spicule pigment deposits, and arteriolar attenuation (Fig. 18.1a) [5]. Fundus autofluorescence may show abnormal macular hyperautofluorescence and peripheral hypoautofluorescence in areas of RPE atrophy (Fig. 18.1b). Goldmann visual fields may demonstrate scotomas or concentric constriction of peripheral fields.

Full-field electroretinogram (ERG) results are typically severely reduced or nonrecordable on initial presentation, or there may be a negative waveform present for the maximal/mixed response [4, 6]. Reduced cone flicker, non-recordable scotopic parameters, and normal responses have also been reported [6].

CLN3-related non-syndromic retinal degeneration follows an autosomal recessive pattern of inheritance. Patients display features more consistent with retinitis pigmentosa, with peripheral pigment mottling and ellipsoid zone loss outside the fovea on OCT [1]. One family with cone-rod degeneration has also been described [1].

S. Zahid et al., *Retinal Dystrophy Gene Atlas*, https://doi.org/10.1007/978-3-319-10867-4_18

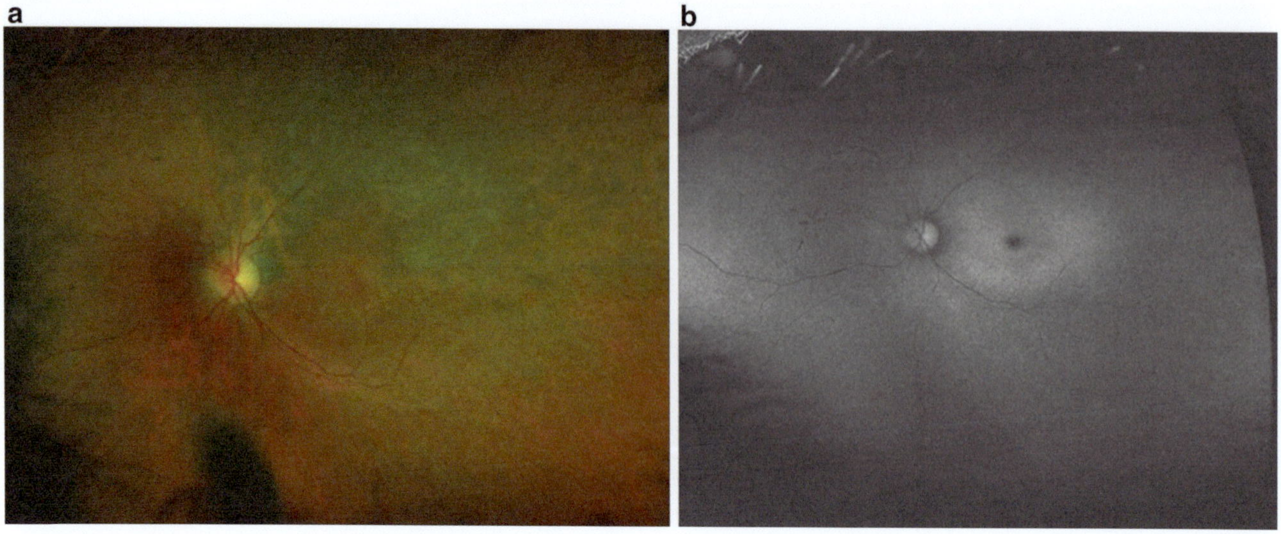

Fig. 18.1 Case summary: 9-year-old male with Batten disease with *CLN3* mutations. (**a**) Wide-field color fundus photograph of the left eye showing RPE macular changes with scant bone spicule pigment deposition in the mid-periphery. (**b**) Wide-field fundus autofluorescence of the left eye showing elevated abnormal parafoveal autofluorescence and hypoautofluorescence in areas of scant pigment deposition in the mid-periphery.

References

1. Wang F, Wang H, Tuan HF, Nguyen DH, Sun V, Keser V, et al. Next generation sequencing-based molecular diagnosis of retinitis pigmentosa: identification of a novel genotype-phenotype correlation and clinical refinements. Hum Genet. 2014;133(3):331–45.
2. Jarvela I, Autti T, Lamminranta S, Aberg L, Raininko R, Santavuori P. Clinical and magnetic resonance imaging findings in Batten disease: analysis of the major mutation (1.02-kb deletion). Ann Neurol. 1997;42(5):799–802.
3. Drack AV, Miller JN, Pearce DA. A novel c.1135_1138delCTGT mutation in CLN3 leads to juvenile neuronal ceroid lipofuscinosis. J Child Neurol. 2013;28(9):1112–6.
4. Horiguchi M, Miyake Y. Batten disease--deteriorating course of ocular findings. Jpn J Ophthalmol. 1992;36(1):91–6.
5. Spalton DJ, Taylor DS, Sanders MD. Juvenile Batten's disease: an ophthalmological assessment of 26 patients. Br J Ophthalmol. 1980;64(10):726–32.
6. Collins J, Holder GE, Herbert H, Adams GG. Batten disease: features to facilitate early diagnosis. Br J Ophthalmol. 2006;90(9):1119–24.

19 CLRN1

CLRN1 encodes Clarin-1, expressed in the ribbon synapses of the cochlea and retina. Although its function in the human retina is unknown, mutations in the gene are associated with Usher syndrome type 3A (USH3A) and non-syndromic retinitis pigmentosa/rod-cone dystrophy.

Mutations in *CLRN1* are associated with hearing loss and retinitis pigmentosa, with or without vestibular dysfunction. Patients with *CLRN1* mutations comprise a larger proportion of patients with Usher syndrome in Finnish and Ashkenazi Jewish populations due to founder effects [1, 2]. Individuals first present with bilateral sensorineural hearing impairment, which ranges from normal to moderate at younger ages and may be profound at later ages [3]. Onset is typically postlingual, and hearing loss is progressive, in contrast to other types of Usher syndrome [4]. Individuals present with visual symptoms, which include nyctalopia or constricted visual fields, from the first to sixth decade, with an average age of diagnosis of retinitis pigmentosa in the second decade [5]. Other visual symptoms include hyperopia, astigmatism, and cataracts. Individuals may have progressive loss of visual acuity with age-related severity similar to that of other types of Usher syndrome [3]. Fundoscopy may reveal features typical of retinitis pigmentosa, including peripheral bone spicule pigmentation, waxy pallor of the optic disc, arteriole attenuation, and loss of retinal pigment epithelium (Figs. 19.1a and 19.2a) [6]. Optical coherence tomography (OCT) may show distorted foveal architecture, normal or reduced parafoveal retinal thickness, and disruption of the ellipsoid zone (more prominent outside the fovea), which tend to be worse in older patients (Figs. 19.1c and 19.2c) [6–8]. Near-infrared reduced-illuminance autofluorescence imaging may reveal a ring of parafoveal hyperautofluorescence (Figs. 19.1b and 19.2b) [6]. Full-field electroretinogram (ERG) is typically consistent with a rod-cone pattern of degeneration and may be non-recordable [6, 8]. GVF testing tends to show ring scotomas and progressive peripheral losses [8, 9]. Adaptive optics may reveal reduced photoreceptor densities in areas outside the fovea, and microperimetry may show elevated response thresholds, both of which tend be more pronounced in advanced stages of disease [8].

CLRN1-related non-syndromic RP follows an autosomal recessive pattern of inheritance. Patients present with symptoms of RP without evidence of hearing loss/impairment. Fundoscopy may demonstrate typical findings of retinitis pigmentosa, such as arteriole attenuation, waxy disc pallor, and peripheral bone spicule pigmentation [10]. ERG may reveal a rod-cone pattern of degeneration [10].

S. Zahid et al., *Retinal Dystrophy Gene Atlas*, https://doi.org/10.1007/978-3-319-10867-4_19

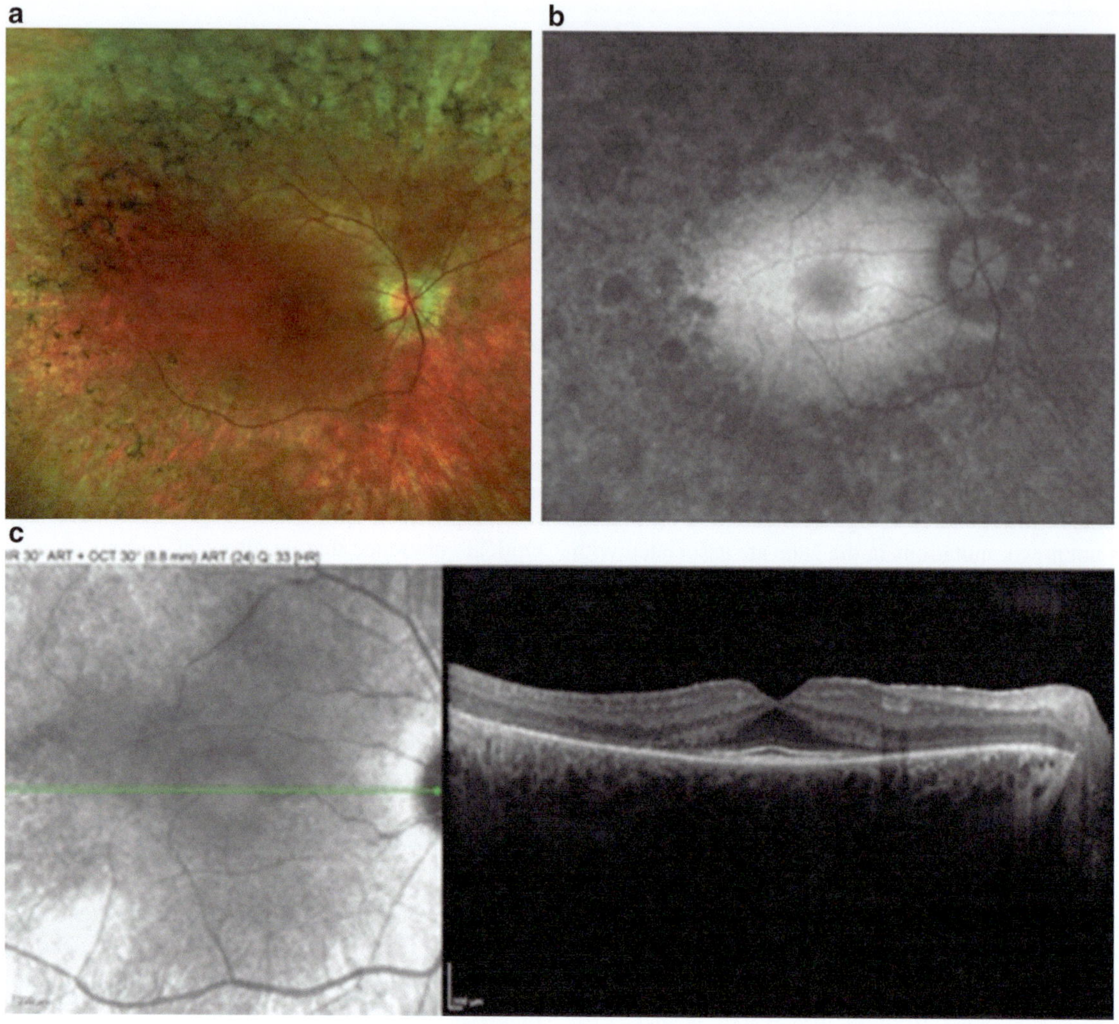

Fig. 19.1 Case summary: 24-year-old male with RP and mild hearing loss since childhood. (**a**) Wide-field color fundus photograph of the right eye showing mid-peripheral RPE atrophy and bone spicule pigmentation. There is also RPE atrophy in the macula with peripapillary atrophy. (**b**) Wide-field fundus autofluorescence of the right eye showing a faint ring of hyperautofluorescence surrounding the fovea and islands of hypoautofluorescence in areas of RPE atrophy in the mid-periphery and along the vascular arcades. (**c**) Spectral domain optical coherence tomography showing extrafoveal loss of the ellipsoid zone and outer nuclear layer.

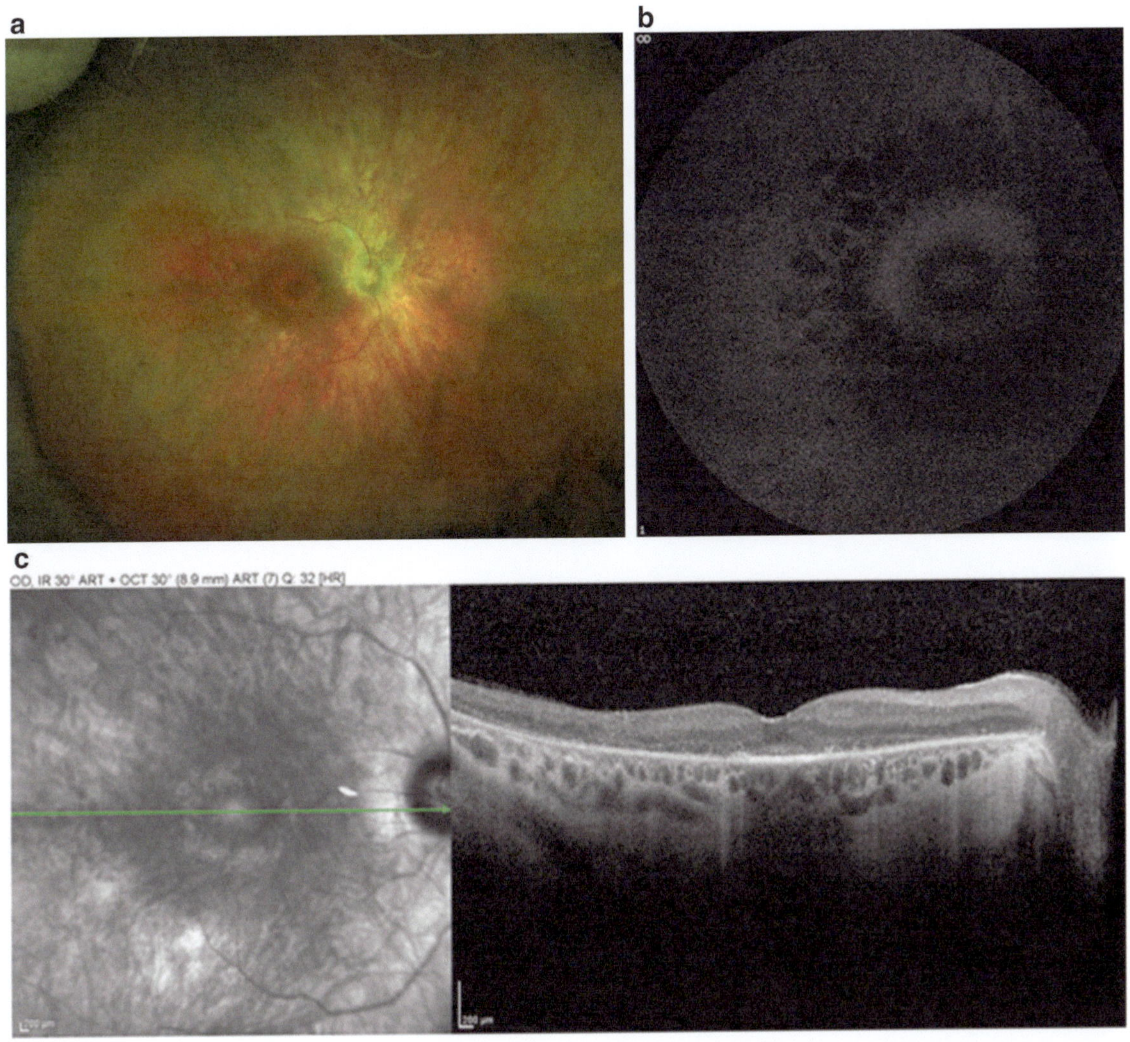

Fig. 19.2 Case summary: 43-year old female with Usher Syndrome. (**a**) Wide-field color fundus photograph of the right eye showing mid-peripheral RPE atrophy, scant bone spicule pigmentation, and a bull's-eye maculopathy with peripapillary atrophy. (**b**) Fundus autofluorescence of the right eye showing a ring of hypoautofluorescence surrounding the fovea (corresponding to the bull's-eye lesion seen in Fig. 19.2a) and islands of hypoautofluorescence in areas of RPE atrophy in the mid-periphery. (**c**) Spectral domain optical coherence tomography showing extensive loss of the ellipsoid zone and outer nuclear layer with thinning of the RPE band surrounding the foveola.

References

1. Ness SL, Ben-Yosef T, Bar-Lev A, Madeo AC, Brewer CC, Avraham KB, et al. Genetic homogeneity and phenotypic variability among Ashkenazi Jews with Usher syndrome type III. J Med Genet. 2003;40(10):767–72.
2. Fields RR, Zhou G, Huang D, Davis JR, Möller C, Jacobson SG, et al. Usher syndrome type III: revised genomic structure of the USH3 gene and identification of novel mutations. Am J Hum Genet. 2002;71(3):607–17.
3. Plantinga RF, Pennings RJ, Huygen PL, Sankila EM, Tuppurainen K, Kleemola L, et al. Visual impairment in Finnish Usher syndrome type III. Acta Ophthalmol Scand. 2006;84(1):36–41.
4. Ebermann I, Wilke R, Lauhoff T, Lubben D, Zrenner E, Bolz HJ. Two truncating USH3A mutations, including one novel, in a German family with Usher syndrome. Mol Vis. 2007;13:1539–47.
5. Pakarinen L, Karjalainen S, Simola KO, Laippala P, Kaitalo H. Usher's syndrome type 3 in Finland. Laryngoscope. 1995;105(6):613–7.
6. Herrera W, Aleman TS, Cideciyan AV, Roman AJ, Banin E, Ben-Yosef T, et al. Retinal disease in Usher syndrome III caused by mutations in the clarin-1 gene. Invest Ophthalmol Vis Sci. 2008;49(6):2651–60.
7. Malm E, Ponjavic V, Moller C, Kimberling WJ, Andreasson S. Phenotypes in defined genotypes including siblings with Usher syndrome. Ophthalmic Genet. 2011;32(2):65–74.
8. Ratnam K, Vastinsalo H, Roorda A, Sankila EM, Duncan JL. Cone structure in patients with usher syndrome type III and mutations in the Clarin 1 gene. JAMA Ophthalmol. 2013;131(1):67–74.
9. Garcia-Garcia G, Aparisi MJ, Rodrigo R, Sequedo MD, Espinós C, Rosell J, et al. Two novel disease-causing mutations in the CLRN1 gene in patients with Usher syndrome type 3. Mol Vis. 2012;18:3070–8.
10. Khan MI, Kersten FF, Azam M, Collin RW, Hussain A, Shah ST, et al. CLRN1 mutations cause nonsyndromic retinitis pigmentosa. Ophthalmology. 2011;118(7):1444–8.

CNGA3 20

CNGA3 encodes the alpha-subunit of the cone photoreceptor cGMP-gated channel involved in phototransduction. *CNGA3* mutations are associated with approximately 25% of autosomal recessive achromatopsia (rod monochromacy) [1–3]. Similarly to patients with mutations in *CNGB3*, patients with achromatopsia caused by mutations in *CNGA3* usually present in their first decade with poor visual acuity (20/200), photophobia, nonspecific color vision deficits, and nystagmus [4, 5]. VA remains stable in some patients but can also deteriorate with time. Fundoscopic examination usually reveals a normal fundus in childhood (60%), while adult patients tend to exhibit loss of foveal structure, pigmentary changes, or bull's-eye macular atrophy. Fundus autofluorescence may reveal foveal and parafoveal hyperfluorescence with normal cross-sectional retinal architecture on OCT in younger patients (Fig. 20.1). Older patients may exhibit focal foveal atrophy on FAF and OCT (Fig. 20.2). However, foveal abnormalities, such as hypolucency or loss of the ellipsoid zone, have also been reported in patients as young as 8 months of age [6]. The macular thickness is reduced, with the reduction typically resulting from outer retinal loss in the context of a maintained inner retina [6]. Electroretinography (ERG) usually shows diminished or absent photopic responses, while scotopic responses are usually normal [6, 7].

S. Zahid et al., *Retinal Dystrophy Gene Atlas*, https://doi.org/10.1007/978-3-319-10867-4_20

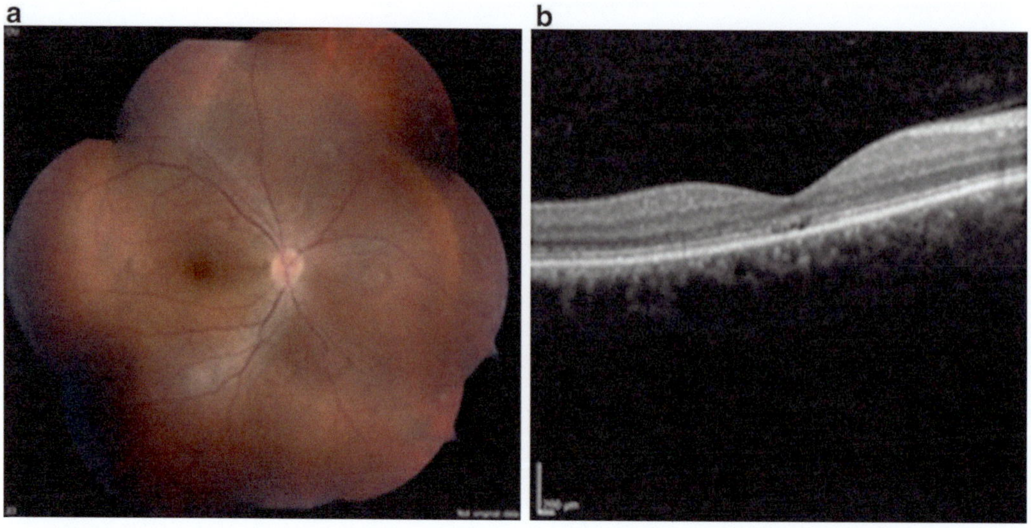

Fig. 20.2 Case summary: 33-year-old woman with autosomal recessive achromatopsia with *CNGA3* mutations. (**a**) Montage color fundus photograph of the right eye showing a normal fundus appearance. (**b**) Spectral domain optical coherence tomography of the right eye showing foveal ellipsoid zone disruption with outer retinal foveal cavitation.

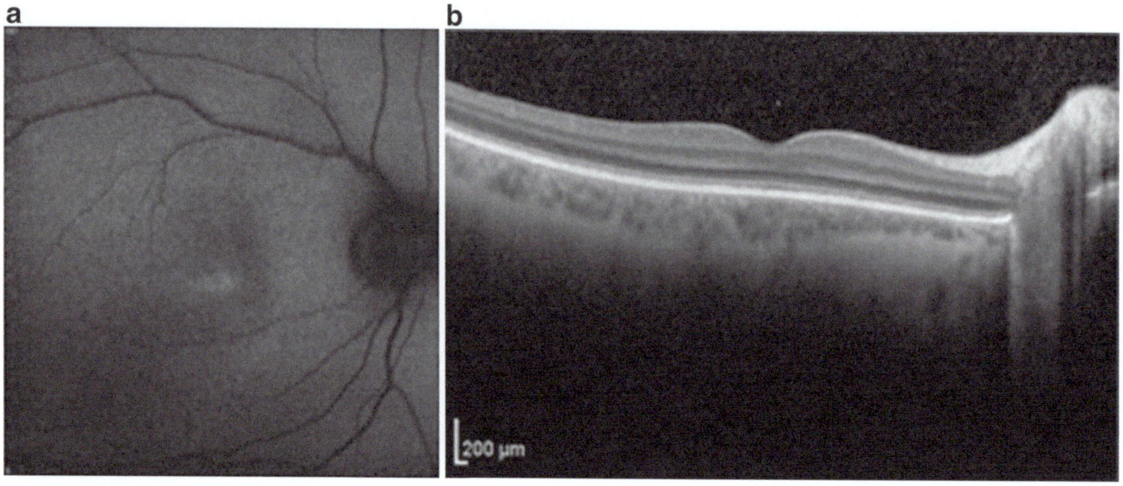

Fig. 20.1 Case summary: 24-year-old male with autosomal recessive achromatopsia with *CNGA3* mutations. (**a**) Fundus autofluorescence of the right eye showing foveal hyperautofluorescence. (**b**) Spectral domain optical coherence tomography of the right eye showing thinning of the ONL and retention of inner retinal layers.

References

1. Kohl S, Varsanyi B, Antunes GA, Baumann B, Hoyng CB, Jägle H, et al. CNGB3 mutations account for 50% of all cases with autosomal recessive achromatopsia. Eur J Hum Genet. 2005;13(3):302–8.
2. Wissinger B, Gamer D, Jagle H, Giorda R, Marx T, Mayer S, et al. CNGA3 mutations in hereditary cone photoreceptor disorders. Am J Hum Genet. 2001;69(4):722–37.
3. Kohl S, Marx T, Giddings I, Jägle H, Jacobson SG, Apfelstedt-Sylla E, et al. Total colourblindness is caused by mutations in the gene encoding the alpha-subunit of the cone photoreceptor cGMP-gated cation channel. Nat Genet. 1998;19(3):257–9.
4. Thiadens AA, Slingerland NW, Roosing S, van Schooneveld MJ, van Lith-Verhoeven JJ, van Moll-Ramirez N, et al. Genetic etiology and clinical consequences of complete and incomplete achromatopsia. Ophthalmology. 2009;116(10):1984–9. e1981
5. Nishiguchi KM, Sandberg MA, Gorji N, Berson EL, Dryja TP. Cone cGMP-gated channel mutations and clinical findings in patients with achromatopsia, macular degeneration, and other hereditary cone diseases. Hum Mutat. 2005;25(3):248–58.
6. Yang P, Michaels KV, Courtney RJ, Wen Y, Greninger DA, Reznick L, et al. Retinal morphology of patients with achromatopsia during early childhood: implications for gene therapy. JAMA Ophthalmol. 2014;132(7):823–31.
7. Fahim AT, Khan NW, Zahid S, Schachar IH, Branham K, Kohl S, et al. Diagnostic fundus autofluorescence patterns in achromatopsia. Am J Ophthalmol. 2013;156(6):1211–9.e1212.

21 *CNGB1*

CNGB1 encodes one of the two subunits (the other is encoded by *CNGA1*) of the rod cyclic nucleotide-gated (CNG) channel. These CNG channels in the rod plasma membrane respond to light-mediated concentration changes in cGMP by causing an influx of calcium, creating calcium-gated voltage signals [1, 2]. Mutations in *CNGB1* cause autosomal recessive retinitis pigmentosa (RP) [1].

CNGB1 mutations are responsible for about 4% of autosomal recessive RP cases [1]. While Bareil et al. [3] described patients with *CNGB1* mutations as having a severe form of RP, others have described patients with *CNGB1* mutations as having less severe phenotypes, with later ages of onset of symptoms [4, 5]. As expected with RP, patients demonstrate night blindness, which may occur in early childhood [3], and a progressively restricted visual field. Significantly reduced visual acuity or legal blindness has been noted in later adult years [4, 5]. Fundus exam, as expected for RP, reveals bony spicule-shaped pigment deposits (Fig. 21.1a, b) [3–5]. Fundus autofluorescence demonstrates hypoautofluorescence corresponding to the areas of atrophy and pigment deposition and may exhibit a hyperautofluorescent ring around the fovea (Fig. 21.1c, d). Optical coherence tomography shows the extent of photoreceptor loss, with progressive loss of the ellipsoid zone extending centrally from the periphery (Fig. 21.1e, f). ERG is eventually nonresponsive, but the age at which this is observed varies. Bareil et al. [3] noted a lack of rod response on ERG in his patient at age 30, while Bocquet et al. [4] noticed nonresponsive ERG at age 44 and Kondo et al. [5] at age 55.

S. Zahid et al., *Retinal Dystrophy Gene Atlas*, https://doi.org/10.1007/978-3-319-10867-4_21

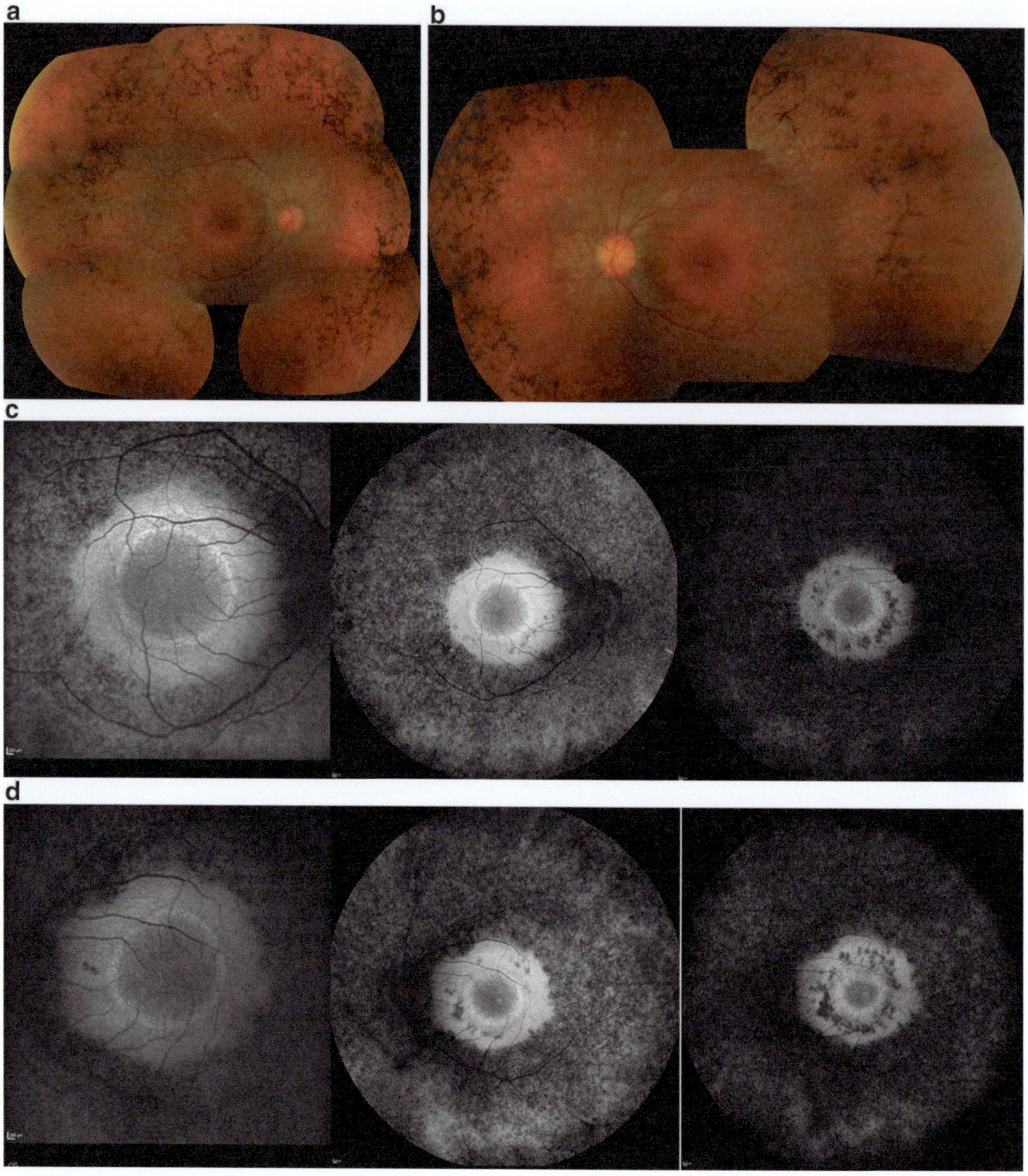

Fig. 21.1 Case summary: 48-year-old female with autosomal recessive retinitis pigmentosa with homozygous mutations in *CNGB1* (c.2544dupG) with best-corrected visual acuity of 20/20 in both eyes that declined to 20/30 in the right eye and 20/40 in the left eye over the course of 3 years. (**a**, **b**) Color fundus photograph montages of the right and left eyes showing mid-peripheral bone spicule pigment deposits and RPE changes in the macula. (**c**, **d**) Fundus autofluorescence of the right and left eyes showing a hyperautofluorescent ring in the parafovea that gradually shrinks over the course of 10 years (three panels show time points at 0, 5, and 10 years). There is also dense patchy hypoautofluorescence within an outside the arcades. As the hyperautofluorescent rings shrink with time, the areas surrounding the rings are gradually filled in by areas of hypoautofluorescence suggestive of atrophy. (**e**, **f**) Spectral domain optical coherence tomography of the right and left eyes showing progressive loss of the foveal ellipsoid zone in both eyes over the course of 6 years with the formation of a pseudo hole in the left eye.

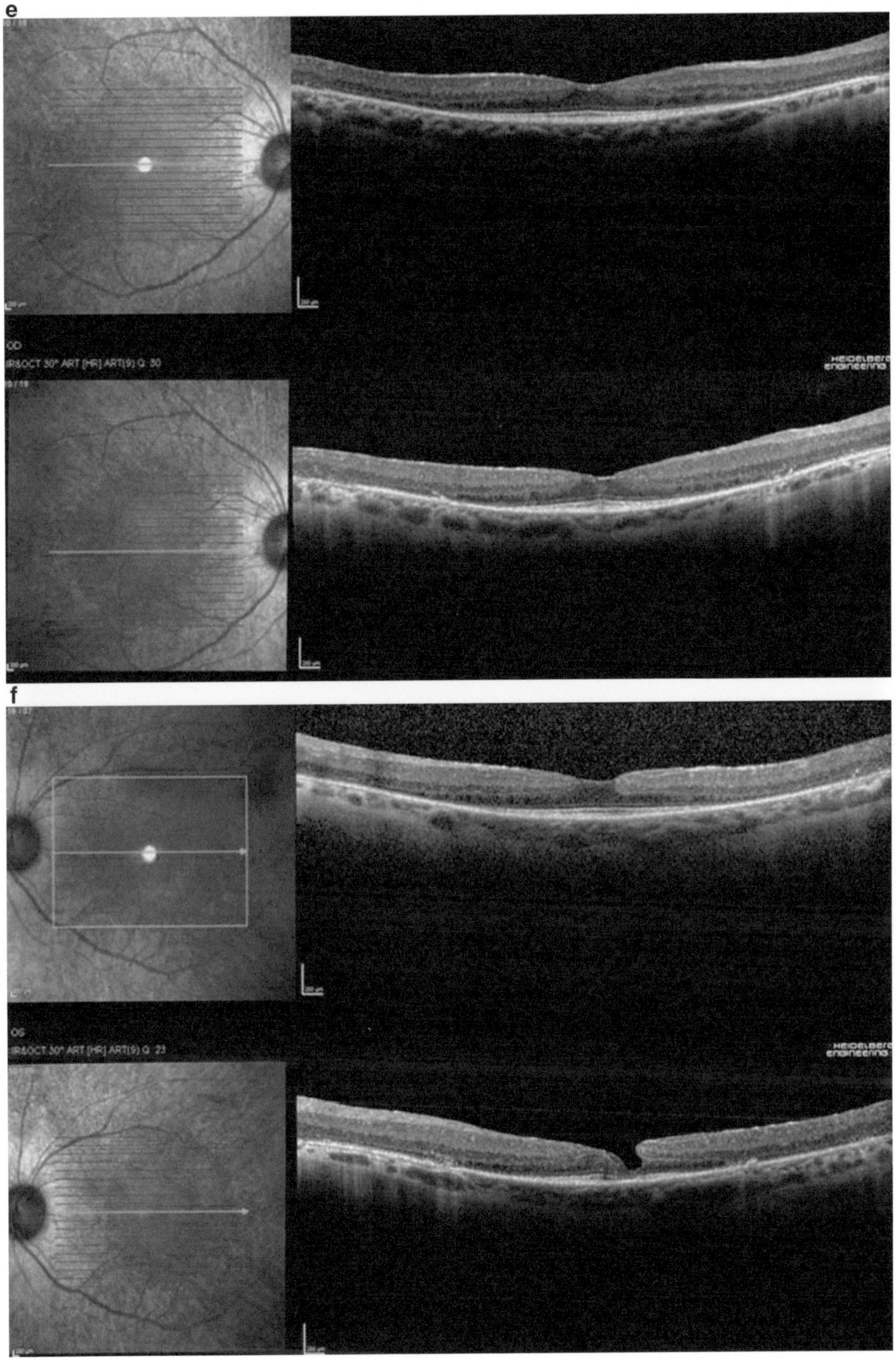

Fig. 21.1 (continued)

References

1. Koch S, Sothilingam V, Garcia Garrido M, Tanimoto N, Becirovic E, Koch F, et al. Gene therapy restores vision and delays degeneration in the CNGB1(−/−) mouse model of retinitis pigmentosa. Hum Mol Genet. 2012;21(20):4486–96.
2. Paquet-Durand F, Beck S, Michalakis S, Goldmann T, Huber G, Mühlfriedel R, et al. A key role for cyclic nucleotide gated (CNG) channels in cGMP-related retinitis pigmentosa. Hum Mol Genet. 2011;20(5):941–7.
3. Bareil C, Hamel CP, Delague V, Arnaud B, Demaille J, Claustres M. Segregation of a mutation in CNGB1 encoding the beta-subunit of the rod cGMP-gated channel in a family with autosomal recessive retinitis pigmentosa. Hum Genet. 2001;108(4):328–34.
4. Bocquet B, Marzouka NA, Hebrard M, Manes G, Sénéchal A, Meunier I, et al. Homozygosity mapping in autosomal recessive retinitis pigmentosa families detects novel mutations. Mol Vis. 2013;19:2487–500.
5. Kondo H, Qin M, Mizota A, Kondo M, Hayashi H, Hayashi K, et al. A homozygosity-based search for mutations in patients with autosomal recessive retinitis pigmentosa, using microsatellite markers. Invest Ophthalmol Vis Sci. 2004;45(12):4433–9.

CNGB3

22

CNGB3 encodes the beta-subunit of the cone photoreceptor cGMP-gated channel, which is involved in calcium influx during phototransduction. *CNGB3* mutations cause autosomal recessive achromatopsia (rod monochromatism), which usually presents in childhood, and cone dystrophy, which generally presents in young adulthood. *CNGB3* mutations are the most common cause (>50%) of achromatopsia [1].

Patients typically present in their first decade with poor visual acuity (20/100 to 20/200 or worse), photophobia, nonspecific color vision deficits, and nystagmus. While it was widely believed that visual acuity remains stable in achromatopsia, many patients experience progressive loss of central vision [2, 3]. Young patients usually exhibit normal fundi (>60%), while older patients may show loss of the foveal structure, pigmentary changes, or bull's-eye macular atrophy (Figs. 22.1a, 22.2a) [4]. Fundus autofluorescence may reveal foveal and parafoveal hyperautofluorescence (Figs. 22.3, 22.1b) with normal cross-sectional retinal architecture on OCT in younger patients (Fig. 22.1c), which may be characteristic of achromatopsia. More advanced disease in older patients may exhibit focal foveal atrophy and "punched-out" outer retinal cavitation on FAF and OCT (Fig. 22.2b, c). However, foveal abnormalities, such as hypolucency or loss of the ellipsoid zone, have also been reported in patients as young as 8 months old [5]. Macular thickness is reduced, with the reduction typically resulting from outer retinal loss in the context of a maintained inner retina [5]. Electroretinography (ERG) exhibits diminished or absent photopic responses, which show progressive loss in some patients [6]. Scotopic ERG responses are usually subnormal but generally do not decline over time [7].

Autosomal recessive cone dystrophy caused by mutations in *CNGB3* is characterized by progressive deterioration of visual acuity and abnormal color vision, which usually begin in the second decade of life [8]. Nystagmus is less common than in achromatopsia. Funduscopic findings are variable and may be normal or include RPE pigmentary changes or bull's-eye maculopathy. ERG reveals a characteristic progressive deterioration of photopic ERG parameters with scotopic parameters in the normal range [7].

S. Zahid et al., *Retinal Dystrophy Gene Atlas*, https://doi.org/10.1007/978-3-319-10867-4_22

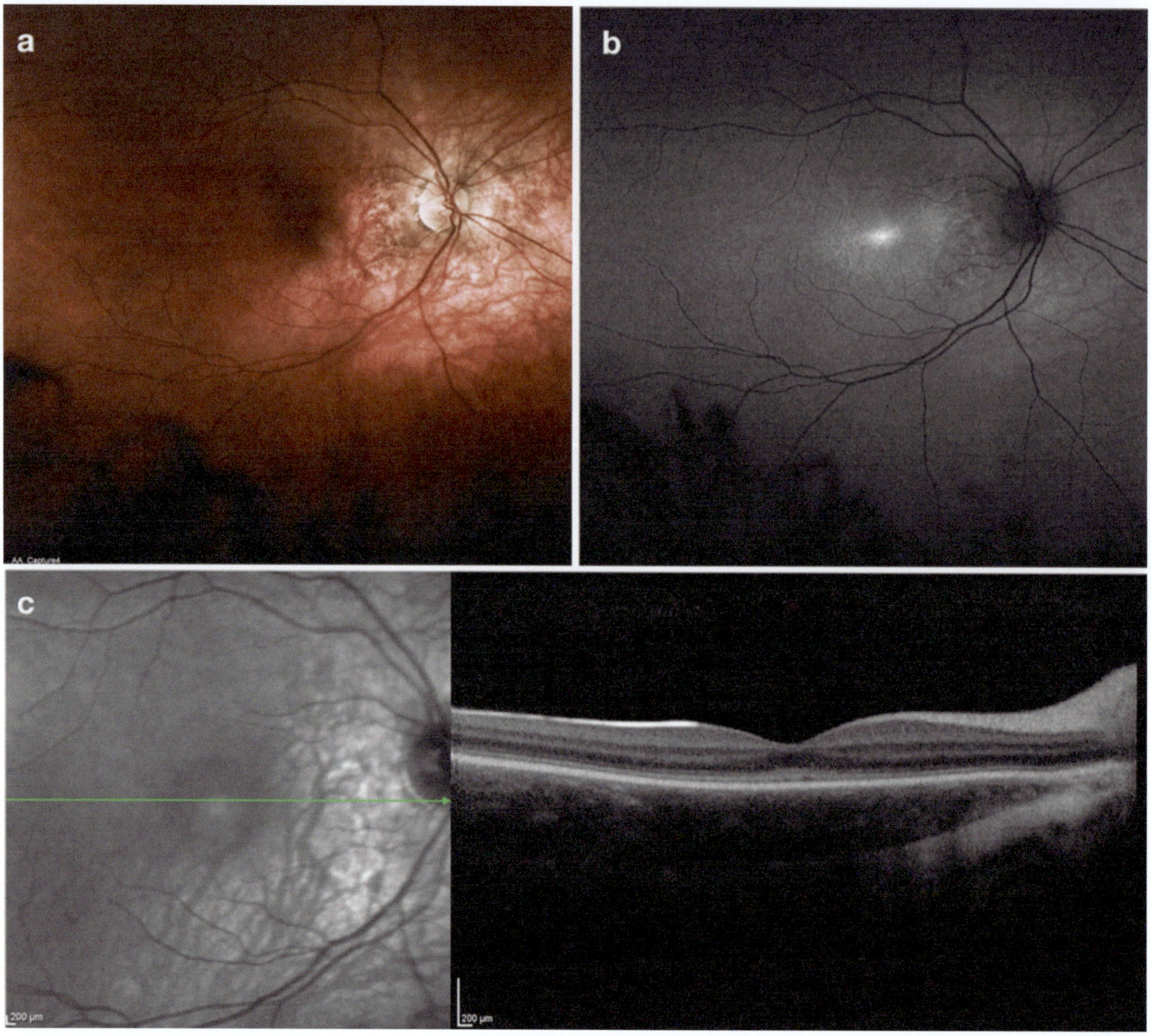

Fig. 22.1 Case summary: 59-year-old woman with achromatopsia. (**a**) Color fundus photograph of the right eye showing foveal hyperpigmentation and atrophy. (**b**) Fundus autofluorescence of the right eye showing foveal hypoautofluorescence corresponding to the area of foveal atrophy. (**c**) Spectral-domain OCT showing outer retinal cavitation at the fovea with loss of the ellipsoid zone at the foveola.

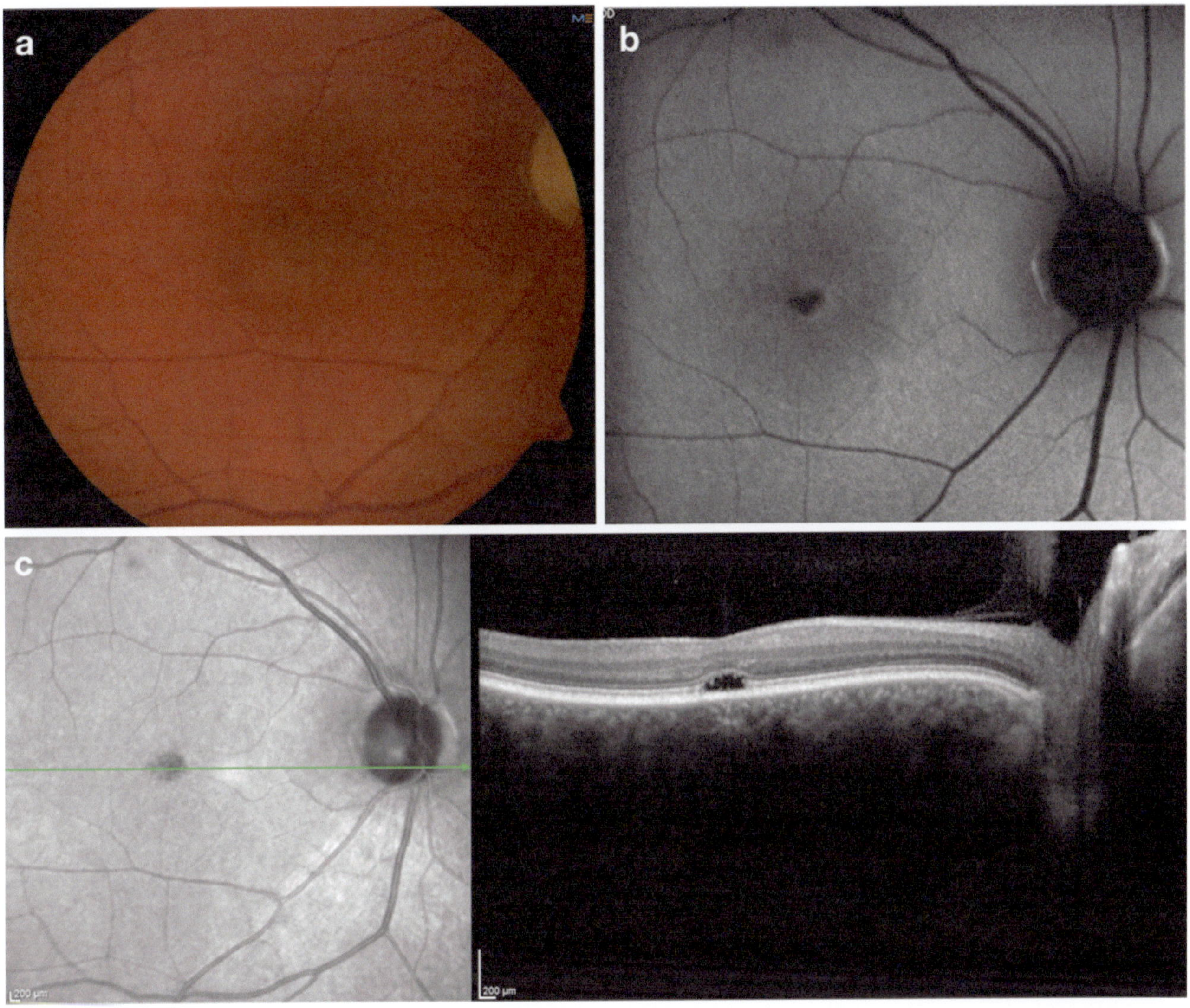

Fig. 22.2 Case summary: 11-year-old girl with achromatopsia. (**a**) Color fundus photograph of the right eye showing a normal macular appearance. (**b**) Wide-field fundus autofluorescence of the right eye showing foveal hyperautofluorescence. (**c**) Spectral-domain optical coherence tomography (OCT) showing a normal foveal architecture.

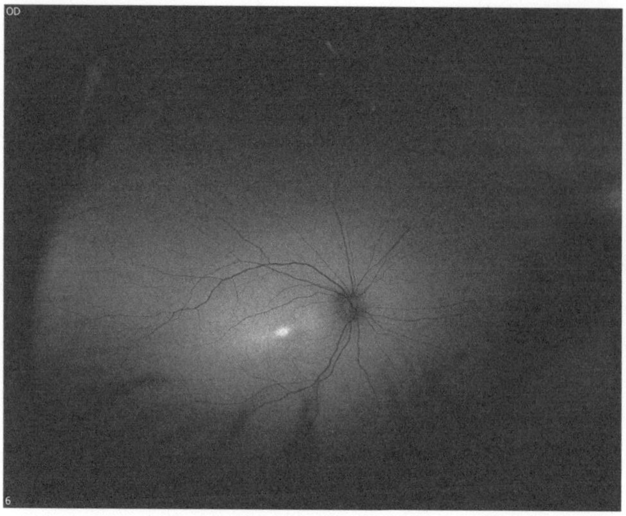

Fig. 22.3 Wide-field fundus autofluorescence of the right eye from a 4-year-old girl with foveal hyperautofluorescence.

References

1. Kohl S, Varsanyi B, Antunes GA, Baumann B, Hoyng CB, Jägle H, et al. CNGB3 mutations account for 50% of all cases with autosomal recessive achromatopsia. Eur J Hum Genet. 2005;13(3):302–8.
2. Nishiguchi KM, Sandberg MA, Gorji N, Berson EL, Dryja TP. Cone cGMP-gated channel mutations and clinical findings in patients with achromatopsia, macular degeneration, and other hereditary cone diseases. Hum Mutat. 2005;25(3):248–58.
3. Wiszniewski W, Lewis RA, Lupski JR. Achromatopsia: the CNGB3 p.T383fsX mutation results from a founder effect and is responsible for the visual phenotype in the original report of uniparental disomy 14. Hum Genet. 2007;121(3–4):433–9.
4. Thiadens AA, Slingerland NW, Roosing S, van Schooneveld MJ, van Lith-Verhoeven JJ, van Moll-Ramirez N, et al. Genetic etiology and clinical consequences of complete and incomplete achromatopsia. Ophthalmology. 2009;116(10):1984–9.
5. Yang P, Michaels KV, Courtney RJ, Wen Y, Greninger DA, Reznick L, et al. Retinal morphology of patients with achromatopsia during early childhood: implications for gene therapy. JAMA Ophthalmol. 2014;132(7):823–31.
6. Khan NW, Wissinger B, Kohl S, Sieving PA. CNGB3 achromatopsia with progressive loss of residual cone function and impaired rod-mediated function. Invest Ophthalmol Vis Sci. 2007;48(8):3864–71.
7. Wang I, Khan NW, Branham K, Wissinger B, Kohl S, Heckenlively JR. Establishing baseline rod electroretinogram values in achromatopsia and cone dystrophy. Doc Ophthalmol. 2012;125(3):229–33.
8. Michaelides M, Aligianis IA, Ainsworth JR, Good P, Mollon JD, Maher ER, et al. Progressive cone dystrophy associated with mutation in CNGB3. Invest Ophthalmol Vis Sci. 2004;45(6):1975–82.

23 CRB1

CRB1 encodes a transmembrane protein involved in retinal development and organization. Mutations are responsible for Leber's congenital amaurosis (LCA) and retinitis pigmentosa (RP). *CRB1* has been reported to be associated with RP with retinal telengiectasias and exudation (Coats-like vasculopathy), RP with preservation of the para-arteriolar retinal pigment epithelium (PPRPE), and dominant pigmented paravenous chorioretinal atrophy [1–5].

LCA caused by *CRB1* mutations is characterized by visual dysfunction at a very young age [6]. Patients typically present before the age of 5 with visual acuities worse than 20/200, night blindness, photophobia, hyperopia, aberrant color vision, and nystagmus [4, 7, 8]. Keratoconus has also been reported in some studies [8, 9]. In the first 5 years, ERGs may be non-recordable or show a cone-rod or rod-cone pattern of dysfunction [10, 11]. Funduscopic and tomographic appearances may be variable, but certain features are suggestive of mutations in *CRB1* (Figs. 23.1a, 23.2, 23.3, 23.4, and 23.5), including white dots at the RPE level in younger patients and mid-peripheral nummular pigmentation (Fig. 23.3) (also seen in patients with *NR2E3*, *NRL*, and *TULP1* mutations) in older patients [10]. Macular atrophy has been reported in about 50% of patients in some studies. OCT may show intraretinal cystic spaces, cystoid macular edema, or an overall increase in foveal thickness (Fig. 23.4b) [10]; Jacobson et al. [12] have reported thick unlaminated retinal architecture in LCA patients with *CRB1* mutations. The most common mutation, C948Y, has been reported to result in LCA when in a homozygous state and to be more likely to be associated with RP when in a compound heterozygous state with another missense allele (Fig. 23.3) [3, 4]. However, another study was unable to recapitulate these findings, though they did report that LCA was more commonly associated with one or two null alleles [2]. Fundus autofluorescence may show loss of autofluorescence signal in areas of retinal pigment epithelium atrophy (Figs. 23.1b and 23.5b).

S. Zahid et al., *Retinal Dystrophy Gene Atlas*, https://doi.org/10.1007/978-3-319-10867-4_23

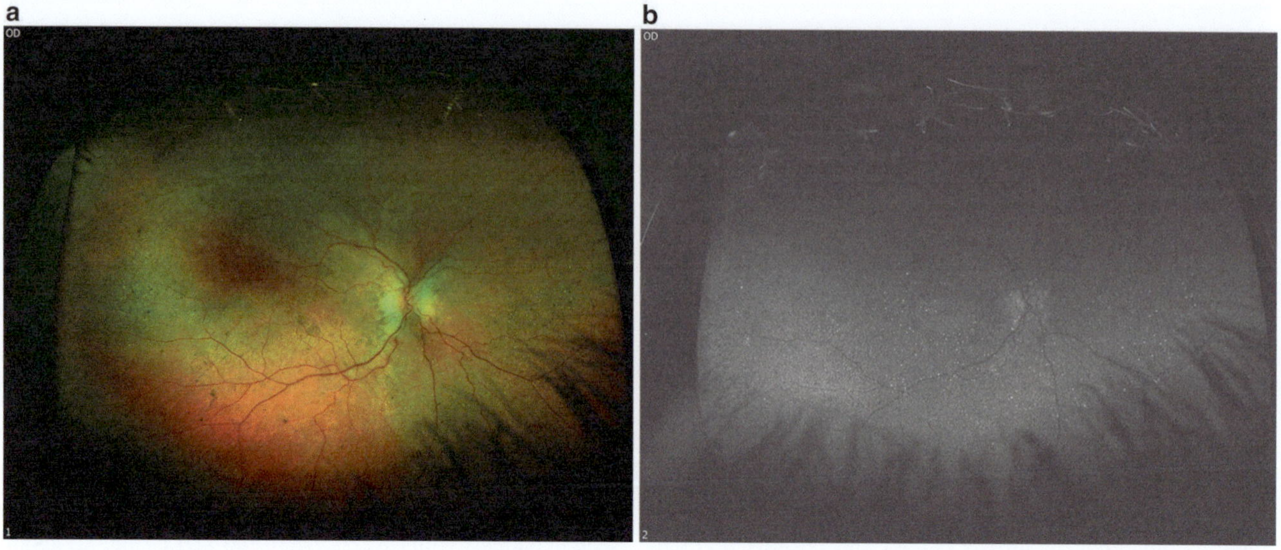

Fig. 23.1 Case summary: An 8-year-old boy with Leber's congenital amaurosis (LCA). (**a**) Color fundus photograph of the right eye showing diffuse retinal pigment epithelium (RPE) atrophy within and outside the vascular arcades associated with pigmentary changes and peripapillary atrophy. (**b**) Fundus autofluorescence of the right eye showing diffuse loss of autofluorescence, with focal pinpoint areas of autofluorescence throughout the fundus.

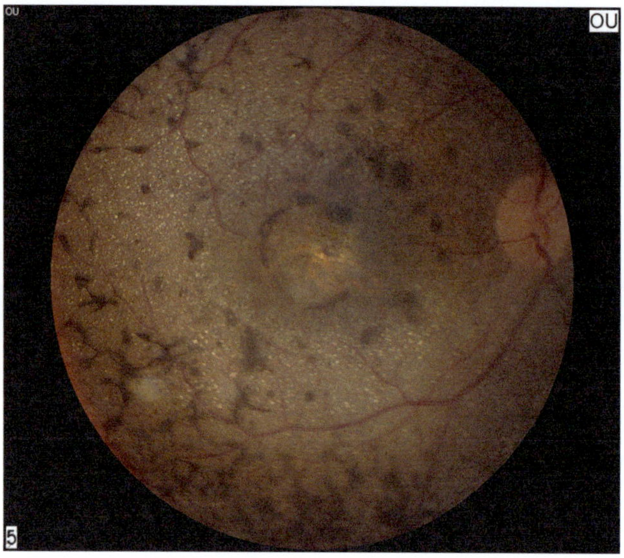

Fig. 23.2 Color fundus photograph of the right eye from a 31-year-old woman with LCA, showing diffuse RPE atrophy with dense bone-spicule pigment deposits throughout the posterior pole.

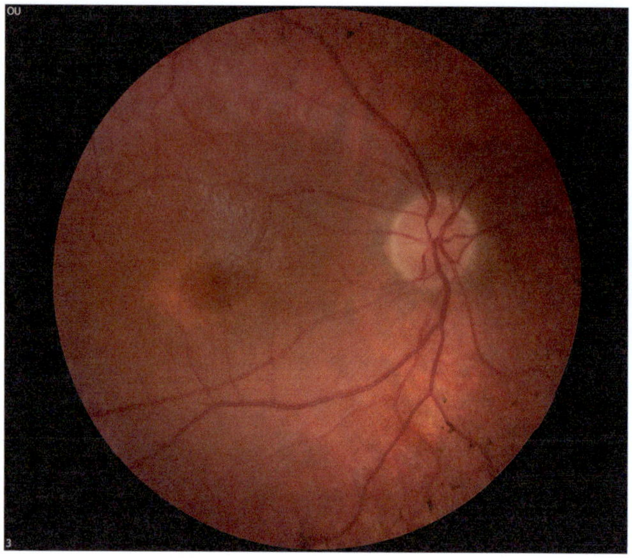

Fig. 23.3 Color fundus photograph of the right eye from an 18-year-old man with rod-cone dystrophy (retinitis pigmentosa), showing RPE atrophy outside the arcades with sparse pigment deposits.

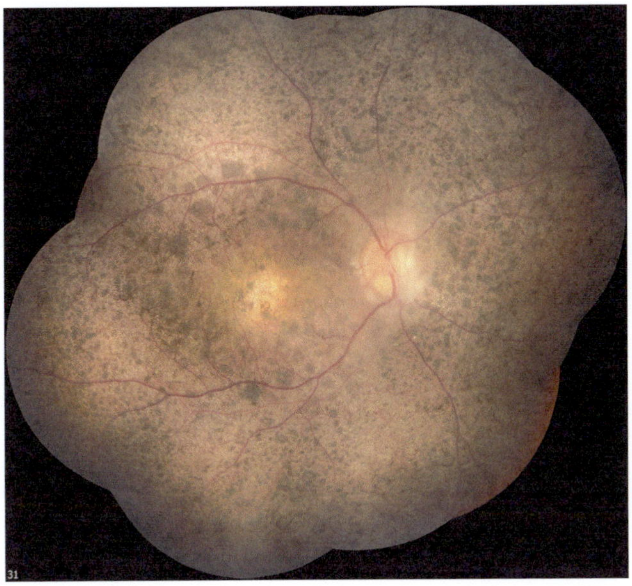

Fig. 23.4 Color fundus photograph of the right eye from a 28-year-old man, showing nummular pigment deposits with diffuse RPE and macular atrophy with peripapillary atrophy.

Up to 7% of recessive RP is caused by mutations in *CRB1* [13]. Patients usually present in the second decade of life with night blindness and reduced visual acuity (ranging from 20/50 to LP in some studies), though in some patients, central visual deficits and photosensitivity predominate. Hyperopia is often observed, while nystagmus is uncommon. These patients often exhibit a variable funduscopic phenotype, with both bone-spicule pattern or clumped nummular pigmentary deposits possible (Figs. 23.3, 23.4, 23.5a, and 23.6). Other findings with *CRB1* include PPRPE and Coats-like vasculopathy, which are commonly observed in the context of RP [2, 3, 5, 15, 16]. Most patients exhibit a maculopathy, with up to 50% of patients exhibiting CME (Fig. 23.5b) [2]. Some patients have been reported to develop angle-closure glaucoma and pupillary block as a result of peripheral telengietasias [10]. Nanophthalmos with RP has been reported [14].

Dominantly inherited pigmented paravenous chorioretinal atrophy has also been reported to be associated with mutations in *CRB1* [17]. McKay et al. [17] reported that the

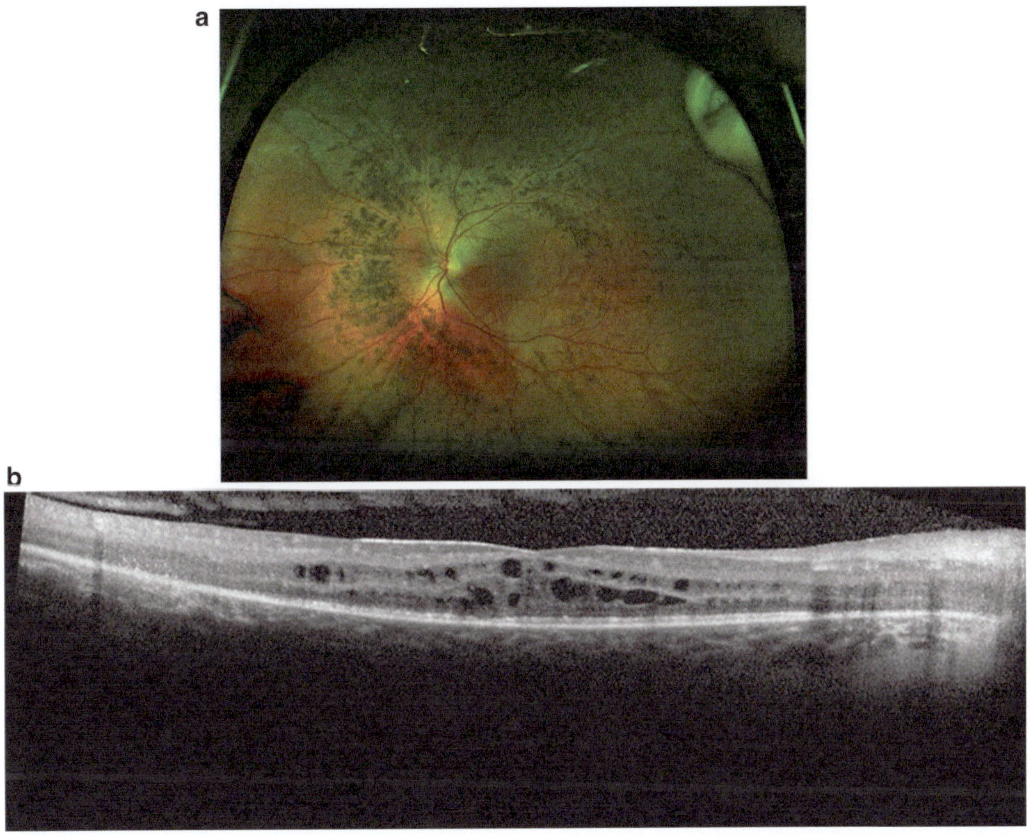

Fig. 23.5 Case summary: 8-year-old female (CEI28492) with Leber's congenital amaurosis/Severe Early Childhood Onset Retinal Dystrophy (SECORD) with heterozygous mutations in *CRB1*. (**a**) Wide-field color fundus photograph of the left eye showing RPE atrophy with pigmentary changes along the arcades. (**b**) Spectral-domain optical coherence tomography showing extensive loss of the ellipsoid zone with foveal-sparing and cystoid macular edema.

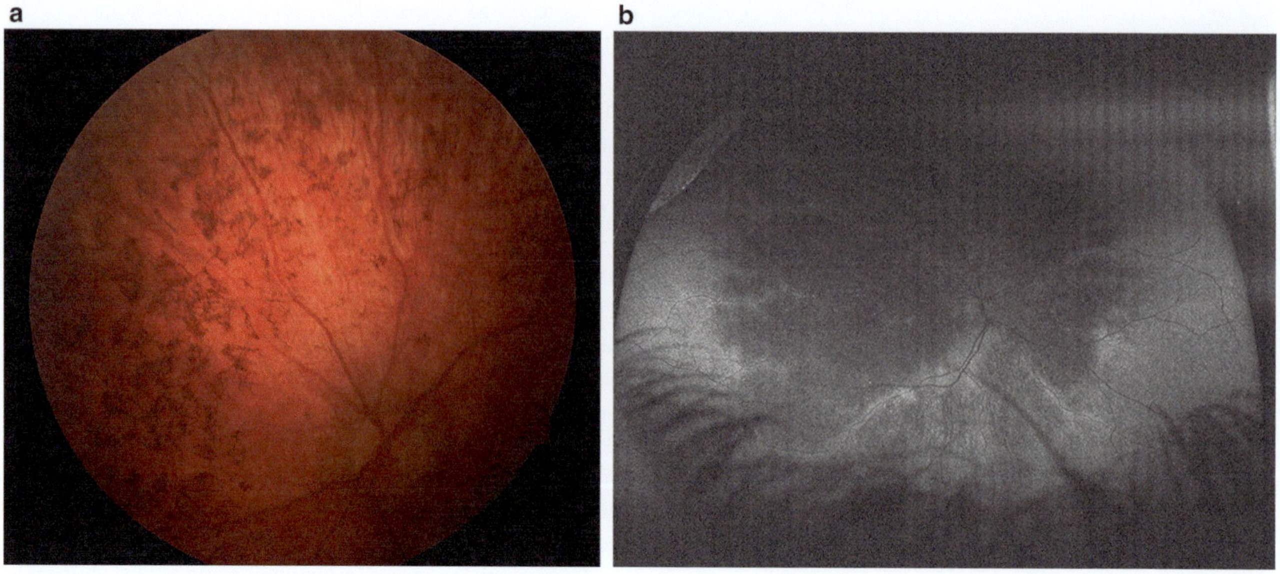

Fig. 23.6 Case summary: 6-year-old female (CEI26281) with Leber's congenital amaurosis/Severe Early Childhood Onset Retinal Dystrophy (SECORD) with compound heterozygous mutations in *CRB1*. (**a**) Color fundus photograph of the left eye showing RPE atrophy with pigmentary changes along the arcades. (**b**) Wide-field fundus autofluorescence of the right eye showing dense and confluent dropout of autofluorescence signal in the posterior pole, suggestive of RPE atrophy.

initial sign of this disease was symmetric chorioretinal atrophy, which progressed to paravenous pigmentation that begins peripherally and extends centrally.

References

1. den Hollander AI, Davis J, van der Velde-Visser SD, Zonneveld MN, Pierrottet CO, Koenekoop RK, et al. CRB1 mutation spectrum in inherited retinal dystrophies. Hum Mutat. 2004;24(5):355–69.
2. Bujakowska K, Audo I, Mohand-Said S, Lancelot ME, Antonio A, Germain A, et al. CRB1 mutations in inherited retinal dystrophies. Hum Mutat. 2012;33(2):306–15.
3. den Hollander AI, Heckenlively JR, van den Born LI, de Kok YJ, van der Velde-Visser SD, Kellner U, et al. Leber congenital amaurosis and retinitis pigmentosa with Coats-like exudative vasculopathy are associated with mutations in the crumbs homologue 1 (CRB1) gene. Am J Hum Genet. 2001;69(1):198–203.
4. Lotery AJ, Jacobson SG, Fishman GA, Weleber RG, Fulton AB, Namperumalsamy P, et al. Mutations in the CRB1 gene cause Leber congenital amaurosis. Arch Ophthalmol. 2001;119(3):415–20.
5. Heckenlively JR. Preserved para-arteriole retinal pigment epithelium (PPRPE) in retinitis pigmentosa. Birth Defects Orig Artic Ser. 1982;18(6):193–6.
6. Weleber RG, Francis PJ, Trzupek KM, Beattie C. Leber congenital amaurosis. In: Pagon RA, Adam MP, Ardinger HH, Wallace SE, Amemiya A, LJH B, et al., editors. GeneReviews® [Internet]. Seattle: University of Washington; 1993–2016; 2004 [2013]. https://www.ncbi.nlm.nih.gov/books/NBK1298/. Accessed 11 Jan 2017.
7. Abouzeid H, Li Y, Maumence IH, Dharmaraj S, Sundin O. A G1103R mutation in CRB1 is co-inherited with high hyperopia and Leber congenital amaurosis. Ophthalmic Genet. 2006;27(1):15–20.
8. McKibbin M, Ali M, Mohamed MD, Booth AP, Bishop F, Pal B, et al. Genotype-phenotype correlation for leber congenital amaurosis in Northern Pakistan. Arch Ophthalmol. 2010;128(1):107–13.
9. McMahon TT, Kim LS, Fishman GA, Stone EM, Zhao XC, Yee RW, et al. CRB1 gene mutations are associated with keratoconus in patients with leber congenital amaurosis. Invest Ophthalmol Vis Sci. 2009;50(7):3185–7.
10. Henderson RH, Mackay DS, Li Z, Moradi P, Sergouniotis P, Russell-Eggitt I, et al. Phenotypic variability in patients with retinal dystrophies due to mutations in CRB1. Br J Ophthalmol. 2011;95(6):811–7.
11. Hanein S, Perrault I, Gerber S, Tanguy G, Barbet F, Ducroq D, et al. Leber congenital amaurosis: comprehensive survey of the genetic heterogeneity, refinement of the clinical definition, and genotype-phenotype correlations as a strategy for molecular diagnosis. Hum Mutat. 2004;23(4):306–17.
12. Jacobson SG, Cideciyan AV, Aleman TS, Pianta MJ, Sumaroka A, Schwartz SB, et al. Crumbs homolog 1 (CRB1) mutations result in a thick human retina with abnormal lamination. Hum Mol Genet. 2003;12(9):1073–8.
13. Fahim AT, Daiger SP, Weleber RG. Retinitis pigmentosa overview. In: Pagon RA, Adam MP, Ardinger HH, Wallace SE, Amemiya A, LJH B, et al., editors. GeneReviews® [Internet]. Seattle: University of Washington; 1993–2016; 2000 [Updated 2013]. https://www.ncbi.nlm.nih.gov/books/NBK1417/. Accessed 11 Jan 2017.
14. Zenteno JC, Buentello-Volante B, Ayala-Ramirez R, Villanueva-Mendoza C. Homozygosity mapping identifies the Crumbs homologue 1 (Crb1) gene as responsible for a recessive syndrome of retinitis pigmentosa and nanophthalmos. Am J Med Genet A. 2011;155A(5):1001–6.
15. Heckenlively JR. Preserved para-arteriole retinal pigment epithelium (PPRPE) in retinitis pigmentosa. Br J Ophthalmol. 1982;66(1):26–30.
16. den Hollander AI, ten Brink JB, de Kok YJ, van Soest S, van den Born LI, van Driel MA, et al. Mutations in a human homologue of Drosophila crumbs cause retinitis pigmentosa (RP12). Nat Genet. 1999;23(2):217–21.
17. McKay GJ, Clarke S, Davis JA, Simpson DA, Silvestri G. Pigmented paravenous chorioretinal atrophy is associated with a mutation within the crumbs homolog 1 (CRB1) gene. Invest Ophthalmol Vis Sci. 2005;46(1):322–8.

24 CRX

CRX encodes a transcription factor involved in the differentiation of photoreceptor cells. Mutations are responsible for autosomal dominant cone-rod dystrophy, adult-onset dominant retinitis pigmentosa (RP), and Leber's congenital amaurosis (LCA) [1–5].

CRX mutations are responsible for about 5% of cone-rod dystrophy [3, 4, 6]. Patients typically present in the first-to-third decades of life with progressively worsening visual acuity (20/25 to <20/200), poor color vision, and, commonly, nystagmus, photosensitivity, and hyperopia. Patients with certain mutations may have a later onset of visual acuity loss [7]. Night blindness and loss of peripheral vision typically occur later in the disease course. Fundus examination is characterized by progressive maculopathy, ranging from normal to pigment clumping in young patients to choroidal and retinal pigment epithelium (RPE) atrophy in later stages of disease, vessel attenuation, and variable pigment deposition peripherally (Figs. 24.1 and 24.2a) [8]. Fundus autofluorescence (FAF) may reveal macular atrophy and a peri-foveal hyperfluorescent ring (Fig. 24.2b). A progressively deteriorating cone-rod electroretinogram pattern (ERG) pattern is characteristic, with initial cone abnormalities progressing to panretinal dysfunction; one study has also reported a negative ERG in one family [9]. Goldmann visual field typically reveals central scotomata with peripherally constricted fields.

CRX mutations are also responsible for about 3% of LCA, most often in an autosomal dominant manner [6, 10]. Patients present at birth or within the first year of life with visual abnormalities (such as poor visual pursuit and digital ocular signs), nystagmus, and a non-recordable ERG [2, 5]. Even when vision is maintained, visual acuity is usually no better than 20/200; night blindness and hyperopia are very common [11, 12]. Fundus examination may be normal initially (Fig. 24.3) but often exhibits features of retinal degeneration, such as macular atrophy, vessel attenuation, and peripheral bone-spicule pigment deposits [11]. Visual improvement has been reported in one case [13]. Autosomal recessive inheritance has also been reported in one family [14].

About 1% of retinitis pigmentosa is attributable to mutations in *CRX* [5, 6]. These patients may be asymptomatic until their 50s to 60s, when they present with peripheral visual defects that deteriorate over the course of a decade. Central visual acuity and ERG parameters are generally maintained until late in the disease course. Fundus features may mimic classical RP and contain pigmentary clumping in the periphery with no macular changes. ERG and GVF typically reveal a rod-cone pattern of retinal degeneration.

S. Zahid et al., *Retinal Dystrophy Gene Atlas*, https://doi.org/10.1007/978-3-319-10867-4_24

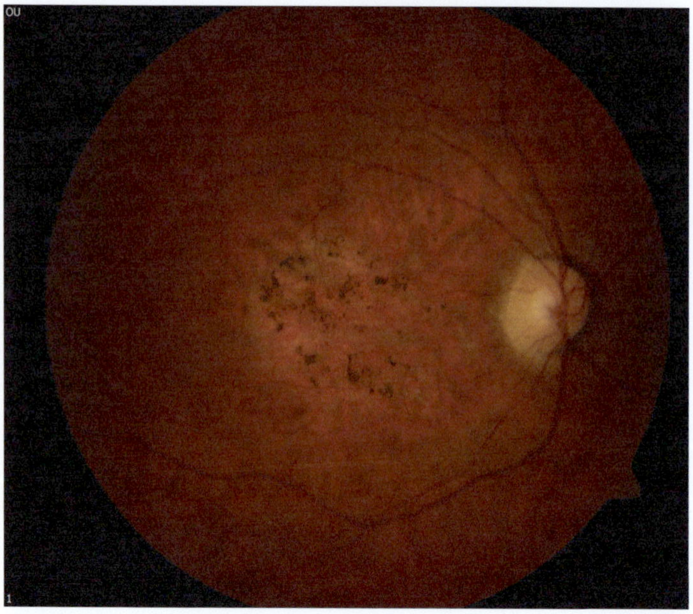

Fig. 24.1 Color fundus photograph of the right eye from a 40-year-old man with isolated cone dysfunction, showing macular atrophy and pigment clumping.

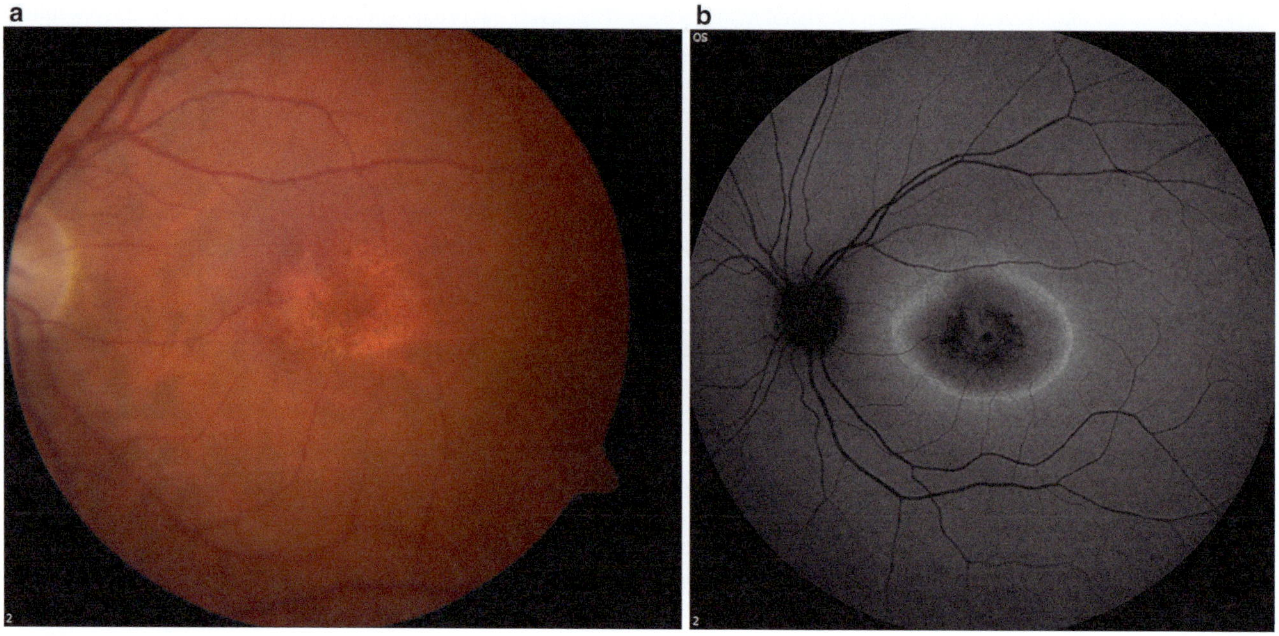

Fig. 24.2 Case summary: A 43-year-old man with a cone-rod dystrophy associated with a mutation in *CRX*. (**a**) Color fundus photograph of the left eye, showing macular atrophy in a partial bull's-eye pattern. (**b**) Fundus autofluorescence of the left eye, showing hypoautofluorescence in the areas of macular atrophy seen in Fig. 3a, surrounded by a hyper-autofluorescent ring.

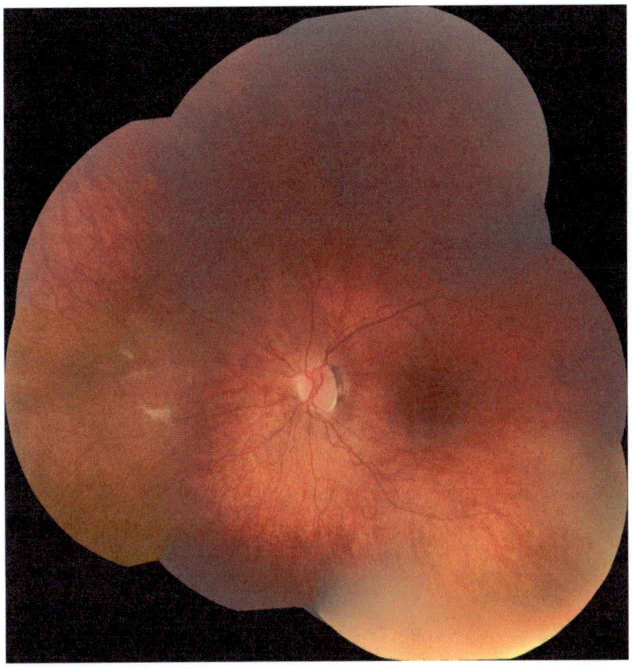

Fig. 24.3 Montage color fundus photograph of the left eye from an 8-year-old female with Leber congenital amaurosis due to mutations in *CRX*, showing no obvious atrophy or pigment deposition.

References

1. Lotery AJ, Namperumalsamy P, Jacobson SG, Weleber RG, Fishman GA, Musarella MA, et al. Mutation analysis of 3 genes in patients with Leber congenital amaurosis. Arch Ophthalmol. 2000;118(4):538–43.
2. Sohocki MM, Sullivan LS, Mintz-Hittner HA, Birch D, Heckenlively JR, Freund CL, et al. A range of clinical phenotypes associated with mutations in CRX, a photoreceptor transcription-factor gene. Am J Hum Genet. 1998;63(5):1307–15.
3. Freund CL, Gregory-Evans CY, Furukawa T, Papaioannou M, Looser J, Ploder L, et al. Cone-rod dystrophy due to mutations in a novel photoreceptor-specific homeobox gene (CRX) essential for maintenance of the photoreceptor. Cell. 1997;91(4):543–53.
4. Swain PK, Chen S, Wang QL, Affatigato LM, Coats CL, Brady KD, et al. Mutations in the cone-rod homeobox gene are associated with the cone-rod dystrophy photoreceptor degeneration. Neuron. 1997;19(6):1329–36.
5. Rivolta C, Berson EL, Dryja TP. Dominant Leber congenital amaurosis, cone-rod degeneration, and retinitis pigmentosa caused by mutant versions of the transcription factor CRX. Hum Mutat. 2001;18(6):488–98.
6. Huang L, Xiao X, Li S, Jia X, Wang P, Guo X, et al. CRX variants in cone-rod dystrophy and mutation overview. Biochem Biophys Res Commun. 2012;426(4):498–503.
7. Paunescu K, Preising MN, Janke B, Wissinger B, Lorenz B. Genotype-phenotype correlation in a German family with a novel complex CRX mutation extending the open reading frame. Ophthalmology. 2007;114(7):1348–57 e1341.
8. Nichols LL 2nd, Alur RP, Boobalan E, Sergeev YV, Caruso RC, Stone EM, et al. Two novel CRX mutant proteins causing autosomal dominant Leber congenital amaurosis interact differently with NRL. Hum Mutat. 2010;31(6):E1472–83.
9. Kitiratschky VB, Nagy D, Zabel T, Zrenner E, Wissinger B, Kohl S, et al. Cone and cone-rod dystrophy segregating in the same pedigree due to the same novel CRX gene mutation. Br J Ophthalmol. 2008;92(8):1086–91.
10. Freund CL, Wang QL, Chen S, Muskat BL, Wiles CD, Sheffield VC, et al. De novo mutations in the CRX homeobox gene associated with Leber congenital amaurosis. Nat Genet. 1998;18(4):311–2.
11. Dharmaraj SR, Silva ER, Pina AL, Li YY, Yang JM, Carter CR, et al. Mutational analysis and clinical correlation in Leber congenital amaurosis. Ophthalmic Genet. 2000;21(3):135–50.
12. Hanein S, Perrault I, Gerber S, Tanguy G, Barbet F, Ducroq D, et al. Leber congenital amaurosis: comprehensive survey of the genetic heterogeneity, refinement of the clinical definition, and genotype-phenotype correlations as a strategy for molecular diagnosis. Hum Mutat. 2004;23(4):306–17.
13. Koenekoop RK, Loyer M, Dembinska O, Beneish R. Visual improvement in Leber congenital amaurosis and the CRX genotype. Ophthalmic Genet. 2002;23(1):49–59.
14. Swaroop A, Wang QL, Wu W, Cook J, Coats C, Xu S, et al. Leber congenital amaurosis caused by a homozygous mutation (R90W) in the homeodomain of the retinal transcription factor CRX: direct evidence for the involvement of CRX in the development of photoreceptor function. Hum Mol Genet. 1999;8(2):299–305.

25 C1QTNF5

C1QTNF5 (previously called *CTRP5*) encodes C1q tumor necrosis factor-related protein and is highly expressed in the retinal pigment epithelium (RPE), lens, and ciliary epithelium. *C1QTNF5* plays an important role in the adhesion of the RPE to the Bruch Membrane, and mutations are thought to impair the adhesion, resulting in sub-RPE deposits. Mutations in *C1QTNF5* are associated with late-onset retinal degeneration (LORD).

C1QTNF5-related LORD follows an autosomal dominant pattern of inheritance. Patients with LORD usually experience a late onset of nyctalopia in the fourth to the sixth decades of life [1]. Best-corrected visual acuity may initially be normal and tends to worsen throughout the disease process to as low as 20/400 [2]. There may be color vision abnormalities. Goldmann visual fields are typically normal early in life and tend to exhibit nasal field loss prior to deficits in the temporal field. Some patients experience central vision loss late in the disease process, usually in their 60s [1]. Choroidal neovascular membrane associated with areas of atrophy may develop late in the disease [1, 3]. Many older patients have ocular hypertension/open-angle glaucoma, though it is unclear whether this is related to the elongated anterior lens zolules [3]. Characteristic ophthalmic findings include peripupillary iris atrophy and elongated anterior lens zonule insertions (Fig. 25.1e) [1–4]. Drusen deposits in the mid- and far-retinal periphery are also common early in the disease process, though the fundus may be normal, and many patients are asymptomatic at this early stage (Fig. 25.1a, b) [3, 4]. Some patients develop scalloped chorioretinal atrophy and bony spicule pigmentary changes in late stages (Fig. 25.2) [1]. Fundus autofluoresence (FAF) imaging may exhibit areas of hypoautofluoresence associated with regions of chorioretinal atrophy, with a surrounding hyperautofluorescent border (Fig. 25.1c) [1, 2]. Similar to other retinal degenerations, spectral domain optical coherence tomography (SD-OCT) may reveal widespread loss of the outer retinal layers, with areas of absence of the ellipsoid zone suggestive of photoreceptor loss and thinning of the outer nuclear layer [1]. Hyper-reflective deposits may be present in the RPE-Bruch's membrane complex, with some patients exhibiting areas of separation in this complex (Fig. 25.1d); choroidal thinning may also be observed [1, 2]. Electroretinography (ERG) may be normal early in the disease state but typically exhibits a rod-cone pattern of degeneration [1, 2]. Pattern or multi-focal ERG may display significant macular involvement in some patients [1]. Abnormal dark adaption may be found early, up to a decade before ophthalmic signs of LORD are exhibited [1, 3].

S. Zahid et al., *Retinal Dystrophy Gene Atlas*, https://doi.org/10.1007/978-3-319-10867-4_25

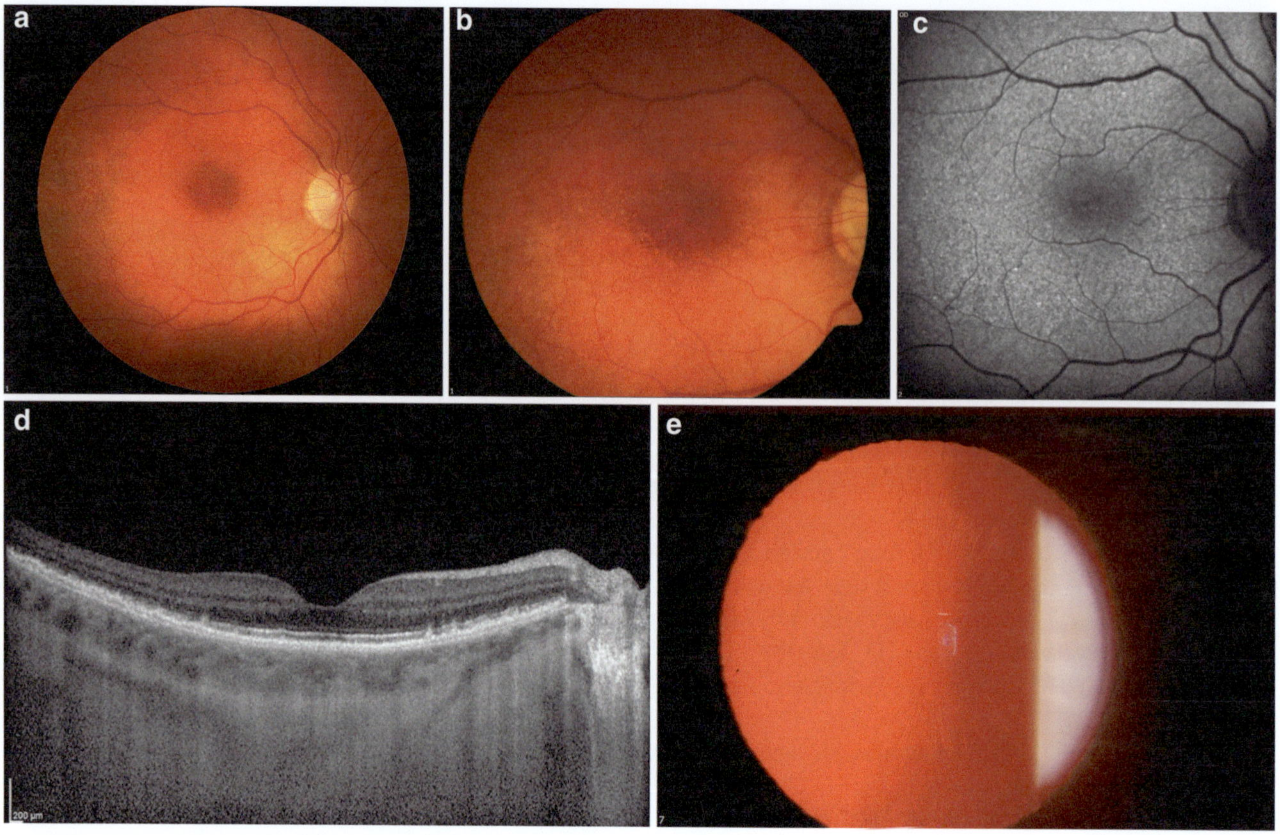

Fig. 25.1 Case summary: 61-year-old female with a mutation in *C1QTNF5*. (**a**) Color fundus photograph of the right eye showing drusen throughout the macula. (**b**) Higher magnification color fundus photograph of the right eye showing drusen throughout the macula. (**c**) Fundus autofluorescence of the right eye showing hyperautofluorescence surrounding hypoautofluorescent drusen throughout the macula. (**d**) Spectral-domain optical coherence tomography showing loss of the ellipsoid zone temporally and drusen. (**e**) Slit lamp photo showing anteriorly-placed lens zonules.

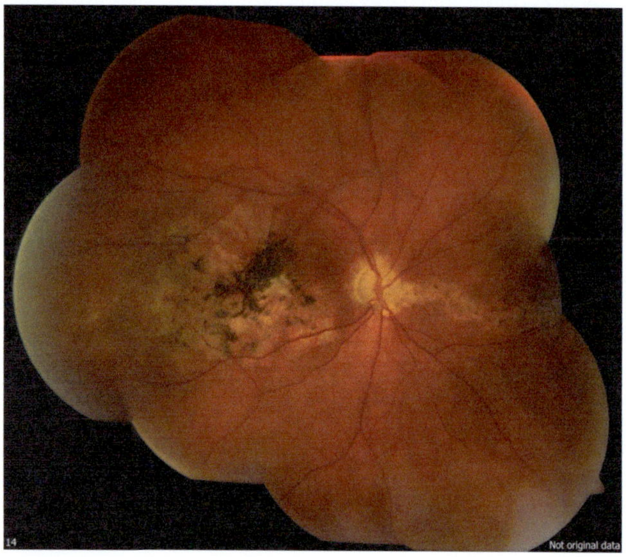

Fig. 25.2 Montage color fundus photograph of the right eye from an 80-year-old woman, showing macular atrophy with pigmentation as well as atrophy nasal to the optic nerve.

References

1. Soumplis V, Sergouniotis PI, Robson AG, Michaelides M, Moore AT, Holder GE, et al. Phenotypic findings in C1QTNF5 retinopathy (late-onset retinal degeneration). Acta Ophthalmol. 2013;91(3):e191–5.
2. Vincent A, Munier FL, Vandenhoven CC, Wright T, Westall CA, Héon E. The characterization of retinal phenotype in a family with C1QTNF5-related late-onset retinal degeneration. Retina. 2012;32(8):1643–51.
3. Ayyagari R, Mandal MN, Karoukis AJ, Chen L, McLaren NC, Lichter M, et al. Late-onset macular degeneration and long anterior lens zonules result from a CTRP5 gene mutation. Invest Ophthalmol Vis Sci. 2005;46(9):3363–71.
4. Subrayan V, Morris B, Armbrecht AM, Wright AF, Dhillon B. Long anterior lens zonules in late-onset retinal degeneration (L-ORD). Am J Ophthalmol. 2005;140(6):1127–9.

26 CYP4V2

CYP4V2 encodes cytochrome P450 4V2, an enzyme responsible for the oxidation of intermediates in the metabolic breakdown of fatty acids. Mutations in *CYP4V2* are associated with Bietti Crystalline Dystrophy (BCD) [1].

BCD follows an autosomal recessive pattern of inheritance, with an onset typically in the second-to-fourth decades of life. The presenting symptoms are variable, but patients experience reduced visual acuity, progressive nyctalopia, visual field constriction, and dyschromatopsia. BCVAs vary widely but tend to worsen with age [2]. Small crystalline deposits may be observed in the peripheral cornea with slit-lamp biomicroscopy (similar crystals may also be seen in peripheral lymphocytes). Fundoscopy reveals crystals in the posterior pole (sometimes extending to the mid-periphery) associated with chorioretinal atrophy (Figs. 26.1a, b and 26.2a) [3]. The crystals, usually in areas of mild degeneration, are less pronounced in areas of chorioretinal atrophy in advanced stages of disease [2, 4, 5]. The crystals localize adjacent to the inner side of retinal pigment epithelium and can be better visualized with SD-OCT (Fig. 26.2b) [6]. Foveal thinning and interruptions in the ellipsoid band may also be seen, with a preservation of the external limiting membrane. In areas of RPE atrophy, presumed photoreceptor rosettes may be observed at the level of Bruch's membrane [2, 4, 6]. ERGs in BCD patients are usually diminished and reflect the severity of the chorioretinal degeneration, ranging from normal to non-recordable photopic and scotopic parameters [7, 8].

S. Zahid et al., *Retinal Dystrophy Gene Atlas*, https://doi.org/10.1007/978-3-319-10867-4_26

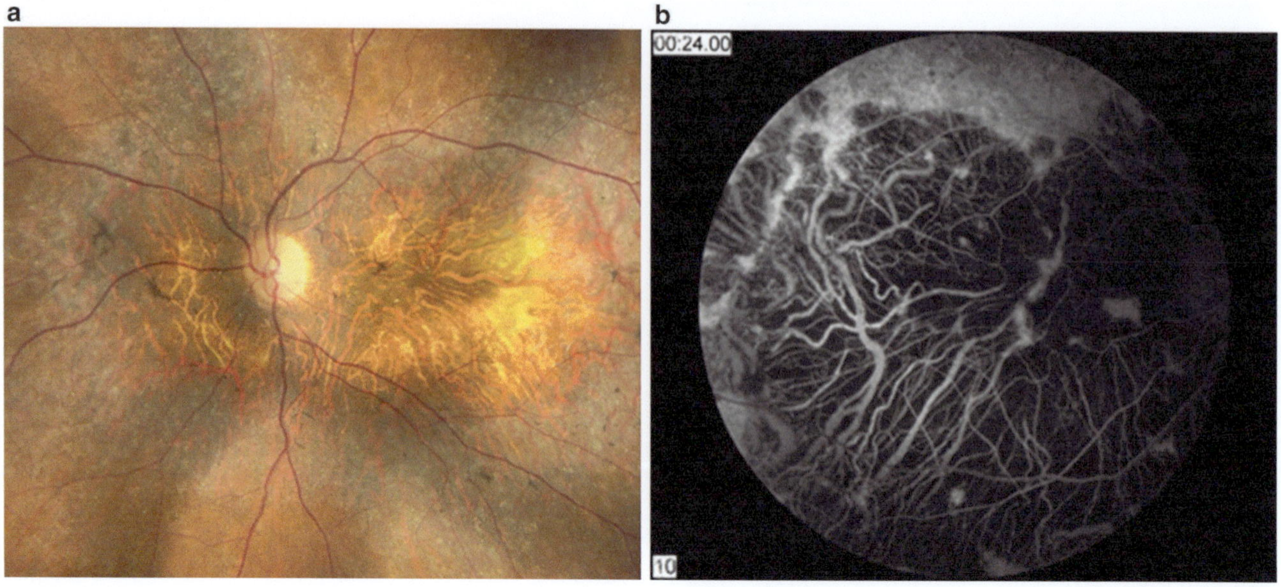

Fig. 26.1 Case summary: 44-year-old man with BCD. (**a**) Color fundus photograph of the left eye, showing chorioretinal atrophy involving the macula and peripapillary regions and crystalline deposits in the macula and along and outside the vascular arcades. (**b**) Fluorescein angiography of the left eye showing severe retinal pigment epithelial and choroidal atrophy, permitting easy visualization of the deep choroidal vasculature.

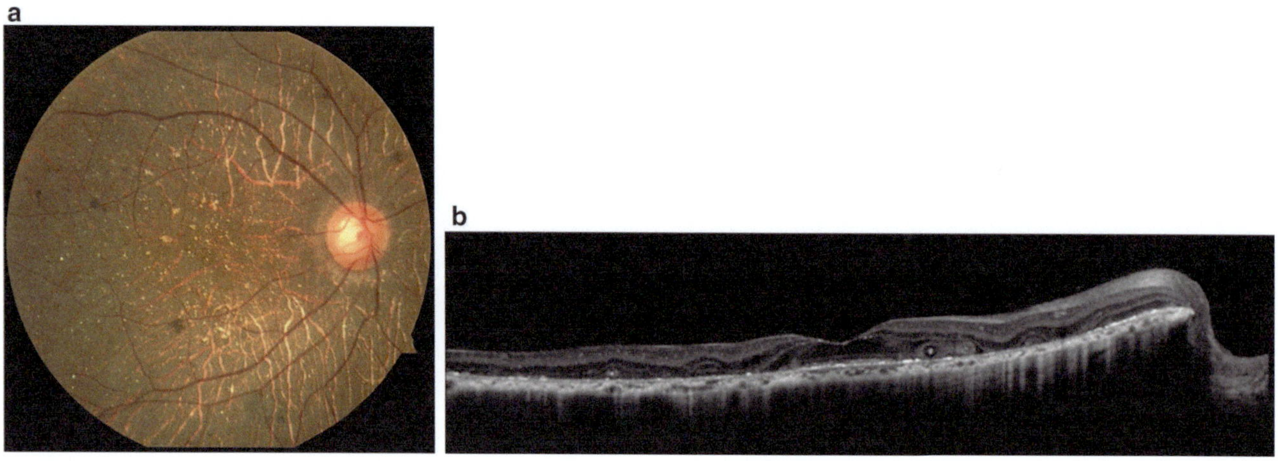

Fig. 26.2 Case summary: 43-year-old male with BCD (CEI25442). (**a**) Color fundus photograph of the right eye, showing chorioretinal atrophy along the arcades and in the macula (sparing the fovea), with scattered crystalline deposits. (**b**) Spectral domain optical coherence tomography of the right eye, showing extrafoveal RPE, ellipsoid zone and outer nuclear layer loss, with hyper-reflective deposits at the level of the RPE (at the outer nuclear layer as well as in the inner retina).

References

1. Okialda KA, Stover NB, Weleber RG, Kelly EJ. Bietti crystalline dystrophy. In: Pagon RA, Adam MP, Ardinger HH, et al., editors. GeneReviews [Internet]. Seattle: University of Washington; 1993–2017; 2012 Apr 12 [Updated 2012]. Available from: https://www.ncbi.nlm.nih.gov/books/NBK91457/. Accessed 23 Jan 2017.
2. Manzouri B, Sergouniotis PI, Robson AG, Webster AR, Moore A. Bietti crystalline retinopathy: report of retinal crystal deposition in male adolescent siblings. Arch Ophthalmol. 2012;130(11):1470–3.
3. Song Y, Mo G, Yin G. A novel mutation in the CYP4V2 gene in a Chinese patient with Bietti's crystalline dystrophy. Int Ophthalmol. 2013;33(3):269–76.
4. Kojima H, Otani A, Ogino K, Nakagawa S, Makiyama Y, Kurimoto M, et al. Outer retinal circular structures in patients with Bietti crystalline retinopathy. Br J Ophthalmol. 2012;96(3):390–3.
5. Chung JK, Shin JH, Jeon BR, Ki CS, Park TK. Optical coherence tomographic findings of crystal deposits in the lens and cornea in Bietti crystalline corneoretinopathy associated with mutation in the CYP4V2 gene. Jpn J Ophthalmol. 2013;57(5):447–50.
6. Pennesi ME, Weleber RG. High-resolution optical coherence tomography shows new aspects of Bietti crystalline retinopathy. Retina. 2010;30(3):531–2.
7. Haddad NM, Waked N, Bejjani R, Khoueir Z, Chouery E, Corbani S, et al. Clinical and molecular findings in three Lebanese families with Bietti crystalline dystrophy: report on a novel mutation. Mol Vis. 2012;18:1182–8.
8. Rossi S, Testa F, Li A, Yaylacioğlu F, Gesualdo C, Hejtmancik JF, et al. Clinical and genetic features in Italian Bietti crystalline dystrophy patients. Br J Ophthalmol. 2013;97(2):174–9.

27 DHDDS

DHDDS encodes dehydrodolichyl diphosphate synthase, an enzyme expressed in many tissues, which catalyzes the production of dolichol, which is a glycosyl carrier lipid required for the synthesis of many types of glycoproteins. Autosomal recessive mutations in *DHDDS* cause retinitis pigmentosa (RP; rod-cone dystrophy). A founder mutation has been described in the Ashkenazi Jewish population, which may account for over 10% of recessive retinitis pigmentosa in this community [1, 2]. Patients tend to exhibit typical RP symptoms with a teenage onset of nyctalopia and peripheral vision loss. Visual acuities may vary widely but tends to be better in younger patients [2]. The rate of disease progression may vary; some patients decline to light perception visual acuity within a decade after exhibiting a non-recordable ERG in their late teens [3]. Fundus findings include characteristic RP findings, such as waxy optic nerve pallor, arteriolar attenuation, and bone spicule-pigment deposition. Macular atrophy has been reported in some patients [2]. Optical coherence tomography (OCT) may reveal preservation of retinal thickness and the photoreceptors at the fovea, which tends to become thinner with increased eccentricity. Some patients exhibit cystoid macular edema [2]. Near-infrared autofluorescence imaging reveals islands of residual retinal pigment epithelium that correspond to areas of preserved photoreceptors visualized on OCT. The electroretinogram usually shows a rod-cone pattern of degeneration, while Goldmann visual field reveals peripheral visual field loss with central islands remaining in older patients [2]. Likewise, dark-adapted static perimetry reveals loss of rod function with age [2].

The chain length of dolichol in plasma and urine have been shown to be altered in patients carrying *DHDDS* mutations [4]. The pathophysiology of retinal dysfunction is not fully understood, but knock-down studies in zebra fish result in photoreceptor degeneration [5].

S. Zahid et al., *Retinal Dystrophy Gene Atlas*, https://doi.org/10.1007/978-3-319-10867-4_27

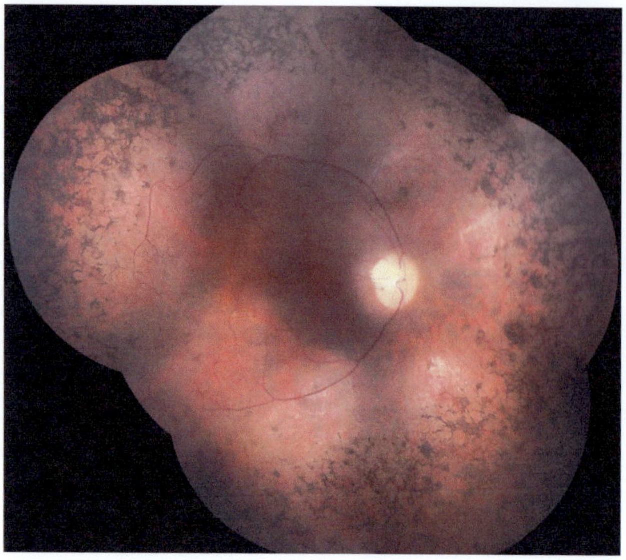

Fig. 27.1 Case summary: 41 year old man with retinitis pigmentosa. Color photo of the right eye, showing optic disc pallor, vascular attenuation, diffuse retinal atrophy, and peripheral bone spicules.

References

1. Züchner S, Dallman J, Wen R, Beecham G, Naj A, Farooq A, et al. Whole-exome sequencing links a variant in DHDDS to retinitis pigmentosa. Am J Hum Genet. 2011;88(2):201–6.
2. Zelinger L, Banin E, Obolensky A, Mizrahi-Meissonnier L, Beryozkin A, Bandah-Rozenfeld D, et al. A missense mutation in DHDDS, encoding dehydrodolichyl diphosphate synthase, is associated with autosomal-recessive retinitis pigmentosa in Ashkenazi Jews. Am J Hum Genet. 2011;88(2):207–15.
3. Lam BL, Zuchner SL, Dallman J, Wen R, Alfonso EC, Vance JM, et al. Mutation K42E in Dehydrodolichol Diphosphate synthase (DHDDS) causes recessive retinitis Pigmentosa. Adv Exp Med Biol. 2014;801:165–70.
4. Wen R, Lam BL, Guan Z. Aberrant dolichol chain lengths as biomarkers for retinitis pigmentosa caused by impaired dolichol biosynthesis. J Lipid Res. 2013;54(12):3516–22.
5. Wen R, Dallman JE, Li Y, Züchner SL, Vance JM, Peričak-Vance MA, et al. Knock-down DHDDS expression induces photoreceptor degeneration in Zebrafish. Adv Exp Med Biol. 2014;801:543–50.

28 EFEMP1

Mutations in *EFEMP1*, which encodes a retinal pigment epithelium (RPE) extracellular matrix glycoprotein of uncertain function, cause autosomal dominant drusen (Doyne's Honeycomb Dystrophy, Malattia Leventinese) [1, 2].

Patients usually present in their 40s to 50s with reduced central acuity and delayed dark adaptation, although many patients are asymptomatic. The rate of visual acuity (VA) deterioration varies, with some patients remaining stable over the course of a decade and others experiencing significant loss of VA. Progressive macular atrophy is the primary cause of vision loss, though choroidal neovascularization is a rare complication that may cause rapid vision loss (Fig. 28.1b). Fundus examination is characterized by bilateral soft drusen throughout the macula, including nasal to the optic disc, which can become confluent (which may give the appearance of retinal fibrosis) and develop into areas of atrophy later in the disease course. The drusen are classically in a radial pattern in the maculae of both eyes (Figs. 28.1a and 28.2a). There are often interocular differences in VA and fundus appearance, but both eyes are almost always affected. The characteristics of the drusen exhibit significant intra- and interfamilial phenotypic variability, but they are typically absent in the periphery. Certain genotypes (e.g., R345W) [3] consistently exhibit peripapillary drusen. Fundus autofluorescence shows hyperautofluorescence in areas of drusen accumulation, while hypofluorescence corresponds to areas of atrophy in later stages of disease. Optical coherence tomography is helpful in imaging the extent and features of the drusen and may also show features of neovascularization. Nonpenetrance of disease has been reported in one patient with an R345W mutation [3].

S. Zahid et al., *Retinal Dystrophy Gene Atlas*, https://doi.org/10.1007/978-3-319-10867-4_28

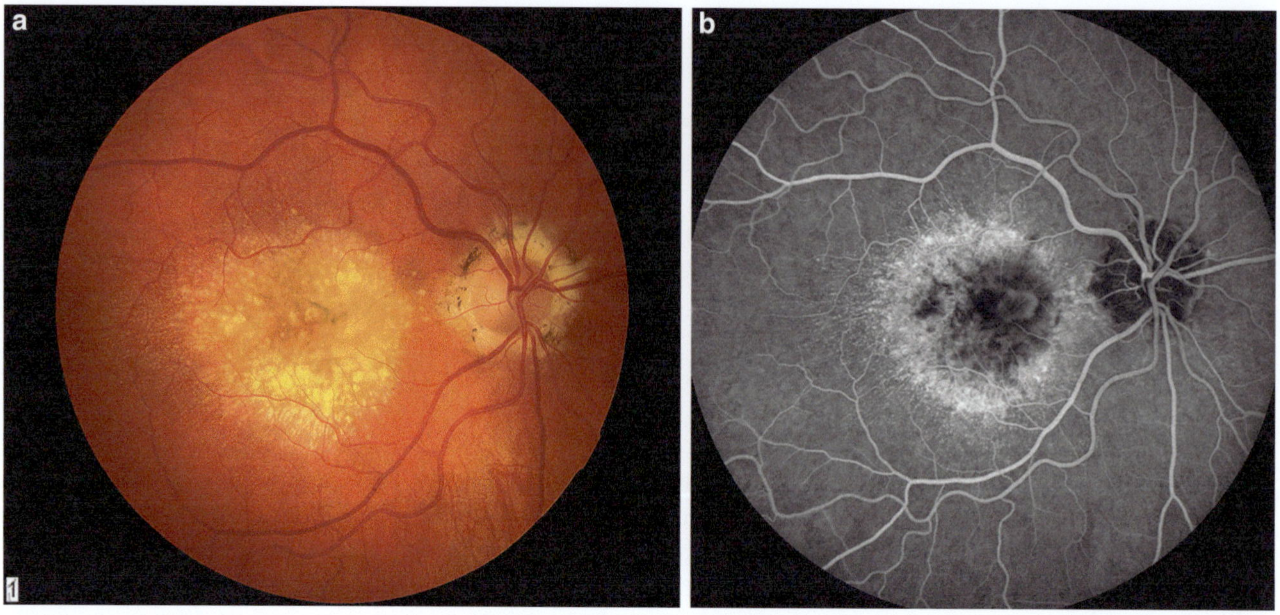

Fig. 28.1 Case summary: 51-year old woman with dominant drusen. (**a**) Color fundus photograph of the right eye showing drusen in a classical radial orientation in the macula. (**b**) Fluorescein angiography of the right eye showing staining of the drusen and a choroidal neovascular membrane in the nasal macula.

a b

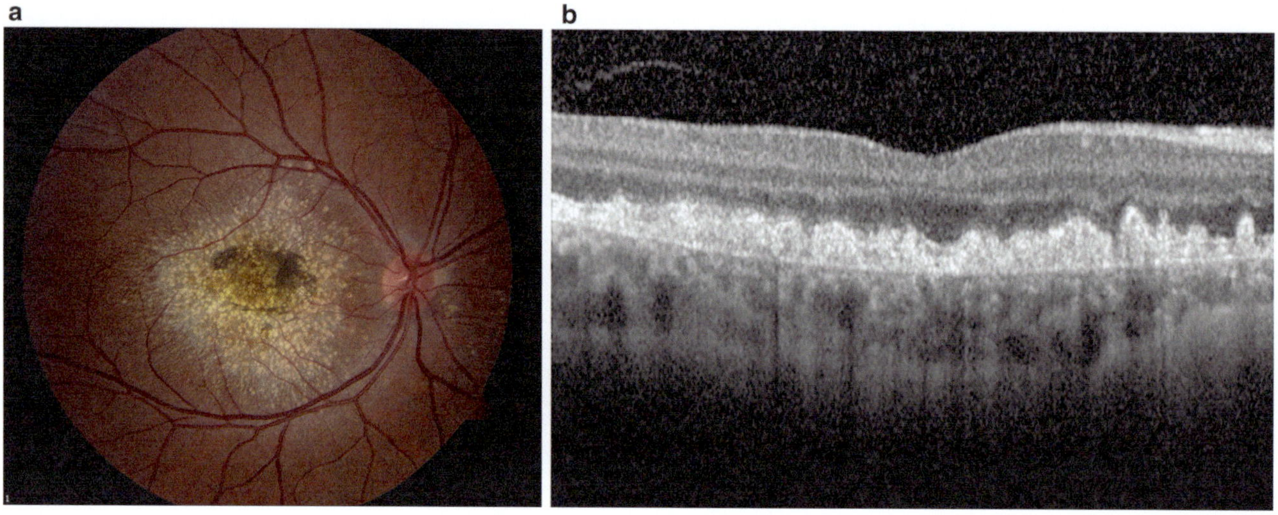

Fig. 28.2 OCT shows extensive drusenoid deposits classical of this condition. Case summary: 27-year-old man. (**a**) Color fundus photograph of the right eye showing drusen in a classical radial orientation in the macula, with hyperpigmentation in areas suggestive of scarring. Also visible are drusen nasal to the optic disc. (**b**) Spectral-domain optical coherence tomography showing extensive macular drusen appearing to be between the retinal pigment epithelium and Bruch's membrane.

References

1. Stone EM, Lotery AJ, Munier FL, Héon E, Piguet B, Guymer RH, et al. A single EFEMP1 mutation associated with both Malattia Leventinese and Doyne honeycomb retinal dystrophy. Nat Genet. 1999;22(2):199–202.
2. Marmorstein LY, Munier FL, Arsenijevic Y, Schorderet DF, McLaughlin PJ, Chung D, et al. Aberrant accumulation of EFEMP1 underlies drusen formation in Malattia Leventinese and age-related macular degeneration. Proc Natl Acad Sci U S A. 2002;99(20):13067–72.
3. Michaelides M, Jenkins SA, Brantley MA Jr, Andrews RM, Waseem N, Luong V, et al. Maculopathy due to the R345W substitution in fibulin-3: distinct clinical features, disease variability, and extent of retinal dysfunction. Invest Ophthalmol Vis Sci. 2006;47(7):3085–97.

29 ELOVL4

Mutations in *ELOVL4*, which is required for the synthesis of fatty acids, cause an autosomal dominant macular dystrophy, also known as "Stargardt-like macular dystrophy" [1–4].

Patients usually present with reduced visual acuity (ranging from 20/50 to 20/200 or worse) as early as the second decade of life, but onset can occur as late as the fifth decade [5]. Patients tend to lose visual acuity with age; color and peripheral vision are usually normal. Fundus examination may be characterized by macular flecks and atrophy similar to those seen in *ABCA4*-related disease, with a normal peripheral retina. However, fundus appearance may exhibit intra- and interfamilial variability, and patients may exhibit macular atrophy with or without flecks, subtle macular retinal pigment epithelium (RPE) disruption, or pattern dystrophy. Full field electroretinography (ERG) is usually normal or mildly decreased, while multifocal ERGs are abnormal. Fluorescein angiography may show macular window defects but has not been reported to exhibit the "dark choroid" characteristic of *ABCA4*-related disease (Fig. 29.1) [5].

S. Zahid et al., *Retinal Dystrophy Gene Atlas*, https://doi.org/10.1007/978-3-319-10867-4_29

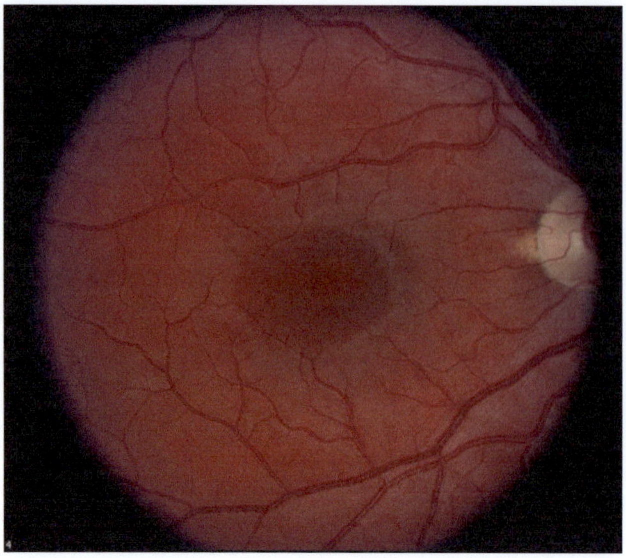

Fig. 29.1 Color fundus photograph from a 21-year-old man, showing subtle macular retinal pigment epithelium disruption.

References

1. Zhang K, Kniazeva M, Han M, Li W, Yu Z, Yang Z, et al. A 5-bp deletion in ELOVL4 is associated with two related forms of autosomal dominant macular dystrophy. Nat Genet. 2001;27(1):89–93.
2. Edwards AO, Miedziak A, Vrabec T, Verhoeven J, Acott TS, Weleber RG, et al. Autosomal dominant Stargardt-like macular dystrophy: I. Clinical characterization, longitudinal follow-up, and evidence for a common ancestry in families linked to chromosome 6q14. Am J Ophthalmol. 1999;127(4):426–35.
3. Vasireddy V, Wong P, Ayyagari R. Genetics and molecular pathology of Stargardt-like macular degeneration. Prog Retin Eye Res. 2010;29(3):191–207.
4. Griesinger IB, Sieving PA, Ayyagari R. Autosomal dominant macular atrophy at 6q14 excludes CORD7 and MCDR1/PBCRA loci. Invest Ophthalmol Vis Sci. 2000;41(1):248–55.
5. Bernstein PS, Tammur J, Singh N, Hutchinson A, Dixon M, Pappas CM, et al. Diverse macular dystrophy phenotype caused by a novel complex mutation in the ELOVL4 gene. Invest Ophthalmol Vis Sci. 2001;42(13):3331–6.

30 EYS

Mutations in *EYS*, which encodes a protein important for photoreceptor morphology, are a common cause of autosomal recessive retinitis pigmentosa (rod-cone dystrophy) and rarely cone-rod dystrophy [1–9]. Patients may present as early as their teens or as late as their forties with night blindness and progressive loss of peripheral field. Visual acuity is usually maintained until late in the disease (often better than 20/50) and fundoscopy reveals optic disc pallor, bone-spicule pigment deposits in the mid-periphery to periphery that increase in density with age, and attenuated vessels. Cataracts have been reported to occur at a younger age (average of 50 years in one study) (Figs. 30.1a and 30.2a) [7]. GVF reveals a rod-cone pattern with progressively constricting fields (Fig. 30.1b), and ERG reveals a rod-cone pattern of degeneration (Fig. 30.1c). One study has shown that patients with homozygous mutations in *EYS* tend to deteriorate with respect to visual acuity and visual fields more rapidly than patients who are compound heterozygotes for pathogenic mutations at the *EYS* locus [7]. Fundus autofluorescence may show hypoautofluorescence in areas of atrophy or hyperautofluorescence at the interface between atrophic and residual (but dysfunctional) retina (Fig. 30.2b). Spectral domain optical coherence tomography may help delineate areas of residual photoreceptor and retinal pigment epithelium (RPE) loss (Fig. 30.2c).

Phenotypic variability has been reported in *EYS* mutations; some patients present with photophobia, night blindness, and reduced visual acuity earlier in the disease course [4]. These patients may exhibit RPE changes or macular atrophy on funduscopy, central scotomata on GVF, and a cone-rod pattern of dysfunction on ERG testing.

S. Zahid et al., *Retinal Dystrophy Gene Atlas*, https://doi.org/10.1007/978-3-319-10867-4_30

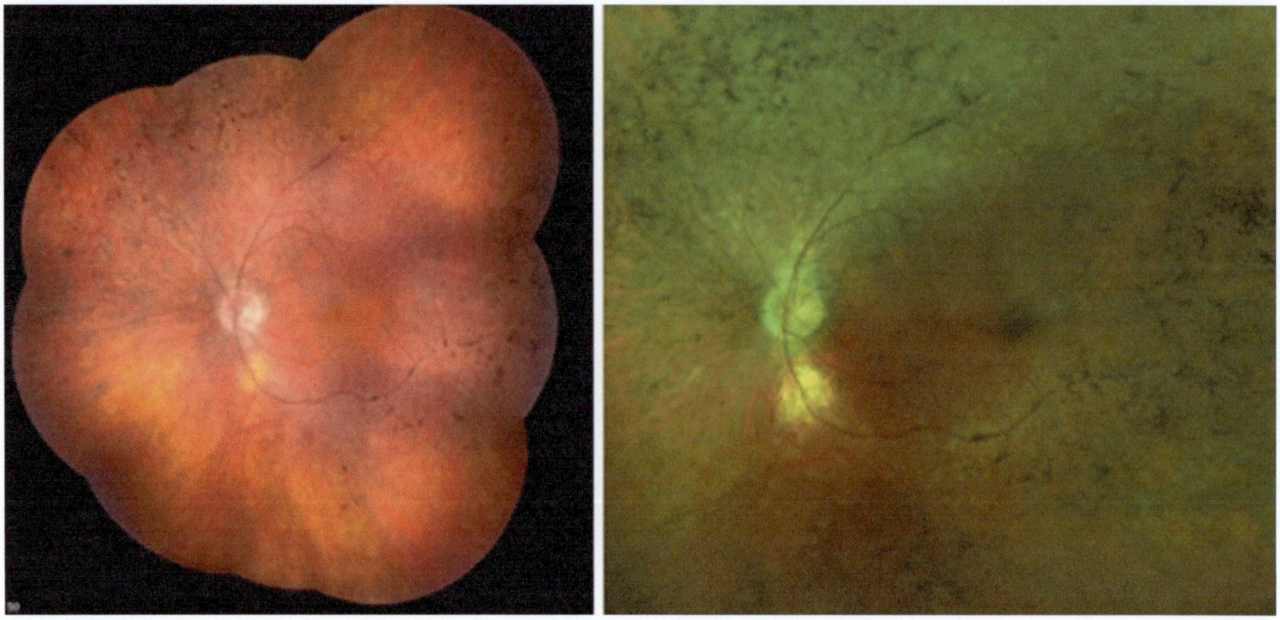

Fig. 30.1 Case summary: 34-year-old man with rod-cone dystrophy with mutations in *EYS*. Color fundus photographs of the left eye at age 34 (left), showing midperipheral RPE atrophy and bone-spicule pigment deposits. Wide-field photograph 7 years later (right), showing an increased density of pigment deposits.

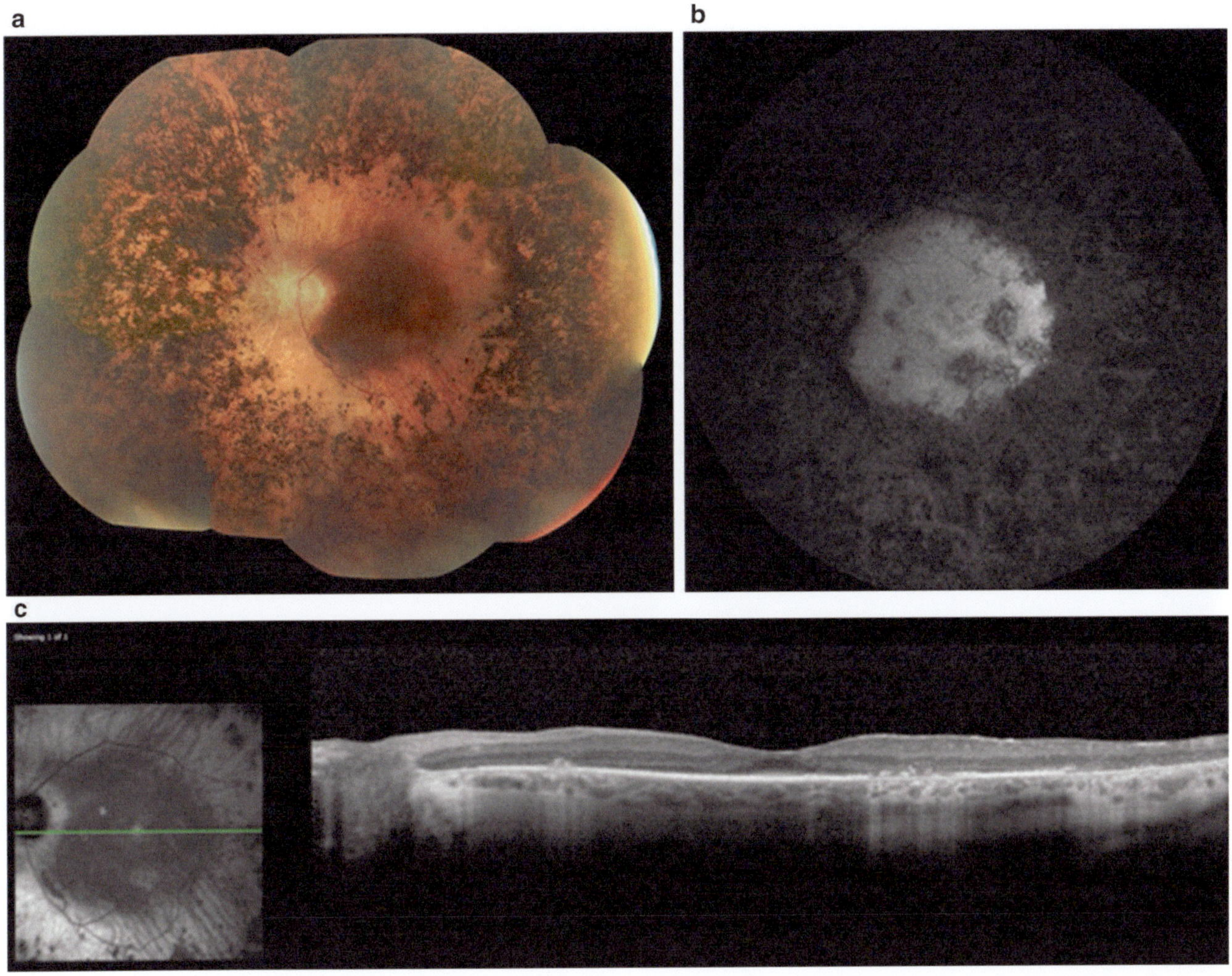

Fig. 30.2 Case summary: 58-year-old male with *EYS* mutations and rod-cone dystrophy. (**a**) Color fundus photograph (montage) of the left eye, showing optic nerve waxy pallor, retinal vessel attenuation, RPE atrophy along the arcades, and dense mid-peripheral bone spicule pigment deposits. (**b**) Fundus autofluorescence of the left eye, showing dense hypoautofluorescence at and outside the arcades corresponding to RPE atrophy and pigmentation. There is hyperautofluorescence at the interface between central residual autofluorescent signal and peripheral hypoautofluorescence. (**c**) Spectral domain optical coherence tomography of the left eye, showing dense ellipsoid zone loss at the macula with a residual central island at the foveola. There are also focal areas of RPE atrophy/loss.

References

1. Katagiri S, Akahori M, Hayashi T, Yoshitake K, Gekka T, Ikeo K, et al. Autosomal recessive cone-rod dystrophy associated with compound heterozygous mutations in the EYS gene. Doc Ophthalmol. 2014;128(3):211–7.
2. Abd El-Aziz MM, Barragan I, O'Driscoll CA, Goodstadt L, Prigmore E, Borrego S, et al. EYS, encoding an ortholog of Drosophila spacemaker, is mutated in autosomal recessive retinitis pigmentosa. Nat Genet. 2008;40(11):1285–7.
3. Abd El-Aziz MM, O'Driscoll CA, Kaye RS, Barragan I, El-Ashry MF, Borrego S, et al. Identification of novel mutations in the ortholog of Drosophila eyes shut gene (EYS) causing autosomal recessive retinitis pigmentosa. Invest Ophthalmol Vis Sci. 2010; 51(8):4266–72.
4. Collin RW, Littink KW, Klevering BJ, van den Born LI, Koenekoop RK, Zonneveld MN, et al. Identification of a 2 Mb human ortholog of Drosophila eyes shut/spacemaker that is mutated in patients with retinitis pigmentosa. Am J Hum Genet. 2008;83(5):594–603.
5. Barragan I, Borrego S, Pieras JI, González-del Pozo M, Santoyo J, Ayuso C, et al. Mutation spectrum of EYS in Spanish patients with autosomal recessive retinitis pigmentosa. Hum Mutat. 2010;31(11):E1772–800.
6. Hosono K, Ishigami C, Takahashi M, Park DH, Hirami Y, Nakanishi H, et al. Two novel mutations in the EYS gene are possible major causes of autosomal recessive retinitis pigmentosa in the Japanese population. PLoS One. 2012;7(2):e31036.
7. Iwanami M, Oshikawa M, Nishida T, Nakadomari S, Kato S. High prevalence of mutations in the EYS gene in Japanese patients with autosomal recessive retinitis pigmentosa. Invest Ophthalmol Vis Sci. 2012;53(2):1033–40.
8. Suto K, Hosono K, Takahashi M, Hirami Y, Arai Y, Nagase Y, et al. Clinical phenotype in ten unrelated Japanese patients with mutations in the EYS gene. Ophthalmic Genet. 2014;35(1):25–34.
9. Audo I, Sahel JA, Mohand-Said S, Lancelot ME, Antonio A, Moskova-Doumanova V, et al. EYS is a major gene for rod-cone dystrophies in France. Hum Mutat. 2010;31(5):E1406–35.

31 FAM161A

FAM161A encodes a ciliary protein that appears to be involved in microtubule stabilization/transport. Mutations in *FAM161A* have been associated with autosomal recessive retinitis pigmentosa (RP) [1–3].

Limited literature is available on patients with mutations in *FAM161A,* but most present with the features of typical RP, although visual acuity may be worse than other mutations. Patients with *FAM161A*-related RP have varying ages of onset, typically from their first-to-third decades of life. Myopia and low visual acuities (ranging from no light perception to 20/200) are common, with count fingers acuity reported as young as age 15. Younger patients in their second decade of life may have better visual acuities, which tends to decline to severe visual handicap by the third and fourth decades of life. Fundoscopy may reveal typical features of retinitis pigmentosa, with arteriole attenuation, bone spicule pigment deposits, waxy optic disc pallor, cataracts, and optic atrophy [2]. There may be grayish dots extending from the arcades to the periphery. OCT imaging shows thinning of the outer nuclear layer with relative preservation under the fovea and may demonstrate the subretinal depositis (Fig. 31.1) [3]. Fundus autofluorescence (FAF) imaging may reveal a ring of hyperautofluorescence around the fovea. Full-field ERGs usually exhibit significantly reduced cone and rod responses and are often nonrecordable, though some patients retain residual cone function at earlier ages [1–3]. GVF typically reveals progressive peripheral field loss [3].

S. Zahid et al., *Retinal Dystrophy Gene Atlas*, https://doi.org/10.1007/978-3-319-10867-4_31

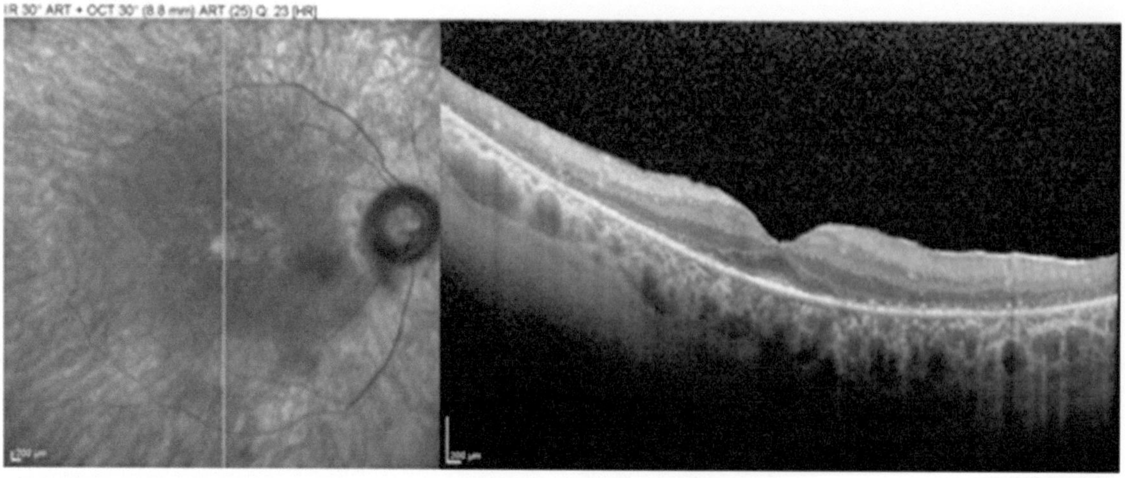

Fig. 31.1 Spectral domain optical coherence tomography of the right eye from a 55-year-old woman with typical RP and gray dots extending from the mid-periphery. There is extensive loss of the ellipsoid zone (EZ) and outer nuclear layer (ONL), with central foveal sparing. Subretinal deposits are also visible the areas of EZ/ONL loss.

References

1. Gu S, Kumaramanickavel G, Srikumari CR, Denton MJ, Gal A. Autosomal recessive retinitis pigmentosa locus RP28 maps between D2S1337 and D2S286 on chromosome 2p11-p15 in an Indian family. J Med Genet. 1999;36(9):705–7.
2. Langmann T, Di Gioia SA, Rau I, Stöhr H, Maksimovic NS, Corbo JC, et al. Nonsense mutations in FAM161A cause RP28-associated recessive retinitis pigmentosa. Am J Hum Genet. 2010;87(3):376–81.
3. Bandah-Rozenfeld D, Mizrahi-Meissonnier L, Farhy C, Obolensky A, Chowers I, Pe'er J, et al. Homozygosity mapping reveals null mutations in FAM161A as a cause of Autosomal-recessive retinitis Pigmentosa. Am J Hum Genet. 2010;87(3):382–91.

32 GNAT1

GNAT1 (Guanine nucleotide-binding protein, alpha-transducing activity polypeptide 1) encodes the alpha subunit of rod transducin. Transducin is the G-protein involved in the phototransduction cascade that facilitates the interaction between rhodopsin and cGMP. Mutations in *GNAT1* have been shown to cause both autosomal recessive and autosomal dominant forms of congenital stationary night blindness (CSNB) and autosomal recessive rod-cone dystrophy [1, 2].

Autosomal dominant CSNB may show non-progressive night blindness from early infancy. Myopia is common, while visual acuities and color vision are typically within normal limits. GVF and fundus appearance are typically normal. The Nougaret type of CSNB, based on the pedigree of Jean Nougaret, demonstrates an electroretinogram (ERG) abnormality in which the rod a-wave is missing [2]. In contrast, a Riggs-type ERG pattern reveals an absent b-wave in response to flashes of dim light and a cone-like response to bright light in scotopic testing conditions. Light-adapted states are typically normal. Dark adaptation testing reveals reduction in rod sensitivities in most patients. Some studies have suggested that these ERG findings reflect a presynaptic defect in rod phototransduction in patients with CSNB [3].

Autosomal recessive CSNB has been reported in one study of a consanguineous family that had many affected family members. Night blindness may start from early childhood, with unaffected visual acuity and color vision. Fundus findings are typically normal, with no signs of arteriolar attenuation or bone spicule changes. ERG recordings may reveal nearly absent a- and b-waves in scotopic conditions with normal photopic parameters [1].

There are a few case reports of patients with homozygous *GNAT1* pathogenic variants associated with late-onset rod-cone dystrophy.

References

1. Naeem MA, Chavali VR, Ali S, Iqbal M, Riazuddin S, Khan SN, et al. GNAT1 associated with autosomal recessive congenital stationary night blindness. Invest Ophthalmol Vis Sci. 2012;53(3):1353–61.
2. Dryja TP, Hahn LB, Reboul T, Arnaud B. Missense mutation in the gene encoding the alpha subunit of rod transducin in the Nougaret form of congenital stationary night blindness. Nat Genet. 1996;13(3):358–60.
3. Szabo V, Kreienkamp HJ, Rosenberg T, Gal A. p.Gln200Glu, a putative constitutively active mutant of rod alpha-transducin (GNAT1) in autosomal dominant congenital stationary night blindness. Hum Mutat. 2007;28(7):741–2.

S. Zahid et al., *Retinal Dystrophy Gene Atlas*, https://doi.org/10.1007/978-3-319-10867-4_32

33 GNAT2

GNAT2 encodes guanine nucleotide-binding protein G(t) subunit alpha-2, which is a part of the transducin complex that amplifies and transmits the visual signal in cone photoreceptors. Autosomal recessive mutations in *GNAT2* cause approximately 1–2% of achromatopsia [1, 2]. Patients with *GNAT2*-related achromatopsia exhibit nystagmus beginning in early infancy, photophobia, abnormal color vision, and poor visual acuity (VA) (usually worse than 20/200–20/400). Progressive deterioration of VA may be observed, while nystagmus may improve in some patients [3]. Color vision testing is usually abnormal, with rod monochromacy observed in many patients, although some patients may retain some color vision [3–5]. One study has suggested that the retention of color vision may be related to splice site mutations that sometimes result in functional protein product [5]. Fundoscopy usually reveals a normal retinal appearance, though some patients exhibit an abnormal foveal reflex or atrophy (Fig. 33.1a–d) [3]. Full-field ERG testing typically reveals varying degrees of abnormal cone function along with normal rod function, although scotopic a-wave amplitudes are reduced in some patients [3–5]. Microperimetry may show central scotomas; SD-OCT usually reveals well-maintained foveal architecture without hypoplasia but may exhibit a hyporeflective zone at the fovea (Fig. 33.1e–f) [6].

S. Zahid et al., *Retinal Dystrophy Gene Atlas*, https://doi.org/10.1007/978-3-319-10867-4_33

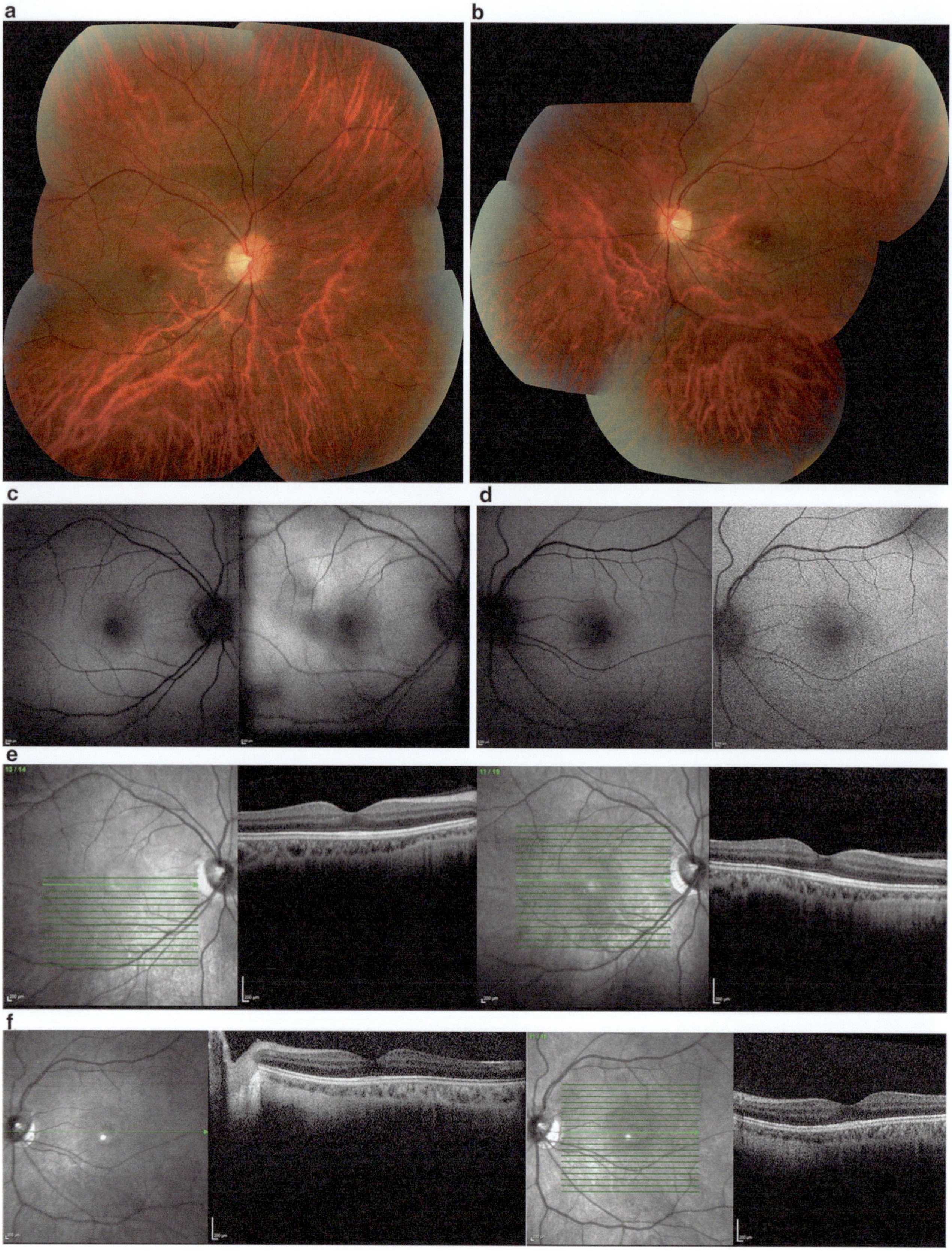

Fig. 33.1 Case summary: 25-year-old male with cone dysfunction syndrome due to homozygous mutations in *GNAT2* (c.139A > G) with best-corrected visual acuity 6/60 in both eyes. (**a**, **b**), Color fundus photographs of the right and left eyes, showing abnormal foveal reflexes, with RPE pigment mottling in both eyes. (**c**, **d**), Fundus autofluorescence of the right and left eyes, showing an essentially unchanged pattern of autofluorescence over 5 years except for a mild increase in certain areas of macular autofluorescence in the right eye. (**e**, **f**), Spectral domain optical coherence tomography of the right and left eyes, showing essentially unremarkable retinal architecture.

References

1. Aligianis IA, Forshew T, Johnson S, Michaelides M, Johnson CA, Trembath RC, et al. Mapping of a novel locus for achromatopsia (ACHM4) to 1p and identification of a germline mutation in the alpha subunit of cone transducin (GNAT2). J Med Genet. 2002;39(9):656–60.
2. Kohl S, Baumann B, Rosenberg T, Kellner U, Lorenz B, Vadalà M, et al. Mutations in the cone photoreceptor G-protein alpha-subunit gene GNAT2 in patients with achromatopsia. Am J Hum Genet. 2002;71(2):422–5.
3. Michaelides M, Aligianis IA, Holder GE, Simunovic M, Mollon JD, Maher ER, et al. Cone dystrophy phenotype associated with a frameshift mutation (M280fsX291) in the alpha-subunit of cone specific transducin (GNAT2). Br J Ophthalmol. 2003; 87(11):1317–20.
4. Ouechtati F, Merdassi A, Bouyacoub Y, Largueche L, Derouiche K, Ouragini H, et al. Clinical and genetic investigation of a large Tunisian family with complete achromatopsia: identification of a new nonsense mutation in GNAT2 gene. J Hum Genet. 2011;56(1):22–8.
5. Rosenberg T, Baumann B, Kohl S, Zrenner E, Jorgensen AL, Wissinger B. Variant phenotypes of incomplete achromatopsia in two cousins with GNAT2 gene mutations. Invest Ophthalmol Vis Sci. 2004;45(12):4256–62.
6. Sundaram V, Wilde C, Aboshiha J, Cowing J, Han C, Langlo CS, et al. Retinal structure and function in achromatopsia: implications for gene therapy. Ophthalmology. 2014;121(1):234–45.

34 GPR98

GPR98 encodes G-protein coupled receptor 98, which is expressed broadly in human cells. Autosomal recessive mutations in *GPR98* cause Usher syndrome type 2C, which is characterized by congenital sensorineural hearing loss and retinitis pigmentosa. These patients tend to exhibit bilateral mild-to-moderate hearing impairment with a downward sloping audiogram, demonstrating more loss at higher frequencies [1, 2]. Visual acuity is maintained until later in the disease course, while nyctalopia and peripheral vision loss typically present between the second and third decades of life [2, 3]. Goldmann visual fields reveal progressive peripheral constriction [2, 4]. Color-vision testing may reveal errors in the Tritan axis [4]. Early-onset bilateral cataracts are also common, although specific subtypes of cataracts have not been described in the literature [2]. Fundoscopy reveals typical findings of retinitis pigmentosa, including bone spicule pigment deposits from the mid-periphery to the periphery, attenuated retinal vasculature, optic nerve pallor, and RPE atrophy; maculopathy is less commonly observed (Figs. 34.1a, 34.2, 34.3 and 34.4) [3, 4]. Fundus autofluorescence reveals hypoautofluorescence in areas corresponding to atrophy, with some patients exhibiting a ring of macular hyperfluorescence (Fig. 34.1b) [4]. Some patients may have cystoid macular edema; patients with normal OCT architecture tend to exhibit a wide range of visual acuity [5]. Increased inner retinal thickness has also been reported in one family [1]. Full-field electroretinography (ERG) tends to reveal a rod-cone pattern of degeneration and is often non-recordable by the fourth decade of life; multifocal ERG tends to reveal maintained function at the macula [1, 4, 5]. There have been two patients reported to exhibit a cone dystrophy on ERG examination in the context of a fundus resembling classical retinitis pigmentosa [1].

Mutations in *GPR98* have also been associated with a subtype of childhood seizures [6].

S. Zahid et al., *Retinal Dystrophy Gene Atlas*, https://doi.org/10.1007/978-3-319-10867-4_34

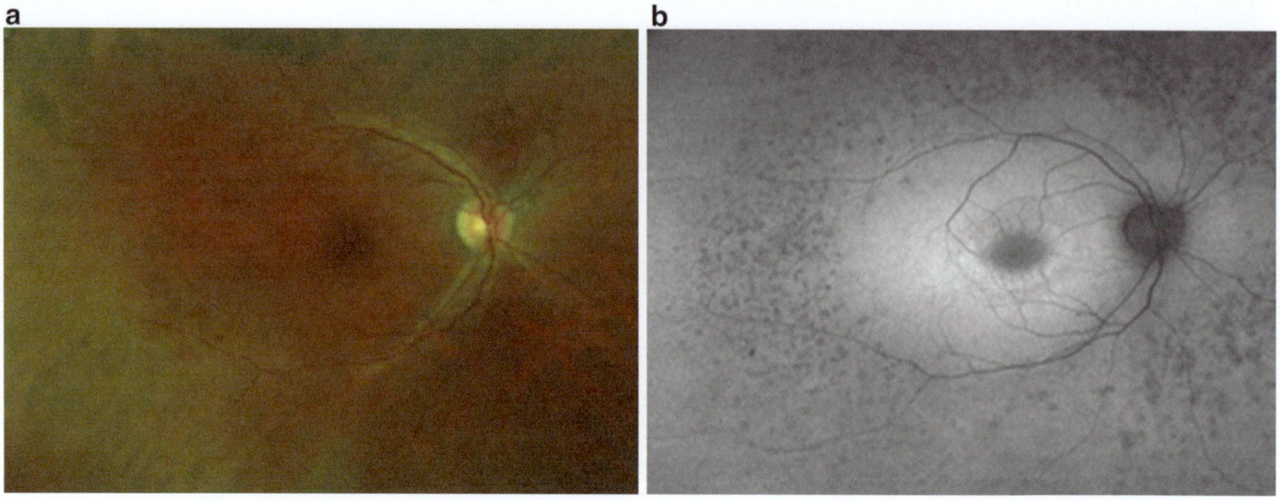

Fig. 34.1 Case summary: 23-year-old man with Usher Syndrome. (**a**) Wide-field color fundus photograph of the right eye showing RPE atrophy in the mid-periphery with scant bone spicule pigmentation. (**b**) Wide-field fundus autofluorescence of the right eye showing a hyperautofluorescent ring surrounding the fovea and areas of hypoautofluorescence in the midperiphery corresponding to areas of RPE atrophy.

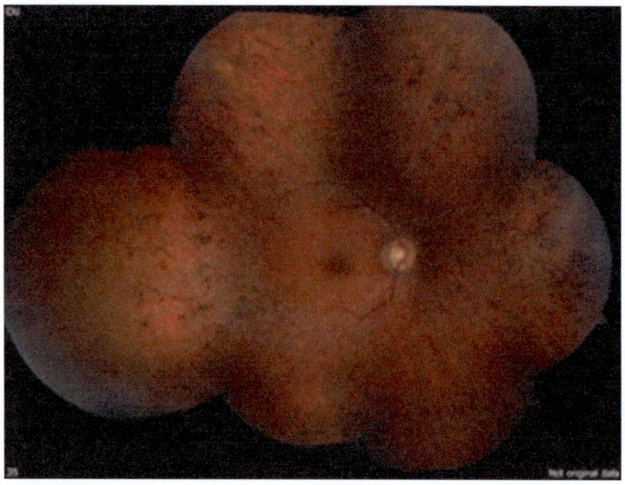

Fig. 34.2 Montage color fundus photograph of the right eye from a 38-year-old man with Usher Syndrome, showing RPE atrophy in the mid-periphery and moderate bone spicule pigmentation.

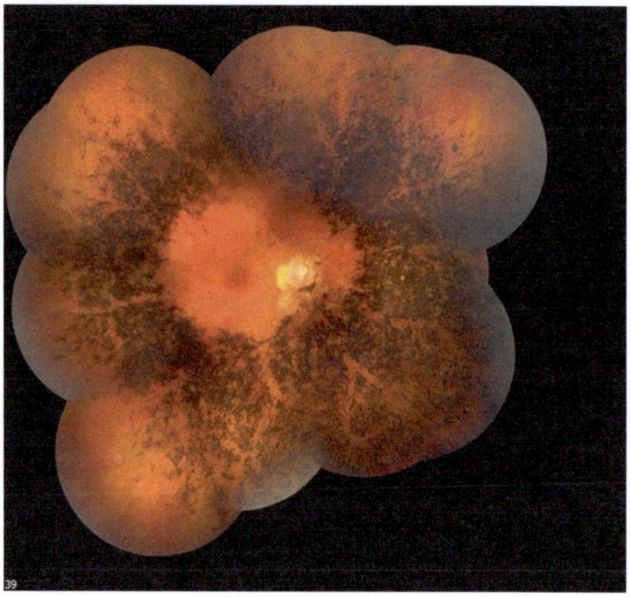

Fig. 34.3 Montage color fundus photograph of the right eye from a 45-year-old woman with Usher Syndrome, showing dense bone spicule pigmentation in the retinal mid-periphery up to the vascular arcades with associated RPE atrophy; there is blunting of the foveal light reflex.

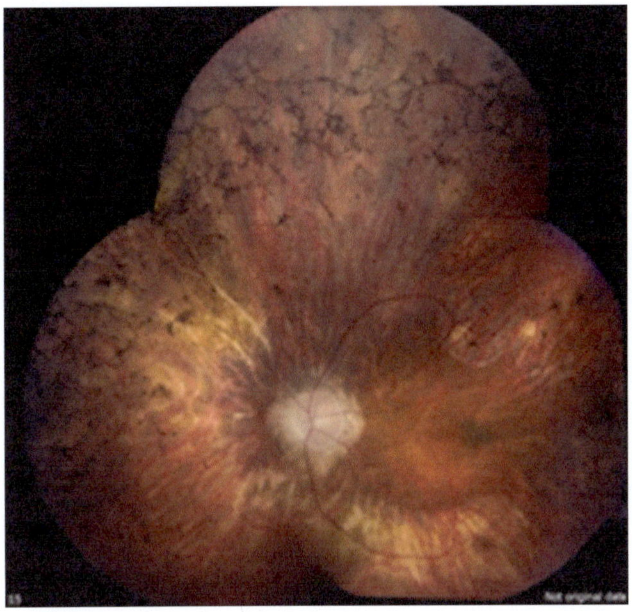

Fig. 34.4 Montage color fundus photograph of the left eye from a 61-year-old man with Usher Syndrome, showing RPE atrophy in the mid-periphery extending to the arcades and moderate bone spicule pigmentation with foveal-sparing.

References

1. Hilgert N, Kahrizi K, Dieltjens N, Bazazzadegan N, Najmabadi H, Smith RJ, et al. A large deletion in GPR98 causes type IIC Usher syndrome in male and female members of an Iranian family. J Med Genet. 2009;46(4):272–6.
2. Garcia-Garcia G, Besnard T, Baux D, Vaché C, Aller E, Malcolm S, et al. The contribution of GPR98 and DFNB31 genes to a Spanish Usher syndrome type 2 cohort. Mol Vis. 2013;19:367–73.
3. Hmani-Aifa M, Benzina Z, Zulfiqar F, Dhouib H, Shahzadi A, Ghorbel A, et al. Identification of two new mutations in the GPR98 and the PDE6B genes segregating in a Tunisian family. Eur J Hum Genet. 2009;17(4):474–82.
4. Ebermann I, Wiesen MH, Zrenner E, Lopez I, Pigeon R, Kohl S, et al. GPR98 mutations cause Usher syndrome type 2 in males. J Med Genet. 2009;46(4):277–80.
5. Malm E, Ponjavic V, Moller C, Kimberling WJ, Andreasson S. Phenotypes in defined genotypes including siblings with Usher syndrome. Ophthalmic Genet. 2011;32(2):65–74.
6. Nakayama J, YH F, Clark AM, Nakahara S, Hamano K, Iwasaki N, et al. A nonsense mutation of the MASS1 gene in a family with febrile and afebrile seizures. Ann Neurol. 2002;52(5):654–7.

35 GUCA1A

GUCA1A encodes guanylate cyclase-activating protein 1A (GCAP1), which is a calcium-binding protein located within the inner segments of the photoreceptors. It regulates guanylyl cyclase 1 by sensing calcium concentrations, which is important for the recovery of rod photoreceptors after light exposure and for the overall phototransduction cascade. Mutations in *GUCA1A* cause autosomal dominant cone and cone-rod dystrophy [1–4].

Onset of visual symptoms for *GUCA1A*-related autosomal dominant cone dystrophy generally occurs after the first two decades of life, between the 20s and 50s. Initial symptoms include reduced visual acuity, loss of color vision, and mild photophobia. Nystagmus is uncommon. Visual acuity usually deteriorates to between 20/200 and count fingers. A range of macular phenotypes may be observed; changes at the level of the retinal pigment epithelium (RPE) at the macula may be observed prior to vision loss. Funduscopic changes are minimal at an early age but may consist of subtle granularity of the RPE. Older patients may exhibit macular atrophy, bone spicule like pigmentation, and retinal vascular attenuation. Goldmann Visual Fields (GVF) reveal full peripheral fields with central scotomas. Full-field electroretinography (ERG) exhibits significant loss of cone function over time, usually in the context of normal rod parameters [1–7]. Some patients may exhibit rod abnormalities later in life. Intra-familial variability has been shown in some studies, with members of some families exhibiting symptoms of cone-rod dystrophy while others exhibit isolated macular dysfunction [3, 4].

Patients with cone-rod dystrophy experience similar symptoms to cone dystrophy patients but are more likely to experience nyctalopia and peripheral vision loss earlier in the disease process. In one study, symptoms (photophobia, poor acuity) were seen within the first decade in a Chinese family. Full-field ERG in these patients revealed a cone-rod pattern of degeneration. Fundus examination may reveal optic disc pallor, attenuated retinal arterioles, macular atrophy, or pigmentary changes in the macula [7, 8].

References

1. Payne AM, Downes SM, Bessant DA, Taylor R, Holder GE, Warren MJ, et al. A mutation in guanylate cyclase activator 1A (GUCA1A) in an autosomal dominant cone dystrophy pedigree mapping to a new locus on chromosome 6p21.1. Hum Mol Genet. 1998;7(2):273–7.
2. Michaelides M, Hardcastle AJ, Hunt DM, Moore AT. Progressive cone and cone-rod dystrophies: phenotypes and underlying molecular genetic basis. Surv Ophthalmol. 2006;51(3):232–58.
3. Downes SM, Holder GE, Fitzke FW, Payne AM, Warren MJ, Bhattacharya SS, et al. Autosomal dominant cone and cone-rod dystrophy with mutations in the guanylate cyclase activator 1A gene-encoding guanylate cyclase activating protein-1. Arch Ophthalmol. 2001;119(1):96–105.
4. Michaelides M, Wilkie SE, Jenkins S, Holder GE, Hunt DM, Moore AT, et al. Mutation in the gene GUCA1A, encoding guanylate cyclase-activating protein 1, causes cone, cone-rod, and macular dystrophy. Ophthalmology. 2005;112(8):1442–7.
5. Sokal I, Dupps WJ, Grassi MA, Brown J Jr, Affatigato LM, Roychowdhury N, et al. A novel GCAP1 missense mutation (L151F) in a large family with autosomal dominant cone-rod dystrophy (adCORD). Invest Ophthalmol Vis Sci. 2005;46(4):1124–32.
6. Jiang L, Katz BJ, Yang Z, Zhao Y, Faulkner N, Hu J, et al. Autosomal dominant cone dystrophy caused by a novel mutation in the GCAP1 gene (GUCA1A). Mol Vis. 2005;11:143–51.
7. Huang L, Li S, Xiao X, Jia X, Sun W, Gao Y, et al. Novel GUCA1A mutation identified in a Chinese family with cone-rod dystrophy. Neurosci Lett. 2013;541:179–83.
8. Kitiratschky VB, Behnen P, Kellner U, Heckenlively JR, Zrenner E, Jägle H, et al. Mutations in the GUCA1A gene involved in hereditary cone dystrophies impair calcium-mediated regulation of guanylate cyclase. Hum Mutat. 2009;30(8):E782–96.

S. Zahid et al., *Retinal Dystrophy Gene Atlas*, https://doi.org/10.1007/978-3-319-10867-4_35

36 GUCA1B

GUCA1B encodes guanylate cyclase activator 1b, which is a calcium-binding protein required for the stimulation of guanylate cyclases in photoreceptors. It is particularly important for rod recovery after light exposure [1]. Mutations in *GUCA1B* cause retinitis pigmentosa (RP).

GUCA1B-related RP follows an autosomal dominant pattern of inheritance. Patients usually have typical features corresponding to RP. Visual acuities may vary from 20/20 to 20/200, with a decline over the course of disease progression; acuity is usually maintained until late in the disease course. Fundoscopy may reveal variable distribution of pigmentary deposition, ranging from the mid-periphery to more diffuse deposition; some patients have been reported to exhibit signs of macular pigment deposition and atrophy [2]. Electroretinogram (ERG) findings may demonstrate severe deterioration of both rod and cone function, with greatly reduced or nonrecordable photopic and scotopic amplitudes [2]. Goldmann Visual Fields (GVF) usually reveal a rod-cone pattern of field loss (progressive visual field constriction). There may be significant intrafamilial variability; some patients with disease-causing mutations have been reported to be asymptomatic and to exhibit a normal fundus [2].

References

1. Makino CL, Peshenko IV, Wen XH, Olshevskaya EV, Barrett R, Dizhoor AM. A role for GCAP2 in regulating the photoresponse. Guanylyl cyclase activation and rod electrophysiology in GUCA1B knock-out mice. J Biol Chem. 2008;283(43):29135–43.
2. Sato M, Nakazawa M, Usui T, Tanimoto N, Abe H, Ohguro H. Mutations in the gene coding for guanylate cyclase-activating protein 2 (GUCA1B gene) in patients with autosomal dominant retinal dystrophies. Graefes Arch Clin Exp Ophthalmol. 2005;243(3):235–42.

S. Zahid et al., *Retinal Dystrophy Gene Atlas*, https://doi.org/10.1007/978-3-319-10867-4_36

37 GUCY2D

GUCY2D encodes guanylyl cyclase 1, which is an enzyme with unknown function expressed in rod and cone photoreceptors. Mutations in *GUCY2D* are associated with autosomal recessive Leber congenital amaurosis (LCA), autosomal recessive cone-rod dystrophy (CORD), and autosomal dominant cone dystrophy (COD).

LCA may be caused by autosomal recessive mutations in *GUCY2D*. These patients usually exhibit nystagmus and nonrecordable ERGs within the first months of life, in addition to other findings in LCA such as poor pursuit and oculodigital sign [1]. Within the first 2 years of life, photophobia and hypermetropia greater than +7.00 D are commonly observed, and visual acuities typically range from count fingers to light perception [1]. Keratoconus may be observed in some patients, possibly secondary to chronic rubbing of the eyes [2]. Fundus examination can appear completely normal or display a "salt-and-pepper" appearance [2]. Older patients have been reported to exhibit early degeneration of the macular and peripheral retina, but it is unclear when this begins to develop and whether it always progresses from an earlier "salt-and-pepper" appearance [1]. Though published data is limited, some patients may exhibit relatively normal FAF imaging in the context of abnormal retinal lamination with normal macular thickness on time-domain OCT [2].

Recessive mutations may also result in a cone-rod dystrophy phenotype [3]. While age of onset may vary, these patients present with nyctalopia in addition to poor visual acuity, dyschromatopsia, and photophobia [3]. In contrast to patients with LCA, these patients tend to retain functional vision during childhood. Fundoscopy may reveal bone spicule pigment deposits, optic disc pallor, and retinal arteriolar attenuation in the context of macular atrophy [3]. Goldmann visual field testing may reveal central scotomas within the first decade of life [4]. Electroretinography (ERG) tends to reveal reduced photopic and scotopic parameters [3, 4].

GUCY2D-related COD typically follows an autosomal dominant pattern of inheritance. Most patients have an onset of photophobia and bilateral visual acuity impairment within the first decade of life. Visual acuities are abnormal at presentation but vary widely from patient to patient, tend to decline with time, and are often less than 20/200 by the third decade of life. Nyctalopia is uncommon in this disease entity, while dyschromatopsia is commonly observed [5, 6]. In children less than 5 years of age, fundus findings may reveal optic disc pallor, macular white deposits, and granular RPE [5]. Fundus findings in adults are typified by macular atrophy, which is often well-defined [7]. Younger patients exhibit pigment mottling in the macula prior to developing perifoveal atrophy [8]. FAF imaging may reveal a ring of hyperautofluorescence surrounding a region of speckled macular hypoautofluorescence [8]. Full-field ERG is characterized by abnormal photopic parameters with normal scotopic function [5, 7]. GVF reveals central scotomas with full peripheral fields [7]. OCT may reveal a foveal loss of the ellipsoid zone early in the disease process, which progresses to retinal thinning [2, 8]. Incomplete penetrance is possible; some patients within the same family and carrying the same disease-causing mutation may not experience symptoms or exhibit any signs of disease [7]. Certain dominantly-inherited mutations of *GUCY2D* have also been reported in families with a central areolar choroidal dystrophy (CACD) phenotype [9].

Cone-rod dystrophies have also been described in patients with autosomal dominant inheritance, although they may be part of the cone dystrophy spectrum described above (Fig. 37.1a) [4, 10, 11]. Notable differences in these patients include the fact that loss of peripheral visual fields is more common, and not all patients experience nyctalopia [10]. While visual acuity may be relatively maintained during the teenage years, most patients have visual acuity worse than 20/200 by age 40; myopia has been reported in 62% of patients in one family [11]. Dark adaptation thresholds are elevated, and some patients may exhibit a negative ERG in the context of both rod and cone ERG abnormalities; multifocal ERG reveals reduced central responses [10]. FAF imaging tends to reveal hypoautofluorescence at the macula in areas of atrophy with a surrounding area of hyperautofluo-

S. Zahid et al., *Retinal Dystrophy Gene Atlas*, https://doi.org/10.1007/978-3-319-10867-4_37

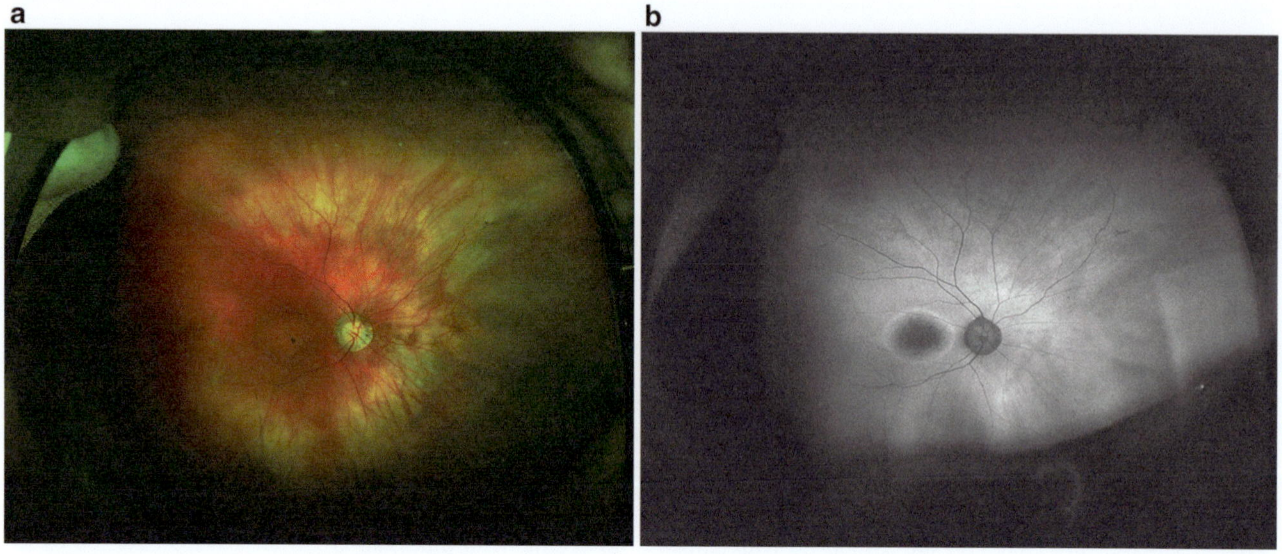

Fig. 37.1 Case summary: 63-year-old female (CEI16027, courtesty of Dr. Richard Weleber) with autosomal dominant cone-rod dystrophy with heterozygous missense mutations in *GUCY2D*. (**a**) Wide-field color fundus photograph of the right eye, showing peripheral retinal pigment epithelium atrophy (with a choroideremia-like appearance of the periphery) as well as central macular atrophy. (**b**) Wide-field fundus autofluorescence, showing central macular hypoautofluorescence corresponding to RPE atrophy, with a surrounding ring of hyperautofluorescence.

rescence, similar to *GUCY2D*-associated cone dystrophy (Fig. 37.1b). OCT findings range from photoreceptor layer thinning with a maintained ellipsoid zone to a punched out localized cavitation with loss of the ellipsoid zone at the fovea [10].

References

1. Hanein S, Perrault I, Gerber S, Tanguy G, Barbet F, Ducroq D, et al. Leber congenital amaurosis: comprehensive survey of the genetic heterogeneity, refinement of the clinical definition, and genotype-phenotype correlations as a strategy for molecular diagnosis. Hum Mutat. 2004;23(4):306–17.
2. Simonelli F, Ziviello C, Testa F, Rossi S, Fazzi E, Bianchi PE, et al. Clinical and molecular genetics of Leber's congenital amaurosis: a multicenter study of Italian patients. Invest Ophthalmol Vis Sci. 2007;48(9):4284–90.
3. Ugur Iseri SA, Durlu YK, Tolun A. A novel recessive GUCY2D mutation causing cone-rod dystrophy and not Leber's congenital amaurosis. Eur J Hum Genet. 2010;18(10):1121–6.
4. Garcia-Hoyos M, Auz-Alexandre CL, Almoguera B, Cantalapiedra D, Riveiro-Alvarez R, Lopez-Martinez MA, et al. Mutation analysis at codon 838 of the Guanylate Cyclase 2D gene in Spanish families with autosomal dominant cone, cone-rod, and macular dystrophies. Mol Vis. 2011;17:1103–9.
5. Xiao X, Guo X, Jia X, Li S, Wang P, Zhang Q. A recurrent mutation in GUCY2D associated with autosomal dominant cone dystrophy in a Chinese family. Mol Vis. 2011;17:3271–8.
6. Zhao X, Ren Y, Zhang X, Chen C, Dong B, Li Y. A novel GUCY2D mutation in a Chinese family with dominant cone dystrophy. Mol Vis. 2013;19:1039–46.
7. Small KW, Silva-Garcia R, Udar N, Nguyen EV, Heckenlively JR. New mutation, P575L, in the GUCY2D gene in a family with autosomal dominant progressive cone degeneration. Arch Ophthalmol. 2008;126(3):397–403.
8. Mukherjee R, Robson AG, Holder GE, Stockman A, Egan CA, Moore AT, et al. A detailed phenotypic description of autosomal dominant cone dystrophy due to a de novo mutation in the GUCY2D gene. Eye (Lond). 2014;28(4):481–7.
9. Hughes AE, Meng W, Lotery AJ, Bradley DT. A novel GUCY2D mutation, V933A, causes central areolar choroidal dystrophy. Invest Ophthalmol Vis Sci. 2012;53(8):4748–53.
10. Zobor D, Zrenner E, Wissinger B, Kohl S, Jagle H. GUCY2D- or GUCA1A-related autosomal dominant cone-rod dystrophy: is there a phenotypic difference? Retina. 2014;34(8):1576–87.
11. Smith M, Whittock N, Searle A, Croft M, Brewer C, Cole M. Phenotype of autosomal dominant cone-rod dystrophy due to the R838C mutation of the GUCY2D gene encoding retinal guanylate cyclase-1. Eye. 2007;21(9):1220–5.

IMPDH1 (RP10)

38

IMPDH1 (RP10) encodes inosine-5-prime-monophosphate dehydrogenase, which plays a key role in the purine biosynthesis pathway. Mutations in *IMPDH1* cause 2–3% of dominant retinitis pigmentosa (ADRP) (rod-cone dystrophy) and rarely cause Leber congenital amaurosis (LCA) [1–8]. While *IMPDH1* is a ubiquitously expressed gene, retina-specific isoforms may be responsible for a phenotype limited to retinal degeneration [9–11].

Patients with ADRP caused by mutations in *IMPDH1* present between the first and third decades of life with night blindness and/or peripheral field loss that progress with time. There is often variability in age of onset even in patients with the same mutations, and symptoms may begin as late as in life as the 40s [3]. Visual acuity may be maintained until later in the disease course but has been shown to be severely reduced at an early age in some patients [6, 12, 13]. Some patients may have color vision deficits [13]. Early-onset posterior subcapsular cataracts are common (average onset of 34 years in one study [5]) [3]. Patients with *IMPDH1* mutations present with typical fundus findings of RP, such as mid-peripheral to peripheral bone-spicule pigment deposits, optic disc pallor, and retinal vessel attenuation; pigmented cells in the vitreous may also be observed (Figs. 38.1a and 38.3). Some patients may develop CME or subretinal fluid, best visualized with OCT [3, 13, 14]. Peripheral/mid-peripheral RPE atrophy develops over time (Figs. 38.1a, 38.2, and 38.3). Some patients develop bull's-eye macular atrophy as well, though this is less commonly observed (Fig. 38.2) [2]. Most patients exhibit cataracts and pigment deposits after the middle of the third decade of life [3]. Fundus autofluorescence shows hypoautofluorescence in areas of RPE atrophy (Fig. 38.1b). The full-field ERG is severely reduced, usually to a similar extent for both rod and cone parameters, but may be recordable in a rod-cone pattern in some younger patients [3, 5, 13, 14]. Multifocal ERG generally shows maintenance of central cone responses, which may be lost with time [14]. Dark adaptation thresholds are frequently elevated. GVF reveals severe progressive constriction of the visual field (Fig. 38.1c) [13].

Some mutations in *IMPDH1* have been associated with dominant LCA (e.g., Arg105Trp and Asn198Lys) [2]. One of these patients presented with roving nystagmus with absent fixation to light before age 1, with a mottled-appearing fundus without pigmentary changes. The other patient presented at about 3 years of age with peripheral vision loss, though her central vision was maintained at 20/40 bilaterally. The fundus of the 3-year old revealed optic disc pallor, diffuse depigmentation of the fundus, and attenuated retinal vessels. More recently, an additional patient with autosomal recessive *IMPDH1*-associated disease presenting within the first few months of life with poor vision and nystagmus [15]. This patient had LP visual acuity and exhibited attenuated retinal vasculature, macular atrophy and pigment deposits in the fundus, and a non-recordable full-field ERG when evaluated at age 23.

S. Zahid et al., *Retinal Dystrophy Gene Atlas*, https://doi.org/10.1007/978-3-319-10867-4_38

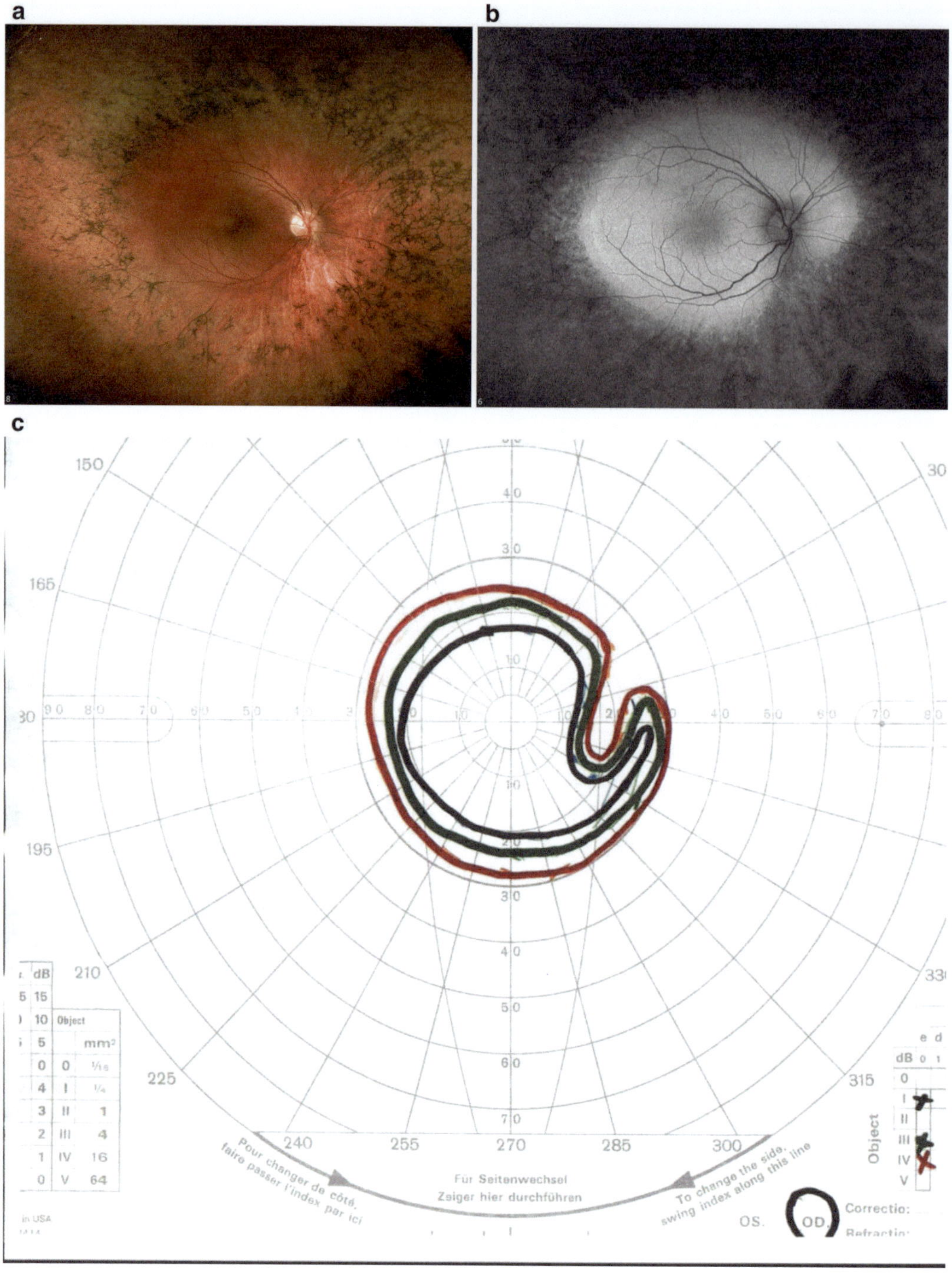

Fig. 38.1 Case summary: 19-year-old woman with rod-cone dystrophy. (**a**) Wide-field color fundus photograph of the right eye, showing typical findings of rod-cone dystrophy, including mid-periphery RPE atrophy with bone spicule pigmentation and sparing of the macula. (**b**) Wide-field fundus autofluorescence of the right eye, showing loss of mid-peripheral autofluorescence in areas with RPE atrophy, with relatively normal appearing macular autofluorescence. (**c**) Goldmann visual field of the right eye, showing constricted fields in all isopters, suggestive of a rod-cone pattern of visual field loss.

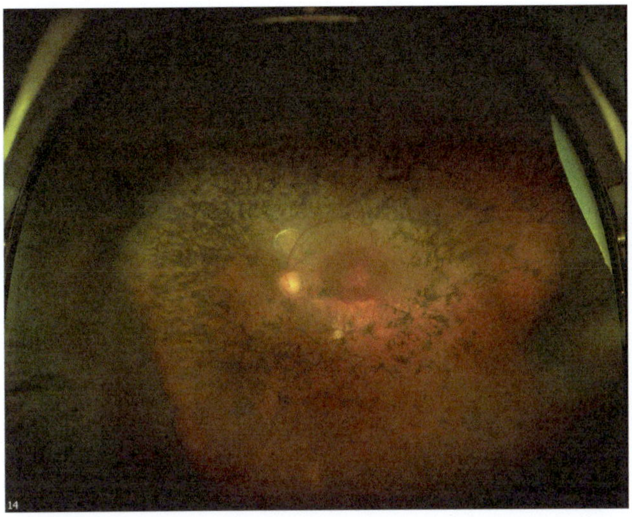

Fig. 38.2 Wide-field color fundus photograph of the left eye from a 56-year-old male with rod-cone dystrophy with a bull's eye lesion in the macula and dense mid-peripheral bone spicule pigment deposits.

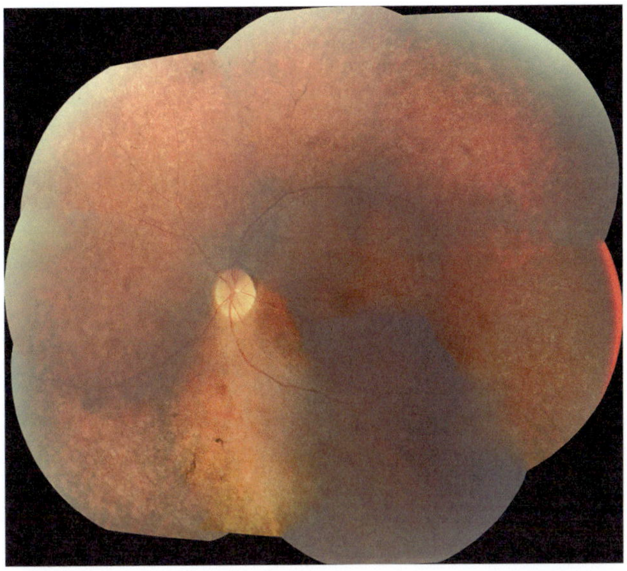

Fig. 38.3 Color fundus photograph from a 20-year-old male (CEI26447) with Leber Congenital Amaurosis/Severe Early Childhood Onset Retinal Dystrophy (SECORD) with heterozygous mutations in IMPDH1, showing diffuse mid-peripheral RPE atrophy with sparse pigmentation.

References

1. Bowne SJ, Sullivan LS, Blanton SH, Cepko CL, Blackshaw S, Birch DG, et al. Mutations in the inosine monophosphate dehydrogenase 1 gene (IMPDH1) cause the RP10 form of autosomal dominant retinitis pigmentosa. Hum Mol Genet. 2002;11(5):559–68.
2. Bowne SJ, Sullivan LS, Mortimer SE, Hedstrom L, Zhu J, Spellicy CJ, et al. Spectrum and frequency of mutations in IMPDH1 associated with autosomal dominant retinitis pigmentosa and leber congenital amaurosis. Invest Ophthalmol Vis Sci. 2006;47(1):34–42.
3. Wada Y, Sandberg MA, McGee TL, Stillberger MA, Berson EL, Dryja TP. Screen of the IMPDH1 gene among patients with dominant retinitis pigmentosa and clinical features associated with the most common mutation, Asp226Asn. Invest Ophthalmol Vis Sci. 2005;46(5):1735–41.
4. McGuire RE, Gannon AM, Sullivan LS, Rodriguez JA, Daiger SP. Evidence for a major gene (RP10) for autosomal dominant retinitis pigmentosa on chromosome 7q: linkage mapping in a second, unrelated family. Hum Genet. 1995;95(1):71–4.
5. Jordan SA, Farrar GJ, Kenna P, Humphries MM, Sheils DM, Kumar-Singh R, et al. Localization of an autosomal dominant retinitis pigmentosa gene to chromosome 7q. Nat Genet. 1993;4(1):54–8.
6. Grover S, Fishman GA, Stone EM. A novel IMPDH1 mutation (Arg231Pro) in a family with a severe form of autosomal dominant retinitis pigmentosa. Ophthalmology. 2004;111(10):1910–6.
7. Shumei L, Xiaoting L, Xiangyun Z, Liqun H, Liang X, Sisi L. Mutation frequency of IMPDH1 gene of Han population in Ganzhou City. Adv Exp Med Biol. 2010;664:293–7.
8. Sullivan LS, Bowne SJ, Birch DG, Hughbanks-Wheaton D, Heckenlively JR, Lewis RA, et al. Prevalence of disease-causing mutations in families with autosomal dominant retinitis pigmentosa: a screen of known genes in 200 families. Invest Ophthalmol Vis Sci. 2006;47(7):3052–64.
9. Spellicy CJ, Xu D, Cobb G, Hedstrom L, Bowne SJ, Sullivan LS, et al. Investigating the mechanism of disease in the RP10 form of retinitis pigmentosa. Adv Exp Med Biol. 2010;664:541–8.
10. Bowne SJ, Liu Q, Sullivan LS, Zhu J, Spellicy CJ, Rickman CB, et al. Why do mutations in the ubiquitously expressed housekeeping gene IMPDH1 cause retina-specific photoreceptor degeneration? Invest Ophthalmol Vis Sci. 2006;47(9):3754–65.
11. McGrew DA, Hedstrom L. Towards a pathological mechanism for IMPDH1-linked retinitis pigmentosa. Adv Exp Med Biol. 2012;723:539–45.
12. Wada Y, Tada A, Itabashi T, Kawamura M, Sato H, Tamai M. Screening for mutations in the IMPDH1 gene in Japanese patients with autosomal dominant retinitis pigmentosa. Am J Ophthalmol. 2005;140(1):163–5.
13. Kozma P, Hughbanks-Wheaton DK, Locke KG, Fish GE, Gire AI, Spellicy CJ, et al. Phenotypic characterization of a large family with RP10 autosomal dominant retinitis pigmentosa: an Asp226Asn mutation in the IMPDH1 gene. Am J Ophthalmol. 2005;140(5):858–67.
14. Schatz P, Ponjavic V, Andreasson S, McGee TL, Dryja TP, Abrahamson M. Clinical phenotype in a Swedish family with a mutation in the IMPDH1 gene. Ophthalmic Genet. 2005;26(3):119–24.
15. Chen Y, Zhang Q, Shen T, Xiao X, Li S, Guan L, et al. Comprehensive mutation analysis by whole-exome sequencing in 41 Chinese families with Leber congenital amaurosis. Invest Ophthalmol Vis Sci. 2013;54(6):4351–7.

39 IMPG2

IMPG2 encodes a component of the retinal extracellular matrix (interphotoreceptor matrix proteoglycan 2), which allows for interaction between photoreceptor cells and between photoreceptor cells and the retinal pigment epithelium (RPE) [1, 2]. It also has calcium-binding potential, which may permit it to have a role in sequestering extracellular calcium released by photoreceptors in response to light [2]. Mutations in *IMPG2* are responsible for autosomal recessive retinitis pigmentosa (RP) with early macular involvement [2, 3].

Thus far, *IMPG2* mutations that have been described are severely pathogenic, leading to nonsense-mediated decay or to a nonfunctional gene product. The mean age of onset of symptoms for these patients is 10.5 years, with night blindness being the most common initial symptom and the next most common being decreased visual acuity [2]. Many patients also have subcapsular posterior cataracts that appear later in life. Visual acuity ranges from 20/30–20/400, and mild-to-high myopia has been reported. Visual fields become progressively constricted with time, along with a gradual decrease in central sensitivity and/or the presence of paracentral scotomas [2]. Fundus exam shows optic disc pallor, attenuated retinal vessels, and bone spicule pigmentation at the periphery and midperiphery [2]. Macular changes range from subtle mottling of macular pigment epithelium to bull's-eye maculopathy to macular chorioretinal atrophy (Fig. 39.1a). In all 17 patients (from 10 families) observed by van Huet et al. [2], fundus autofluorescence (FAF) showed macular involvement, with profound macular hypoautofluorescence observed in later stages of the disease (indicating RPE atrophy) and with hypoautofluorescence in the midperiphery with granularity (Fig. 39.1b). However, in two of the patients observed by van Huet et al. [2], only subtle macular FAF abnormalities were observed. Spectral domain optical coherence tomography shows loss of photoreceptor inner and outer segments (ellipsoid zone) before RPE cell loss, which gives rise to severe outer retinal thinning (Fig. 39.1c). In all 17 patients observed by van Huet et al., ERG was either non-recordable (mean age of 51 years) or demonstrated a severely reduced rod-cone pattern of dysfunction [2].

A hypomorphic missense allele in *IMPG2* has been identified, and the patient carrying this mutation in a homozygous state was found to have mild maculopathy and mildly affected visual function but no diagnosis of RP [2, 3].

S. Zahid et al., *Retinal Dystrophy Gene Atlas*, https://doi.org/10.1007/978-3-319-10867-4_39

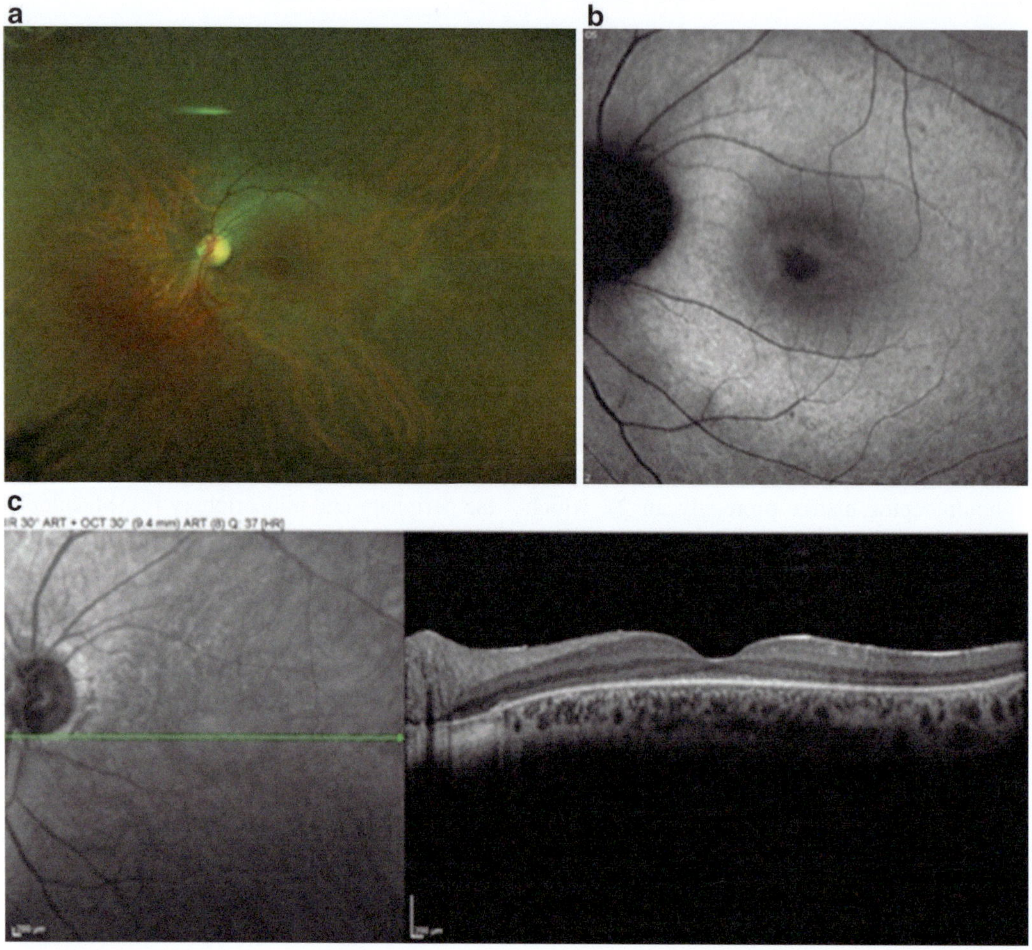

Fig. 39.1 Case summary: 23-year-old female with rod-cone dystrophy. (**a**) Wide-field color fundus photograph of the left eye showing subtle macular RPE abnormalities. (**b**) Fundus autofluorescence of the left eye, showing a subtle ring of macular hyperautofluorescence surrounding the fovea. (**c**) Spectral domain optical coherence tomography of the left eye, showing an extensive extrafoveal ellipsoid zone and outer nuclear layer loss.

References

1. Kelly J, O'Neill MJF. Interphotoreceptor matrix proteoglycan 2; IMPG2. OMIM. 607056. 2002 (updated 2014). http://omim.org/entry/607056. Accessed 24 Jan 2017.
2. van Huet RA, Collin RW, Siemiatkowska AM, Klaver CC, Hoyng CB, Simonelli F, et al. IMPG2-associated retinitis pigmentosa displays relatively early macular involvement. Invest Ophthalmol Vis Sci. 2014;55(6):3939–53.
3. Bandah-Rozenfeld D, Collin RW, Banin E, van den Born LI, Coene KL, Siemiatkowska AM, et al. Mutations in IMPG2, encoding interphotoreceptor matrix proteoglycan 2, cause autosomal-recessive retinitis pigmentosa. Am J Hum Genet. 2010;87(2):199–208.

40 *IQCB1*

IQCB1 encodes IQ-Motif Containing Protein, which is expressed in the outer segment and connecting cilia of photoreceptors and believed to be involved in ciliogenesis. Recessive mutations in *IQCB1* can either cause Senior-Loken Syndrome (SLSN), which is an oculo-renal condition characterized by nephronophthisis (medullary cystic kidney disease) and Leber congenital amaurosis (LCA), or non-syndromic LCA [1].

Patients generally have an early-onset severe LCA phenotype, with pendular nystagmus and poor fixation from birth. Patients may be highly hyperopic and often have poor visual acuity (hand motion to light perception), but in the minority with better acuity, vision is 20/70 or worse. Patients may also have keratoconus or cataracts. It is important to note that while retinal examination of a 1–2 year-old patient is typically normal, one study found prominent retinal changes at 18 months in a mutation-confirmed patient. The fundus may also reveal a "lobular" pattern of subtle alternating hypo- and hyperpigmentation around the vascular arcades or diffuse retinal pigment epithelial changes. Fundus autofluorescence may reveal patchy hyper- and hypoautofluorescence areas throughout the fundus or a hyperautofluorescent ring in the parafoveal region (Fig. 40.1a). Spectral domain optical coherence tomography is useful to demonstrate the extent of photoreceptor loss (Fig. 40.1b). ERGs typically are non-detectable early in the disease course. There is a wide variability in the onset, severity, and presence of renal disease in these patients. When patients do develop nephronophthisis, it typically occurs from the second decade of life onward. Therefore, patients with *IQCB1*-related LCA should be routinely screened for renal disease due to the significant long-term risk of renal failure [2].

S. Zahid et al., *Retinal Dystrophy Gene Atlas*, https://doi.org/10.1007/978-3-319-10867-4_40

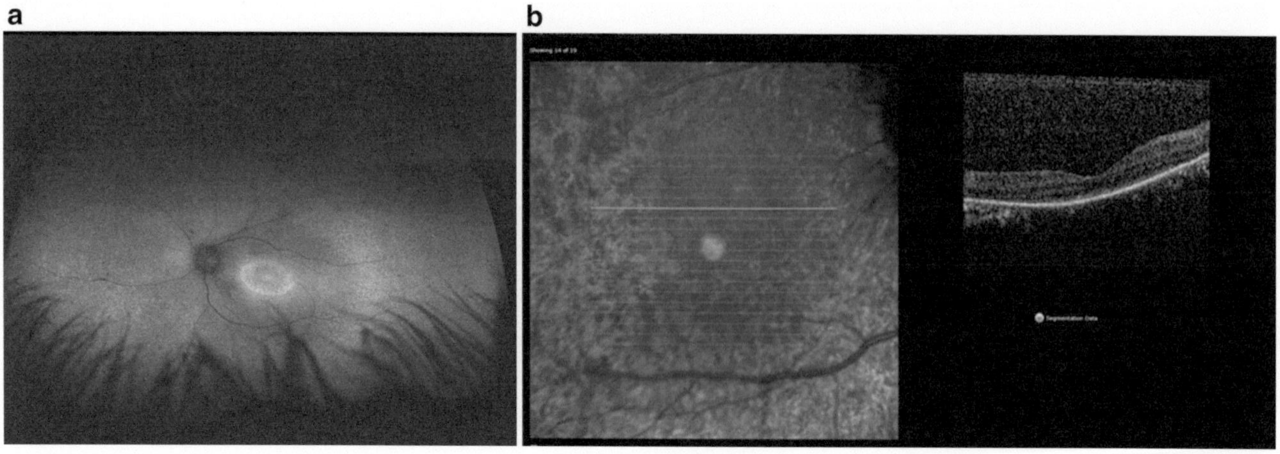

Fig. 40.1 Case summary: 14-year-old Asian female with a history of Leber congenital amaurosis (CEI25377) with a homozygous mutation in *IQCB1* (courtesy of Richard Weleber). (**a**) Wide-field fundus autofluorescence of the left eye, showing patchy hyper- and hypoautofluorescence throughout the fundus, with a hyperautofluorescent ring in the parafoveal region. (**b**) Spectral domain optical coherence tomography of the right eye, showing extensive loss of the ellipsoid zone and the outer nuclear layer.

References

1. Estrada-Cuzcano A, Koenekoop RK, Coppieters F, Kohl S, Lopez I, Collin RW, et al. IQCB1 mutations in patients with leber congenital amaurosis. Invest Ophthalmol Vis Sci. 2011;52(2):834–9.
2. Stone EM, Cideciyan AV, Aleman TS, Scheetz TE, Sumaroka A, Ehlinger MA, et al. Variations in NPHP5 in patients with nonsyndromic leber congenital amaurosis and Senior-Loken syndrome. Arch Ophthalmol. 2011;129(1):81–7.

41 KCNV2

KCNV2 encodes a subunit of a voltage-gated potassium channel expressed in human rod and cone photoreceptors. Autosomal recessive mutations in *KCNV2* are associated with the unique phenotype of cone dystrophy with supernormal rod response (CDSRR), also known as *KCNV2* retinopathy.

Onset is usually during infancy or early childhood, with slow but variable rates of progression, and a greater degree of cone loss over time compared to rod function. Within the first decade of life, patients typically experience reduced visual acuity, abnormal color vision (most commonly in the red-green axis), and mild photophobia with impaired adaptation to bright conditions. Nyctalopia is variable and may be experienced from childhood or develop in later stages of disease [1, 2]. Nystagmus and strabismus may also be present in young patients [3, 4]. Patients often have myopia and varying degrees of astigmatism. Central scotomas are commonly observed; in patients with rod loss, peripheral fields may also constrict over time [4–6]. Best-corrected visual acuity ranges from 20/30 to 20/400, but there is marked variability between patients. Fundus findings are variable but are generally limited to the macula and begin with an impaired foveal reflex and mild retinal pigment epithelium (RPE) changes (Figs. 41.1a, 41.2a, and 41.3a) [7]. Bull's-eye maculopathy may also be observed; this may be more readily visualized on optical coherence tomography (OCT) and fundus autofluorescence (FAF) imaging (Figs. 41.1b and 41.3b) [1, 2]. Some patients exhibit a well-circumscribed area of macular atrophy [1]. Mild optic disc pallor may also be observed in some patients [2].

FAF imaging may reveal a perifoveal ring of increased autofluorescence (AF) (Figs. 41.1b and 41.3b) [1–3, 6, 8]. Some patients may also exhibit increased AF at the fovea, which can also be seen in some other cone/cone-rod dystrophies [6]. OCT findings range from reduced intensity of the foveal EZ without disruption and focal loss of the foveal ellipsoid zone (common finding) to significant loss of outer retinal structure at the fovea (Figs. 41.1c, 41.2b, and 41.3c) [1, 8]. Patients may also have a "hyporeflective zone" on OCT [6, 8].

Dark adaptation thresholds to red and green stimuli are elevated and may be more pronounced in patients with null mutations than in those with missense variants [1]. A unique characteristic observed with full-field electroretinography (ERG) is that the scotopic b-wave in this disorder is delayed and markedly reduced or absent at low flash intensities yet normal or "supernormal" in amplitude at the highest flash intensities [3–10]. The light-adapted and flicker ERGs exhibit reduced amplitudes and prolonged implicit times, consistent with generalized cone system dysfunction [4, 11]. While some patients do not exhibit "supernormal" rod amplitudes, all exhibit delayed implicit times and a notably greater increase in b-wave amplitude with small increases in light intensity. Multifocal ERG usually shows loss of amplitudes and prolonged implicit times that are more prominent in the central rings [1]. Adaptive optics imaging reveals foveal loss of cone photoreceptors [6].

S. Zahid et al., *Retinal Dystrophy Gene Atlas*, https://doi.org/10.1007/978-3-319-10867-4_41

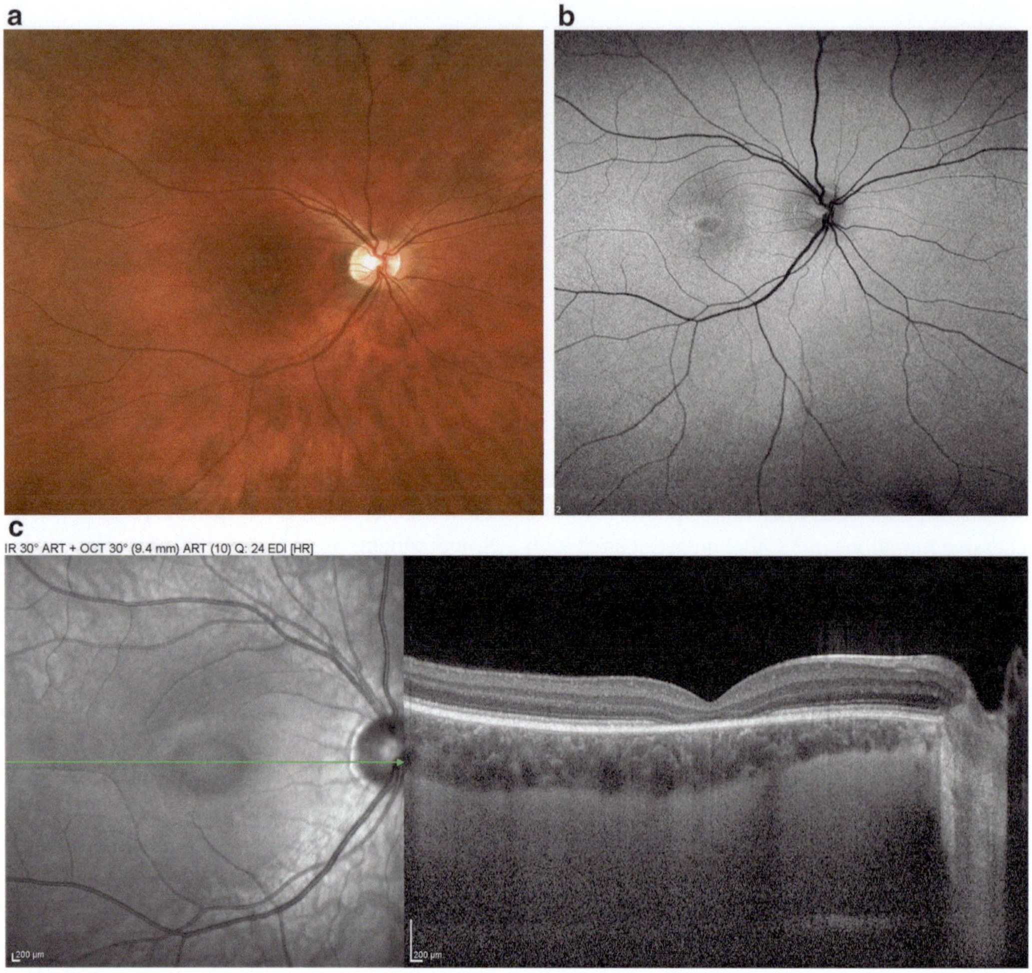

Fig. 41.1 Case summary: 14-year-old boy with *KCNV2* retinopathy and 20/300 vision OU. (**a**) Color fundus photograph of the right eye, showing macular atrophy. (**b**) Fundus autofluorescence of the right eye, showing a small ring of hyperautofluorescence surrounding the fovea. (**c**) Spectral domain-optical coherence tomography, showing loss of the foveal ellipsoid zone and thinning of the outer nuclear layer at age 16.

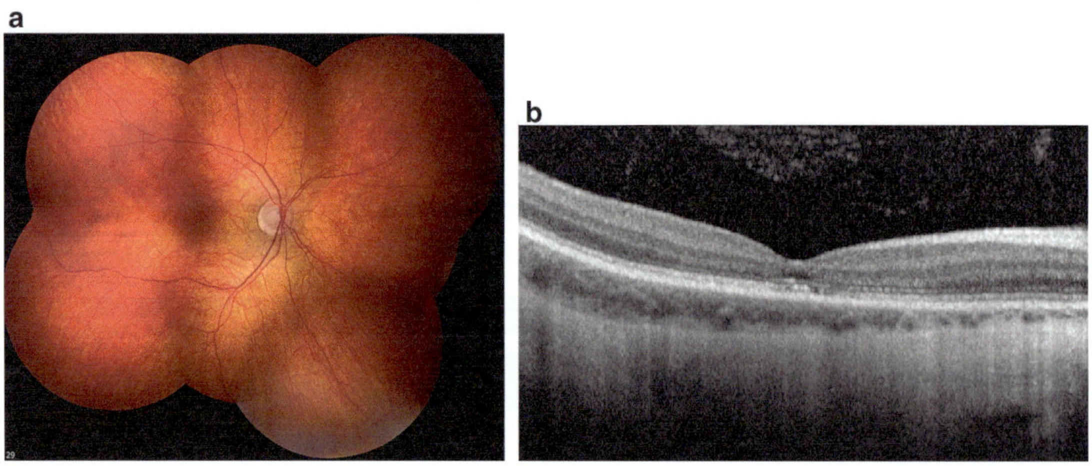

Fig. 41.2 Case summary: 6-year-old girl with *KCNV2* retinopathy and 20/200, 20/300 visual acuity. (**a**) Color fundus photograph of the right eye, showing loss of the foveal reflex. (**b**) Spectral domain-optical coherence tomography, showing disruption of the foveal ellipsoid zone at age 12.

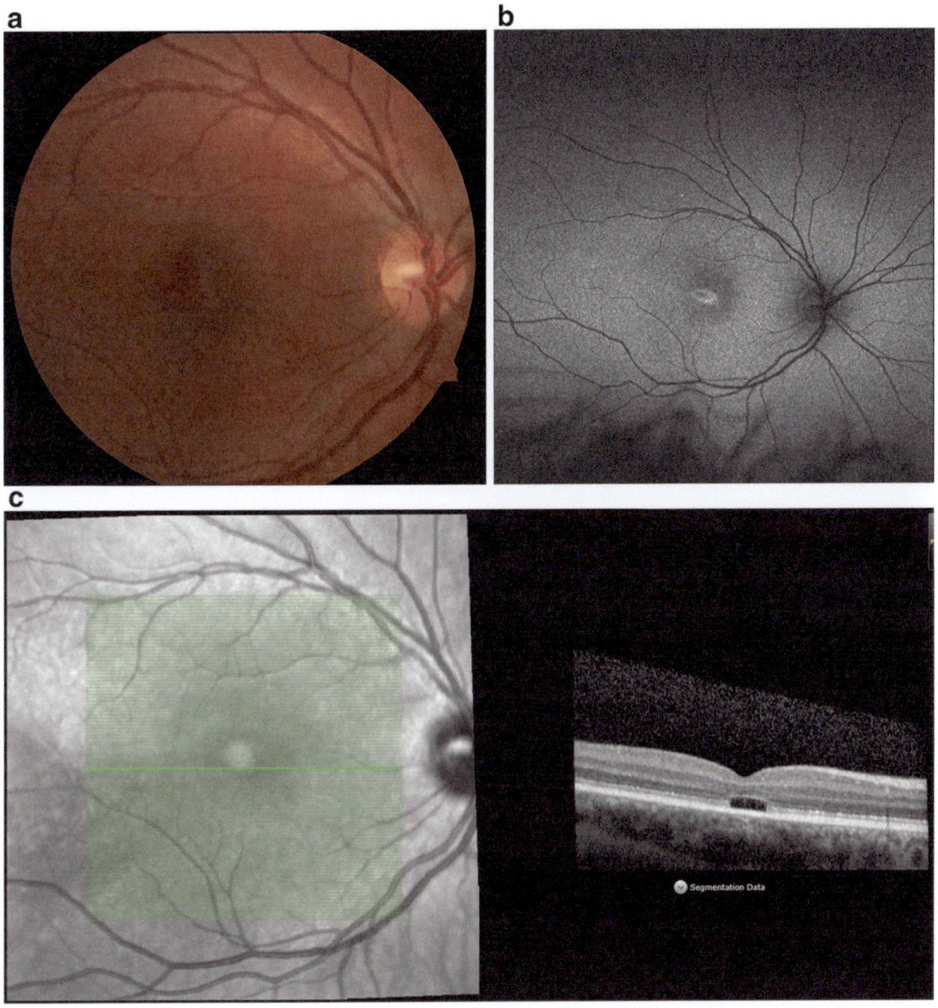

Fig. 41.3 Case summary: 11-year-old girl (CEI26492) KCNV2 mutations. (**a**) Color fundus photograph of the right eye, showing macular atrophy. (**b**) Fundus autofluorescence of the right eye, showing a small ring of hyperautofluorescence surrounding the fovea. (**c**) Spectral domain-optical coherence tomography showing complete loss of the foveal ellipsoid zone.

References

1. Zobor D, Kohl S, Wissinger B, Zrenner E, Jägle H. Rod and cone function in patients with KCNV2 retinopathy. PLoS One. 2012;7(10):e46762.
2. Michaelides M, Holder GE, Webster AR, Hunt DM, Bird AC, Fitzke FW, et al. A detailed phenotypic study of "cone dystrophy with supernormal rod ERG". Br J Ophthalmol. 2005;89(3):332–9.
3. Khan AO, Alrashed M, Alkuraya FS. 'Cone dystrophy with supranormal rod response' in children. Br J Ophthalmol. 2012;96(3):422–6.
4. Wissinger B, Dangel S, Jägle H, Hansen L, Baumann B, Rudolph G, et al. Cone dystrophy with supernormal rod response is strictly associated with mutations in KCNV2. Invest Ophthalmol Vis Sci. 2008;49(2):751–7.
5. Friedburg C, Wissinger B, Schambeck M, Bonin M, Kohl S, Lorenz B. Long-term follow-up of the human phenotype in three siblings with cone dystrophy associated with a homozygous p.G461R mutation of KCNV2. Invest Ophthalmol Vis Sci. 2011;52(12):8621–9.
6. Vincent A, Wright T, Garcia-Sanchez Y, Kisilak M, Campbell M, Westall C, et al. Phenotypic characteristics including in vivo cone photoreceptor mosaic in KCNV2-related "cone dystrophy with supernormal rod electroretinogram". Invest Ophthalmol Vis Sci. 2013;54(1):898–908.
7. Zelinger L, Wissinger B, Eli D, Kohl S, Sharon D, Banin E. Cone dystrophy with supernormal rod response: novel KCNV2 mutations in an underdiagnosed phenotype. Ophthalmology. 2013;120(11):2338–43.
8. Sergouniotis PI, Holder GE, Robson AG, Michaelides M, Webster AR, Moore AT. High-resolution optical coherence tomography imaging in KCNV2 retinopathy. Br J Ophthalmol. 2012;96(2):213–7.
9. Ritter M, Vodopiutz J, Lechner S, Moser E, Schmidt-Erfurth UM, Janecke AR. Coexistence of KCNV2 associated cone dystrophy with supernormal rod electroretinogram and MFRP related oculopathy in a Turkish family. Br J Ophthalmol. 2013;97(2):169–73.
10. Wissinger B, Schaich S, Baumann B, Bonin M, Jägle H, Friedburg C, et al. Large deletions of the KCNV2 gene are common in patients with cone dystrophy with supernormal rod response. Hum Mutat. 2011;32(12):1398–406.
11. Ben Salah S, Kamei S, Senechal A, Lopez S, Bazalgette C, Bazalgette C, et al. Novel KCNV2 mutations in cone dystrophy with supernormal rod electroretinogram. Am J Ophthalmol. 2008;145(6):1099–106.

42 KLHL7

KLHL7 encodes Kelch-like protein 7, which is part of the E3 ubiquitin ligase complex of the proteasomal pathway. Mutations in *KLHL7* cause 1–2% of autosomal dominant retinitis pigmentosa (adRP) (rod-cone dystrophy) [1–3].

Broadly, when compared with adRP caused by mutations in other genes, adRP caused by *KLHL7* mutations exhibits a later age of disease onset, with median age of diagnosis of 50 years, although some patients may exhibit more rapid deterioration of visual function [3]. Interestingly, evaluation in one patient, aged 17 years, revealed a normal fundus with no deterioration in ERG parameters [2]. Initial symptoms are typical for RP, with patients presenting with nyctalopia and decreased peripheral vision. Visual acuity is usually maintained until late in the disease course, when macular atrophy may develop [3].

Fundoscopy may demonstrate a normal fundus in younger patients but usually shows mid-peripheral bone spicules in areas of RPE atrophy, attenuated vasculature, and disc pallor (Fig. 42.1a–d). Full-field ERG reveals a rod-cone pattern of degeneration but exhibits intrafamilial variability [2, 3]. Wen et al. [3] report a 3% rate of yearly decline in the photopic flicker response. Multifocal ERG usually reveals preserved responses until late in the disease course, when there may be macular atrophy. GVF testing reveals constriction of peripheral fields, paracentral scotomata, or normal visual fields in younger patients. Fields are usually limited to 10–20° by age 65, although some patients may retain peripheral islands into their 60s [3]. OCT usually reveals retinal thinning and loss of the ellipsoid zone but with foveal preservation (Fig. 42.1e–f) [3]. CME has also been reported [2, 3].

S. Zahid et al., *Retinal Dystrophy Gene Atlas*, https://doi.org/10.1007/978-3-319-10867-4_42

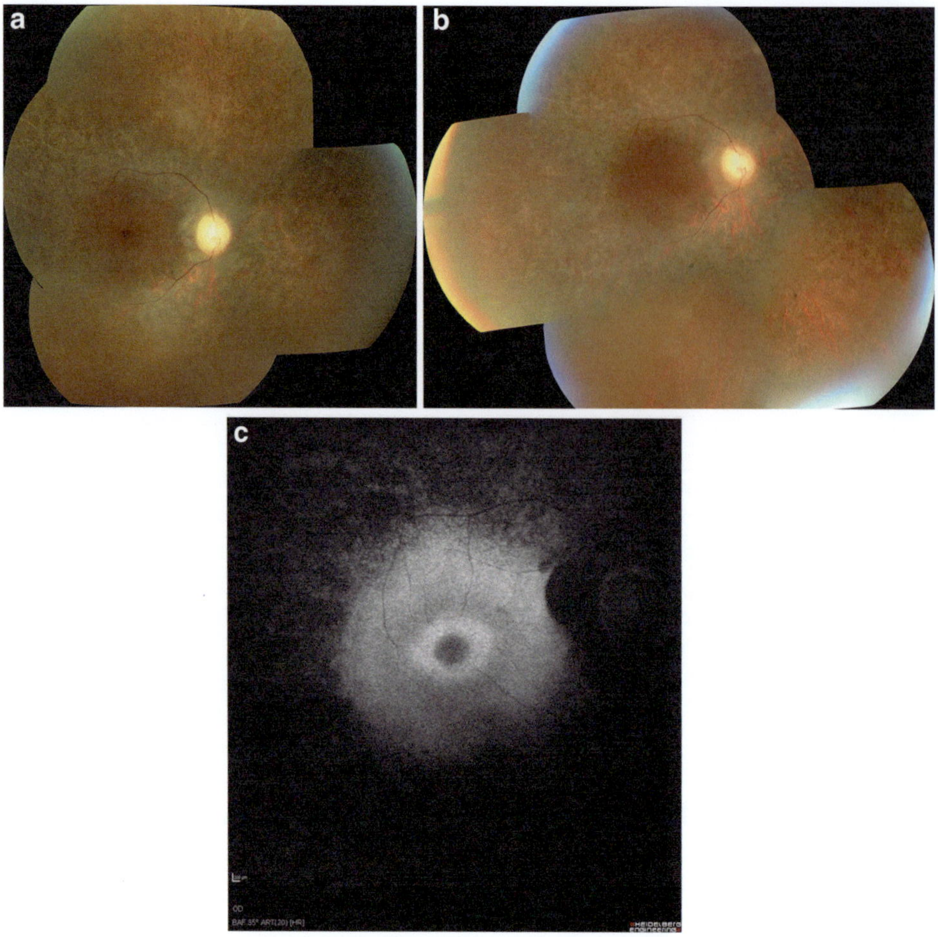

Fig. 42.1 Case summary: 56-year-old female with late-onset rod-cone dystrophy with a mutation in *KLHL7*, with best-corrected visual acuity of 20/40 in both eyes. (**a**, **b**) Color fundus photographs of the right and left eyes, showing RPE atrophy along and outside the arcades. (**c**) Fundus autofluorescence image of the right eye, showing hypoautofluorescent areas along and outside the arcades in areas of RPE atro phy as well as hyperautofluorescent rings surrounding the foveae in both eyes. (**d**, **e**) Spectral domain optical coherence tomography, showing significant ellipsoid zone and outer nuclear layer loss in both eyes, with sparing at the fovea. There are also mild epiretinal membranes in both eyes.

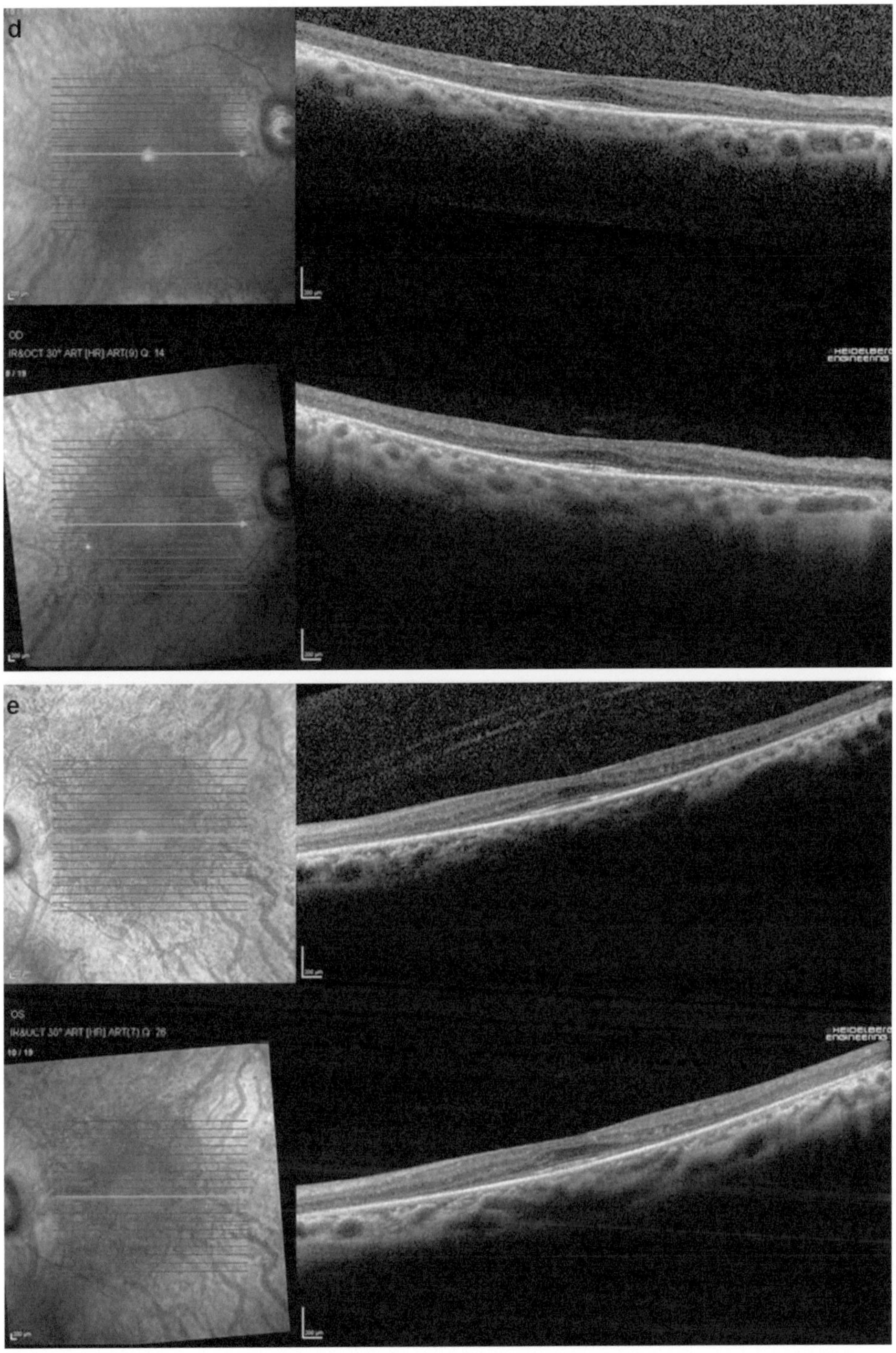

Fig. 42.1 (continued)

References

1. Friedman JS, Ray JW, Waseem N, Johnson K, Brooks MJ, Hugosson T, et al. Mutations in a BTB-Kelch protein, KLHL7, cause autosomal-dominant retinitis pigmentosa. Am J Hum Genet. 2009;84(6):792–800.
2. Hugosson T, Friedman JS, Ponjavic V, Abrahamson M, Swaroop A, Andréasson S. Phenotype associated with mutation in the recently identified autosomal dominant retinitis pigmentosa KLHL7 gene. Arch Ophthalmol. 2010;128(6):772–8.
3. Wen Y, Locke KG, Klein M, Bowne SJ, Sullivan LS, Ray JW, et al. Phenotypic characterization of 3 families with autosomal dominant retinitis pigmentosa due to mutations in KLHL7. Arch Ophthalmol. 2011;129(11):1475–82.

43 *LCA5*

LCA5 encodes lebercilin, which is involved in microtubule transport. Mutations in *LCA5* cause 1–2% of autosomal recessive Leber congenital amaurosis [1–5].

Patients with *LCA5* mutations typically present within the first few months of life with poor pupillary reflexes, roving eye movements, oculodigital sign, high hyperopia, and pendular nystagmus. Given poor visual function and nonrecordable electroretinogram (ERG), pupillary response thresholds using direct transient pupillary light reflex measurements have been used to quantify function and were found to be elevated by over 5.5 log units in one study [6]. Bilateral keratoconus has been reported in one family [5]. Visual acuity is generally very poor and may range from 20/100–20/400 or worse (Mohamed et al. and Jacobson et al. reported LP in all patients from two families [2, 6]). Very young patients may exhibit a normal fundus, but patients eventually develop attenuated vasculature, pigment mottling, and bone spicule deposits (Figs. 43.1 and 43.2a). White dots, posterior staphyloma, macular atrophy, and early-onset cataracts have also been reported in one family; macular atrophy may progress to a coloboma-like appearance [2]. Metallic sheen of the macula [7] and optic disc drusen [1, 6] have also been reported. Hyperopia may progress with age [3]. Fundus autofluorescence may show hyperautofluorescence at the fovea (Fig. 43.2b). The full-field ERG is extinguished at an early age [3]. When recordable, it may show a rod-cone pattern of degeneration [5]. When fields are recordable, Goldmann visual field testing may show small central islands of vision [6]. Jacobson et al. reported that optical coherence tomography (OCT) reveals abnormal retinal lamination that worsens with eccentricity from the fovea; outer retinal structures may be maintained at the fovea (Fig. 43.2c). Infrared autofluorescence may show preserved RPE in younger patients in areas of maintained photoreceptor integrity (as seen on OCT) [6].

S. Zahid et al., *Retinal Dystrophy Gene Atlas*, https://doi.org/10.1007/978-3-319-10867-4_43

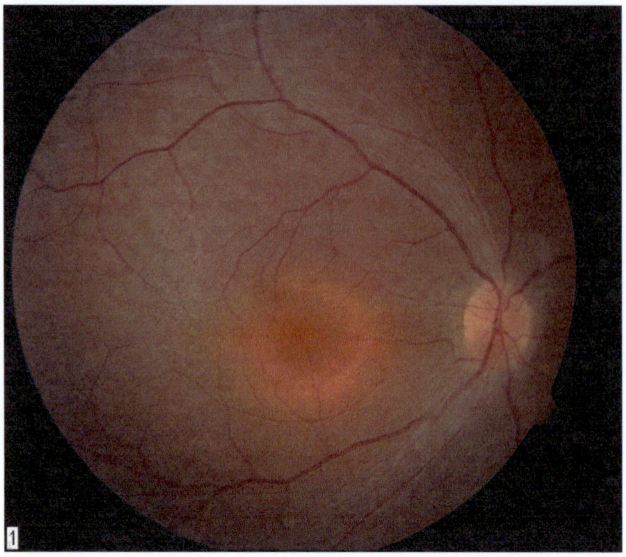

Fig. 43.1 Case summary: 22-year-old man with Leber congenital amaurosis. (**a**) Color fundus photograph of the right eye, showing macular atrophy and midperipheral patchy retinal pigment epithelium changes.

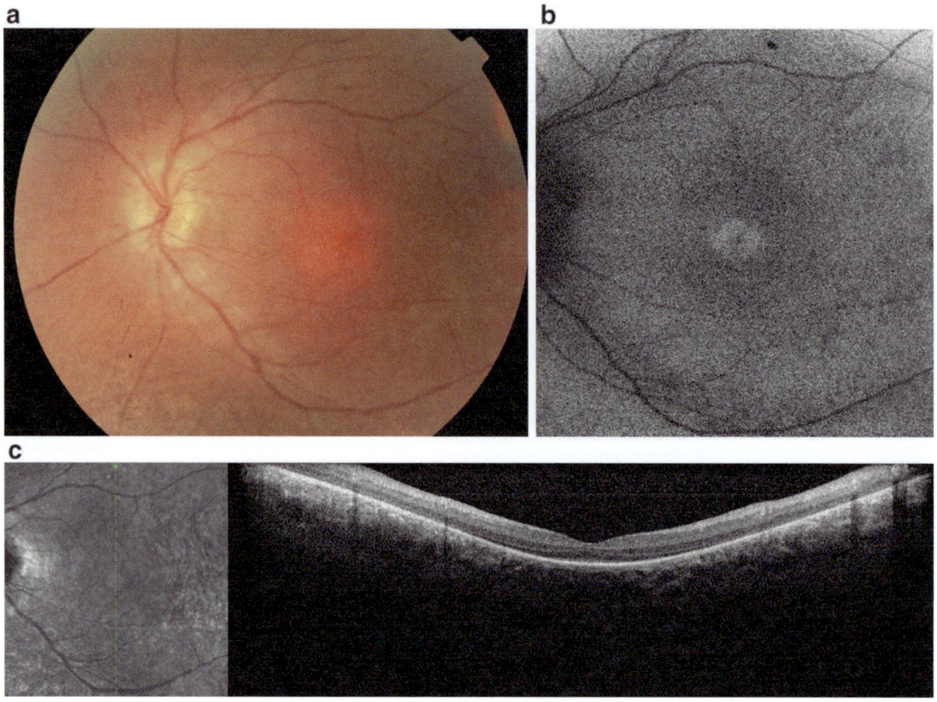

Fig. 43.2 Case summary: 20-year-old with Leber congenital amaurosis, onset at birth, visual acuity 1.3 logMAR (Snellen 20/400). (**a**) Color fundus photograph of the left eye, showing a mildly pale disc, attenuated vessels, and mid-peripheral retinal pigment epithelium mottling in the macula. (**b**) Fundus autofluorescence of the left eye, showing a small central residual hyperautofluorescent island. (**c**) Spectral domain-optical coherence tomography, showing ellipsoid zone loss outside the fovea.

References

1. den Hollander AI, Koenekoop RK, Mohamed MD, Arts HH, Boldt K, Towns KV, et al. Mutations in LCA5, encoding the ciliary protein lebercilin, cause Leber congenital amaurosis. Nat Genet. 2007;39(7):889–95.
2. Mohamed MD, Topping NC, Jafri H, Raashed Y, McKibbin MA, Inglehearn CF. Progression of phenotype in Leber's congenital amaurosis with a mutation at the LCA5 locus. Br J Ophthalmol. 2003;87(4):473–5.
3. Dharmaraj S, Li Y, Robitaille JM, Silva E, Zhu D, Mitchell TN, et al. A novel locus for Leber congenital amaurosis maps to chromosome 6q. Am J Hum Genet. 2000;66(1):319–26.
4. Gerber S, Hanein S, Perrault I, Delphin N, Aboussair N, Leowski C, et al. Mutations in LCA5 are an uncommon cause of Leber congenital amaurosis (LCA) type II. Hum Mutat. 2007;28(12):1245.
5. Ahmad A, Daud S, Kakar N, Nürnberg G, Nürnberg P, Babar ME, et al. Identification of a novel LCA5 mutation in a Pakistani family with Leber congenital amaurosis and cataracts. Mol Vis. 2011;17:1940–5.
6. Jacobson SG, Aleman TS, Cideciyan AV, Sumaroka A, Schwartz SB, Windsor EA, et al. Leber congenital amaurosis caused by Lebercilin (LCA5) mutation: retained photoreceptors adjacent to retinal disorganization. Mol Vis. 2009;15:1098–106.
7. Ramprasad VL, Soumittra N, Nancarrow D, Sen P, McKibbin M, Williams GA, et al. Identification of a novel splice-site mutation in the Lebercilin (LCA5) gene causing Leber congenital amaurosis. Mol Vis. 2008;14:481–6.

44 LRAT

LRAT encodes lecithin retinol acyltransferase, which catalyzes the earlier reactions in the retinoid visual pathway in the retinal pigment epithelium (RPE). Recessive mutations in *LRAT* cause a spectrum of disease that ranges from Leber congenital amaurosis (LCA) to forms of "juvenile" or "early-onset" retinitis pigmentosa (RP) that present slightly later in life [1–3].

Patients with recessive mutations in *LRAT* may present within the first few years of life (often less than 3 years of age) with poor visual acuity, progressive and severe night blindness, impaired dark adaptation, and photophilia; some patients may have nystagmus and abnormal color vision [2, 4]. Fundus findings include retinal vascular attenuation, disc pallor, and bilateral peripheral atrophy; retinal pigmentation or bone-spicule deposits are uncommon. Some patients may have RPE mottling at the macula that extends to the arcades. Epiretinal membranes and asteroid hyalosis have been reported as well. Fundus autofluorescence (FAF) reveals globally reduced signal intensity, reflecting reduced lipofuscin accumulation, though there may be rare patchy increased signal intensity in the macula or around the optic disc. OCT may show a broadened foveal pit and outer retinal hyperreflective deposits, with poorly defined retinal lamination [4]. The inner segment/outer segment (IS/OS) (ellipsoid zone) line, which reflects photoreceptor integrity, may be maintained in younger patients [4]. A "saw-tooth" pattern in the nerve fiber layer was reported in three of four patients with *LRAT* mutations [4]. The visual field is significantly reduced, and the full-field electroretinogram (ERG) is non-recordable at an early age. When the ERG is recordable, it is usually only photopic responses that are detected, corresponding to a rod-cone pattern of degeneration. Goldmann Visual Field (GVF) reveals constricted visual fields in a rod-cone pattern. Further specialized testing, such as static threshold perimetry and dark-adapted spectral sensitivity testing, may reveal the extent of loss of rod and cone function [4].

S. Zahid et al., *Retinal Dystrophy Gene Atlas*, https://doi.org/10.1007/978-3-319-10867-4_44

References

1. Thompson DA, Li Y, McHenry CL, Carlson TJ, Ding X, Sieving PA, et al. Mutations in the gene encoding lecithin retinol acyltransferase are associated with early-onset severe retinal dystrophy. Nat Genet. 2001;28(2):123–4.
2. Senechal A, Humbert G, Surget MO, Bazalgette C, Bazalgette C, Arnaud B, et al. Screening genes of the retinoid metabolism: novel LRAT mutation in leber congenital amaurosis. Am J Ophthalmol. 2006;142(4):702–4.
3. den Hollander AI, Lopez I, Yzer S, Zonneveld MN, Janssen IM, Strom TM, et al. Identification of novel mutations in patients with Leber congenital amaurosis and juvenile RP by genome-wide homozygosity mapping with SNP microarrays. Invest Ophthalmol Vis Sci. 2007;48(12):5690–8.
4. Dev Borman A, Ocaka LA, Mackay DS, Ripamonti C, Henderson RH, Moradi P, et al. Early onset retinal dystrophy due to mutations in LRAT: molecular analysis and detailed phenotypic study. Invest Ophthalmol Vis Sci. 2012;53(7):3927–38.

45 MAK

MAK encodes a protein kinase involved in the regulation of photoreceptor-connecting cilium length in its longer isoform [1], which is present in the inner segments, cell bodies, and axons of rod and cone photoreceptors [1, 2]. Its shorter isoform predominates in the testes [3]. Mutations are responsible for autosomal recessive retinitis pigmentosa (RP).

The most frequently encountered mutation in *MAK* is a 353-bp insertion of an Alu repeat in exon 9 [1, 2], which has a carrier frequency of 1 in 55 in the Ashkenazi Jewish population, suggesting that it would be responsible for about 33% of RP in this group of individuals [1]. Nonsense and missense mutations in *MAK* have been identified in other populations, although at a lower frequency, with homozygous mutations present in 11 of 334 individuals screened with isolated or autosomal recessive RP [4]. Age of onset for individuals with *MAK* mutations varies from 20 to 60 years, and symptoms appear to be less severe than other types of RP. Visual acuity is often 20/50 or better in at least one eye until the 70s [1, 4]. On fundus exam, individuals display typical pigmentary changes in the midperipheral retina, vessel attenuation, and waxy pallor of the optic nerve head (Fig. 45.1a) [1]. Fundus autofluorescence may show areas of macular hyperautofluorescence and hypoautofluorescence in areas of retinal pigment epithelium (RPE) atrophy (Fig. 45.1b). In the population homozygous for the Jewish founder mutation, Optical coherence tomography (OCT) shows decreasing foveal photoreceptor layer thickness with increasing distance from the fovea (Fig. 45.1c), and some patients display hyperthickness of the paracentral inner retina. On electroretinography (ERG) in this same population, only 4 of the 24 patients had detectable rod ERG b-waves, while 13 had a detectable cone flicker. All showed rod-cone dysfunction. On Goldmann visual field testing, visual field was seen to decrease at 11% per year for the large isopter target and 18.4% per year for the smaller target. Early loss was seen in the superior-temporal quadrant, later loss in the superior and midperipheral fields, and only central islands were present at late stages of disease. The nasal field was relatively spared [1]. In populations with other mutations in *MAK*, visual field was also observed to be significantly constricted, with half of the 8 subjects in the study by Ozgul et al. [4] demonstrating tunnel vision of 25° or less. However, two of these patients had only sectoral RP [4].

S. Zahid et al., *Retinal Dystrophy Gene Atlas*, https://doi.org/10.1007/978-3-319-10867-4_45

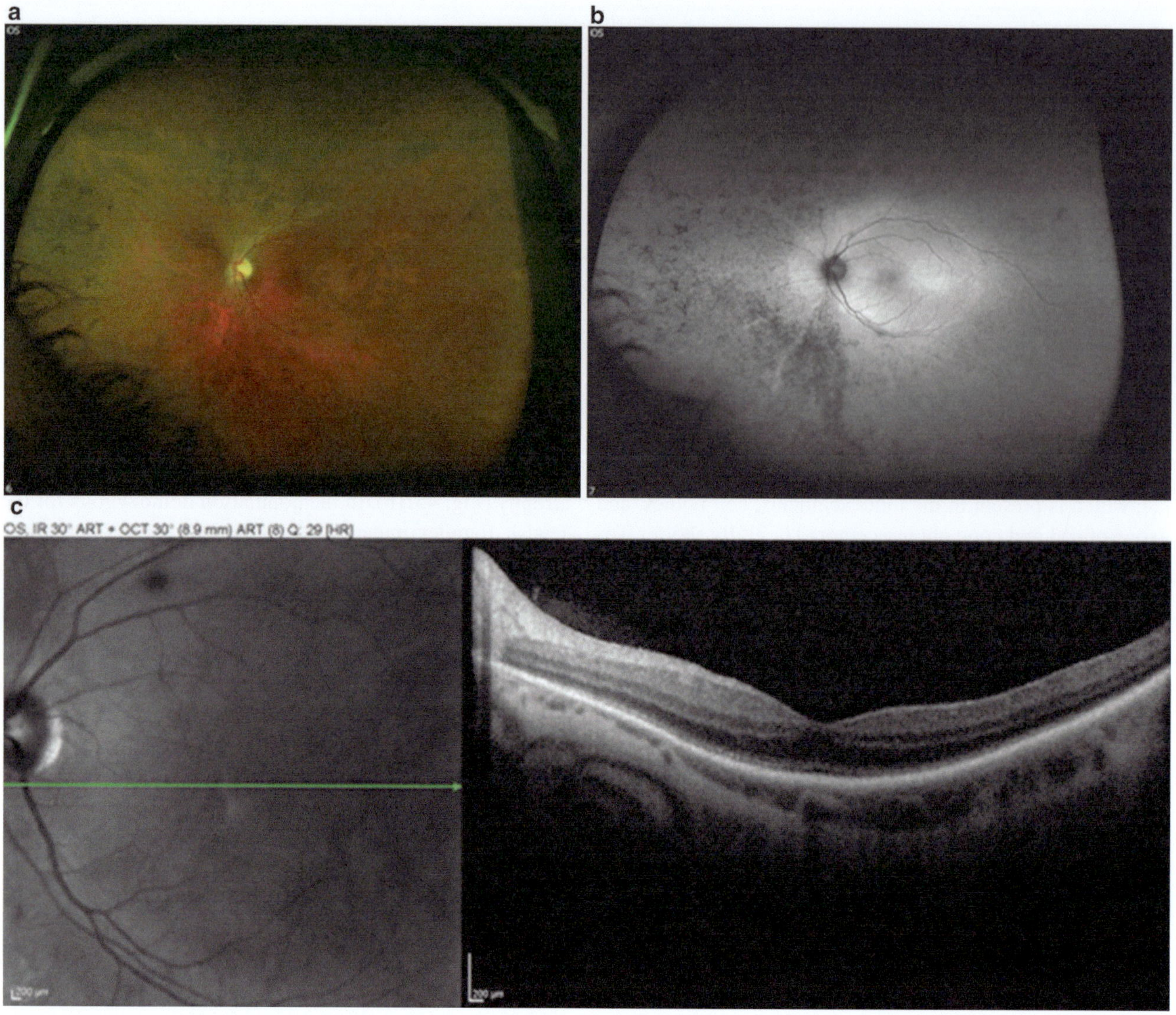

Fig. 45.1 Case summary: 34-year-old man with RP. (**a**) Wide-field color fundus photograph of the left eye, showing nasal RPE atrophy and bone spicule pigmentation prominent in the mid-peripheral retina. (**b**) Wide-field fundus autofluorescence of the left eye, showing areas of abnormal macular hyperautofluorescence and nasal areas of hypoautofluorescence corresponding to RPE atrophy and pigment deposition. (**c**) Spectral domain optical coherence tomography of the left eye, showing essentially normal macular architecture except for temporal loss of the ellipsoid zone.

References

1. Stone EM, Luo X, Héon E, Lam BL, Weleber RG, Halder JA, et al. Autosomal recessive retinitis pigmentosa caused by mutations in the MAK gene. Invest Ophthalmol Vis Sci. 2011;52(13):9665–73.
2. Tucker BA, Scheetz TE, Mullins RF, DeLuca AP, Hoffmann JM, Johnston RM, et al. Exome sequencing and analysis of induced pluripotent stem cells identify the cilia-related gene male germ cell-associated kinase (MAK) as a cause of retinitis pigmentosa. Proc Natl Acad Sci U S A. 2011;108(23):E568–76.
3. McKusick VA, O'Neill MJF. Male germ cell-associated kinase; MAK. OMIM. 154235. 1994 (updated 2011). http://omim.org/entry/154235. Accessed 24 Jan 2017.
4. Ozgül RK, Siemiatkowska AM, Yücel D, Myers CA, Collin RW, Zonneveld MN, et al. Exome sequencing and cis-regulatory mapping identify mutations in MAK, a gene encoding a regulator of ciliary length, as a cause of retinitis pigmentosa. Am J Hum Genet. 2011;89(2):253–64.

46 MERTK

MERTK encodes the widely-expressed tyrosine-protein kinase Mer, which is a receptor tyrosine kinase involved in a signal transduction pathway that regulates numerous cellular processes. In the retina, it is expressed in the RPE and plays a role in the phagocytosis of rod outer segments. Autosomal recessive mutations in *MERTK* cause retinitis pigmentosa (rod-cone dystrophy) [1–4].

Visual symptoms include nyctalopia, progressive constriction of peripheral visual fields, and loss of visual acuity. Symptom onset occurs within the first two decades of life. Visual acuities are usually 20/50 or better before age 16, although in one family with macular atrophy, patients had light perception only vision by age 9; acuity declines progressively and is often light perception only before age 50 [1, 2, 4]. Posterior subcapsular cataracts are common. Fundus examination findings reveal arteriolar attenuation and bone-spicule pigment deposits in the mid-periphery with atrophy. Many patients have been reported to have macular abnormalities, including crystalline deposits, RPE pigment mottling, macular atrophy, and bull's eye maculopathy (Figs. 46.1a and 46.2a). Some patients exhibit a ring of hyperautofluorescence around a hypoautofluorescent fovea (Figs. 46.1b, 46.2b, d, and 46.3a). Areas of macular atrophy are hypoautofluorescent and are sometimes surrounded by a region of hyperautofluorescence similar to that seen in geographic atrophy associated with advanced dry age-related macular degeneration [3, 5]. Optical coherence tomography (OCT) usually reveals thinning of the outer retina, debris-like material in the subneurosensory space, and disruption of the external limiting membrane/ellipsoid zone/RPE (Figs. 46.1c, 46.2c, and 46.3b) [4, 5]. Full-field electroretinography demonstrates a rod-cone pattern of degeneration within the first decade of life and tends to decline with age [1–4]. Goldmann visual field (GVF) testing may be normal in young teenagers but typically illustrates progressive peripheral constriction in a rod-cone pattern.

In one study, a homozygous loss of function of *MERTK* due to uniparental disomy was reported. The ophthalmic phenotypes described in this patient were similar those described above [6].

S. Zahid et al., *Retinal Dystrophy Gene Atlas*, https://doi.org/10.1007/978-3-319-10867-4_46

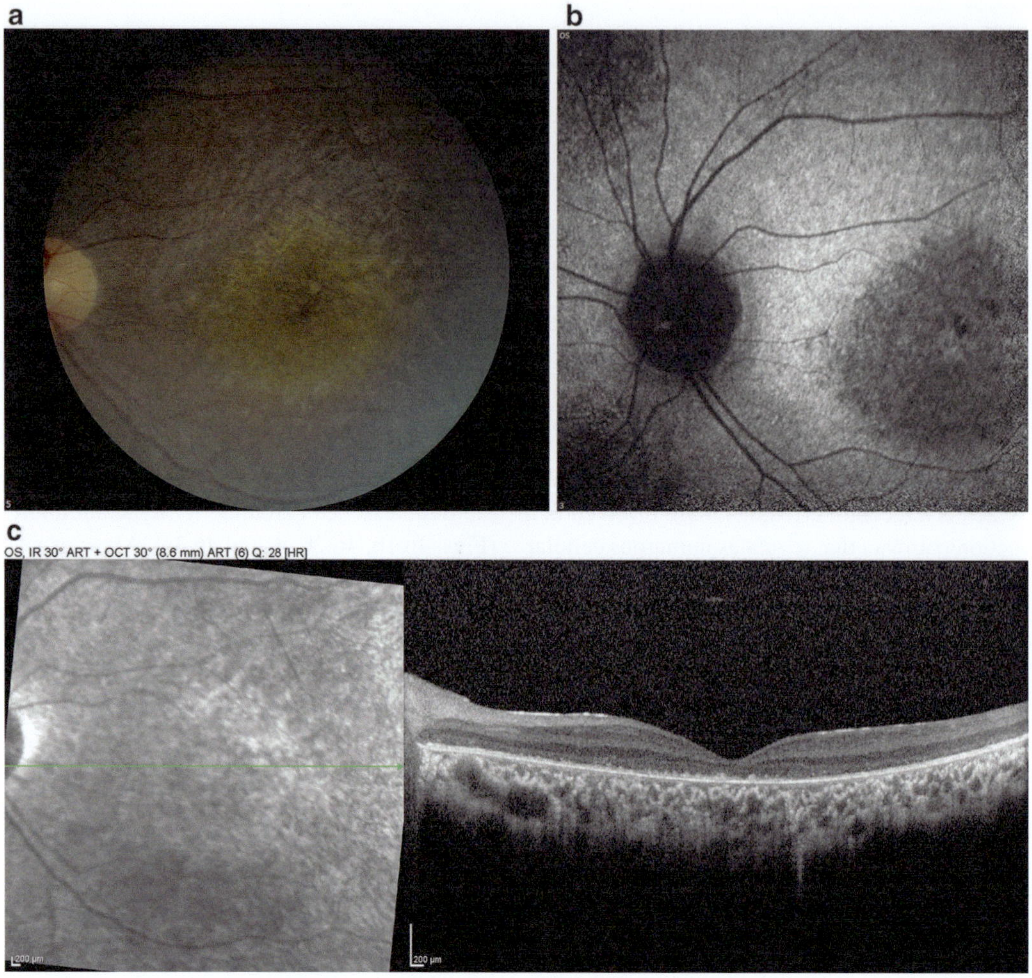

Fig. 46.1 Case summary: 12-year-old male with rod-cone dystrophy associated with mutations in *MERTK*. (**a**) Color fundus photograph of the left eye, showing macular atrophy and retinal pigment epithelium (RPE) changes. (**b**) Fundus autofluorescence, showing macular hypoautofluorescence with surrounding abnormal hyperautofluorescence. (**c**) Spectral domain-optical coherence tomography (SD-OCT), showing significant ellipsoid zone (EZ) loss in the macula.

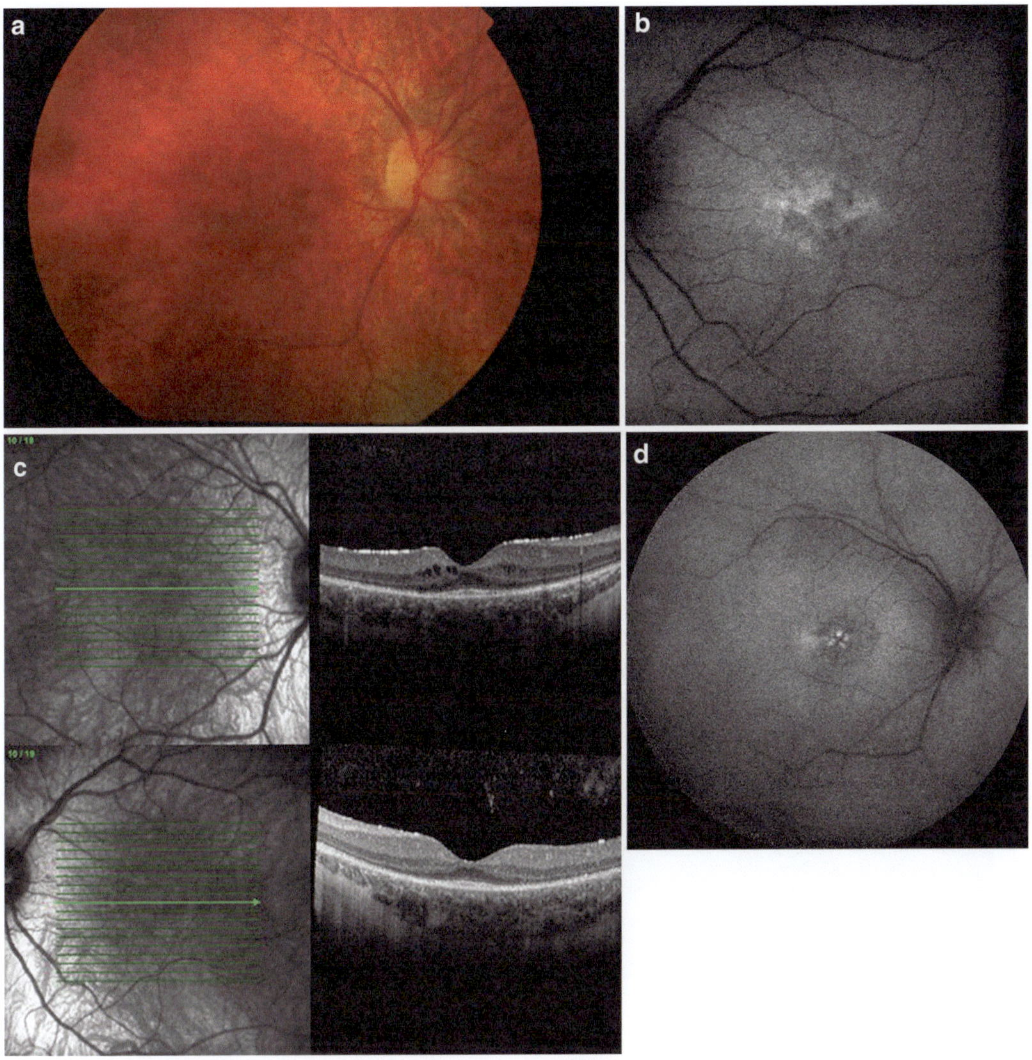

Fig. 46.2 Case summary: An 11-year-old male with *MERTK* retinopathy. (**a**) Color fundus photograph of the right eye, showing RPE mottling and pigment clumping in the macula. (**b**) Fundus autofluorescence of the left eye, showing macular hyperautofluorescent foci. (**c**) Spectral domain-OCT, showing EZ loss with foveal-sparing, with epiretinal membranes in both eyes and cystic changes in the right eye. (**d**) Fundus autofluorescence (55°) of the same patient at age 14, showing marked cystoid macular edema and macular hyperautofluorescent foci.

a

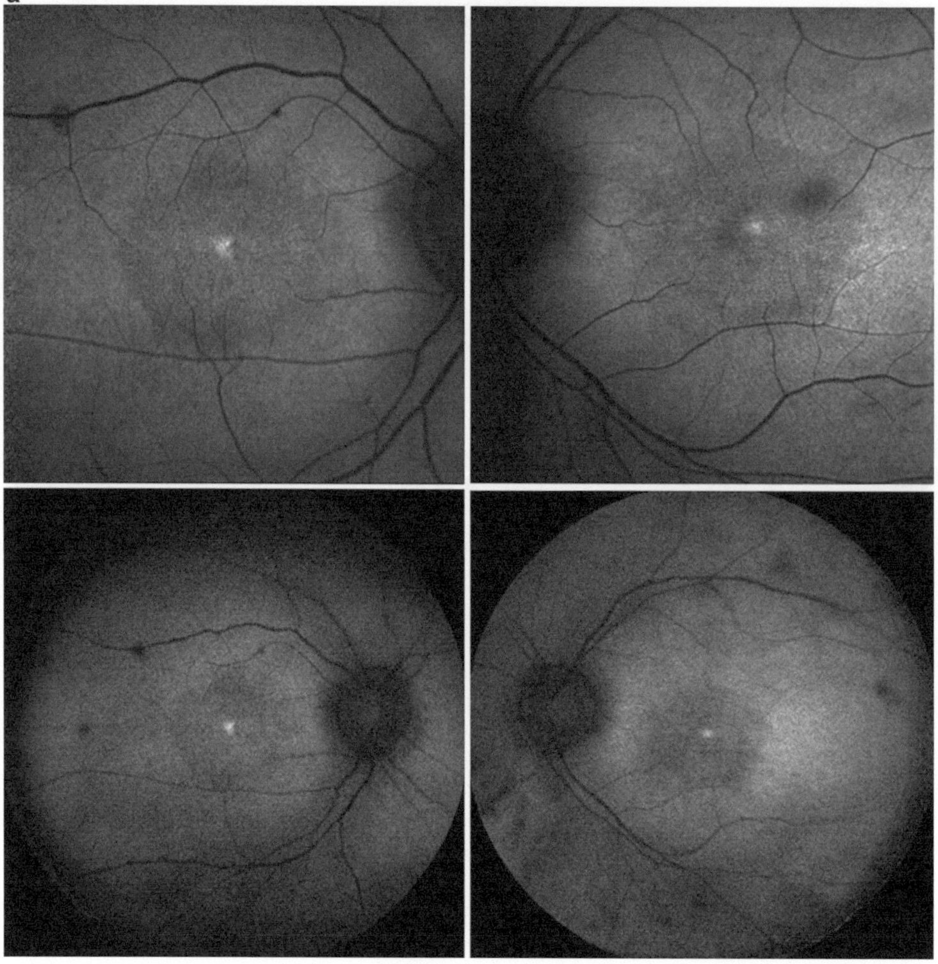

Fig. 46.3 Case summary: A 16-year-old patient with *MERTK*-related disease. (**a**) Fundus autofluorescence of the right and left eyes, showing central hyperautofluorescent foci in both eyes, with hypoautofluorescent spots along the superior arcades in the right eye and superotemporal to the fovea in the left eye. 55-degree autofluorescence demonstrates hyperautofluorescent foci outside the arcades in both eyes. (**b**) Spectral domain-OCT of the right and left eyes, showing epiretinal membranes and diffuse macular EZ loss.

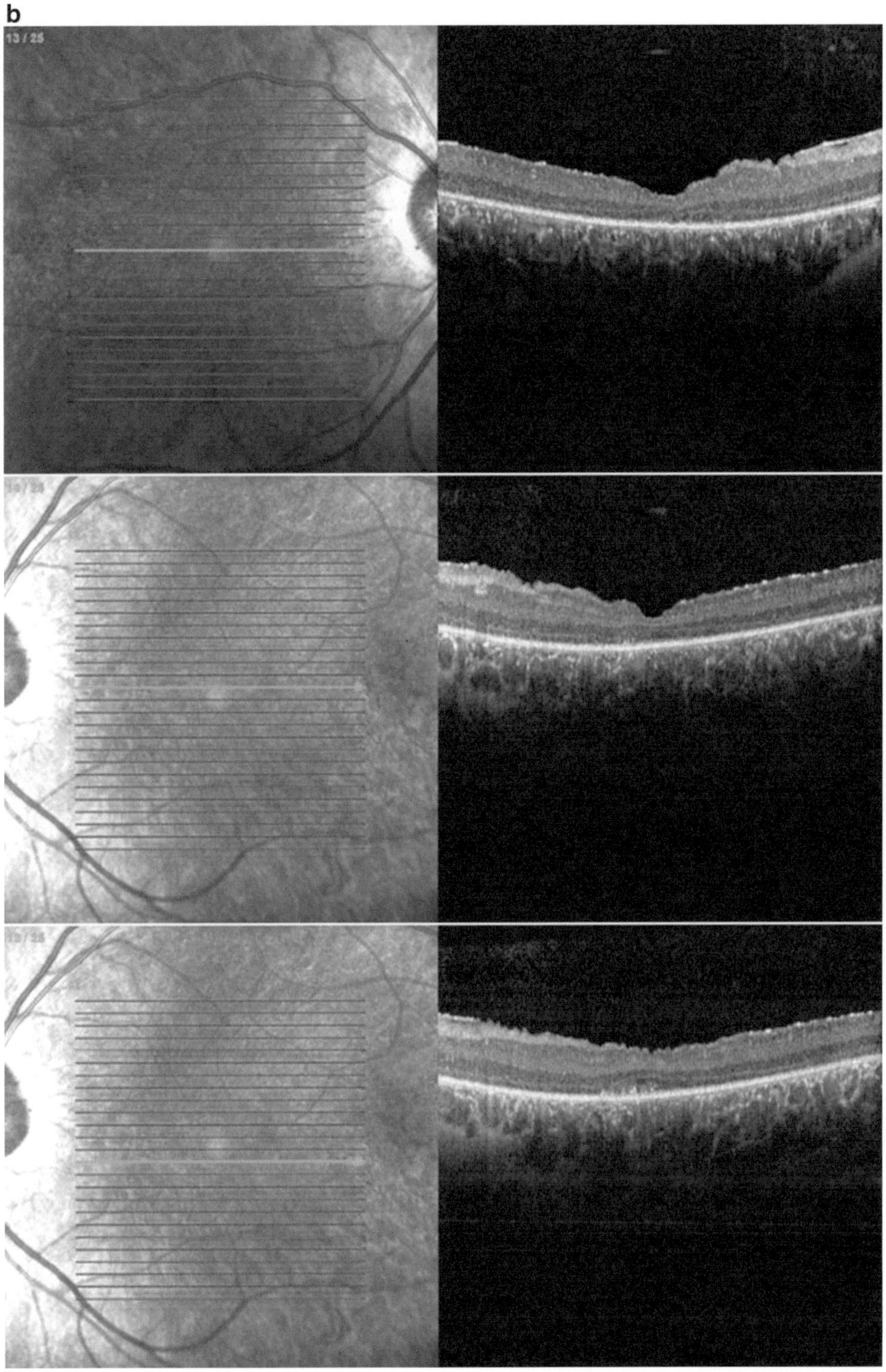

Fig. 46.3 (continued)

References

1. Gal A, Li Y, Thompson DA, Weir J, Orth U, Jacobson SG, et al. Mutations in MERTK, the human orthologue of the RCS rat retinal dystrophy gene, cause retinitis pigmentosa. Nat Genet. 2000;26(3):270–1.
2. Shahzadi A, Riazuddin SA, Ali S, Li D, Khan SN, Husnain T, et al. Nonsense mutation in MERTK causes autosomal recessive retinitis pigmentosa in a consanguineous Pakistani family. Br J Ophthalmol. 2010;94(8):1094–9.
3. Tschernutter M, Jenkins SA, Waseem NH, Saihan Z, Holder GE, Bird AC, et al. Clinical characterisation of a family with retinal dystrophy caused by mutation in the Mertk gene. Br J Ophthalmol. 2006;90(6):718–23.
4. Mackay DS, Henderson RH, Sergouniotis PI, Li Z, Moradi P, Holder GE, et al. Novel mutations in MERTK associated with childhood onset rod-cone dystrophy. Mol Vis. 2010;16:369–77.
5. Charbel Issa P, Bolz HJ, Ebermann I, Domeier E, Holz FG, Scholl HP. Characterisation of severe rod-cone dystrophy in a consanguineous family with a splice site mutation in the MERTK gene. Br J Ophthalmol. 2009;93(7):920–5.
6. Thompson DA, McHenry CL, Li Y, Richards JE, Othman MI, Schwinger E, et al. Retinal dystrophy due to paternal isodisomy for chromosome 1 or chromosome 2, with homoallelism for mutations in RPE65 or MERTK, respectively. Am J Hum Genet. 2002;70(1):224–9.

47 MYO7A

MYO7A encodes an unconventional myosin, which acts as an ATPase-driven motor protein to transport melanosomes and phagosomes along actin filaments in the RPE and opsin and other phototransduction proteins in photoreceptors [1]. Mutations in *MYO7A* are associated with Usher Syndrome type 1B (USH1B).

MYO7A-related Usher syndrome type 1B follows an autosomal recessive pattern of inheritance. Type 1 Usher syndrome is characterized by severe-to-profound non-progressive sensorineural hearing loss (SNHL), pre-adolescent onset retinitis pigmentosa (RP), and often vestibular areflexia [2–4]. Visual acuities are typically better than 20/60 in the first two decades of life [2]. Visual fields in USH1B patients start with mid-peripheral loss and progress to residual small central islands, with a small temporal peripheral field in the most advanced stages of the disease. Funduscopy reveals arteriolar attenuation and RPE atrophy with bone-spicule like pigmentation (Figs. 47.1, 47.2a, and 47.3) [4–7]. Fundus autofluorescence may show a ring of hyperautofluorescence in the macula (Fig. 47.4a). Optical coherence tomography (OCT) reveals loss of outer retinal structure, sparing the fovea, and cystoid macular edema is frequently present (Figs. 47.2b and 47.4b). Full-field electroretinogram (ERG) shows severely reduced or nonrecordable parameters.

S. Zahid et al., *Retinal Dystrophy Gene Atlas*, https://doi.org/10.1007/978-3-319-10867-4_47

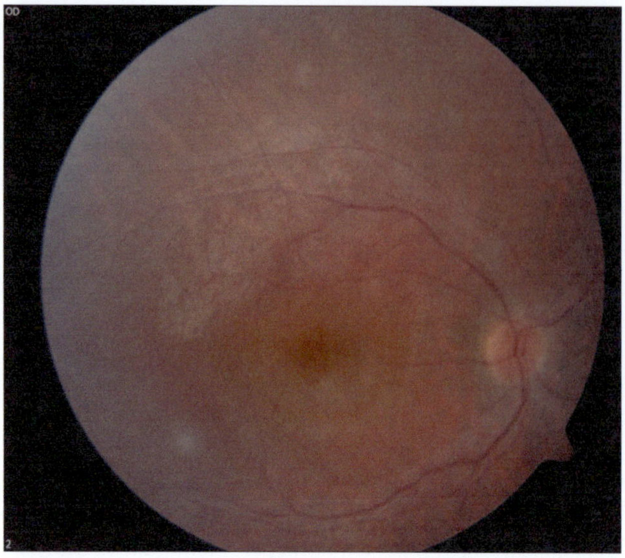

Fig. 47.1 Color fundus photograph of the right eye from a 15-year-old male with Usher Syndrome, showing RPE atrophy outside and along the arcades, with macular-sparing.

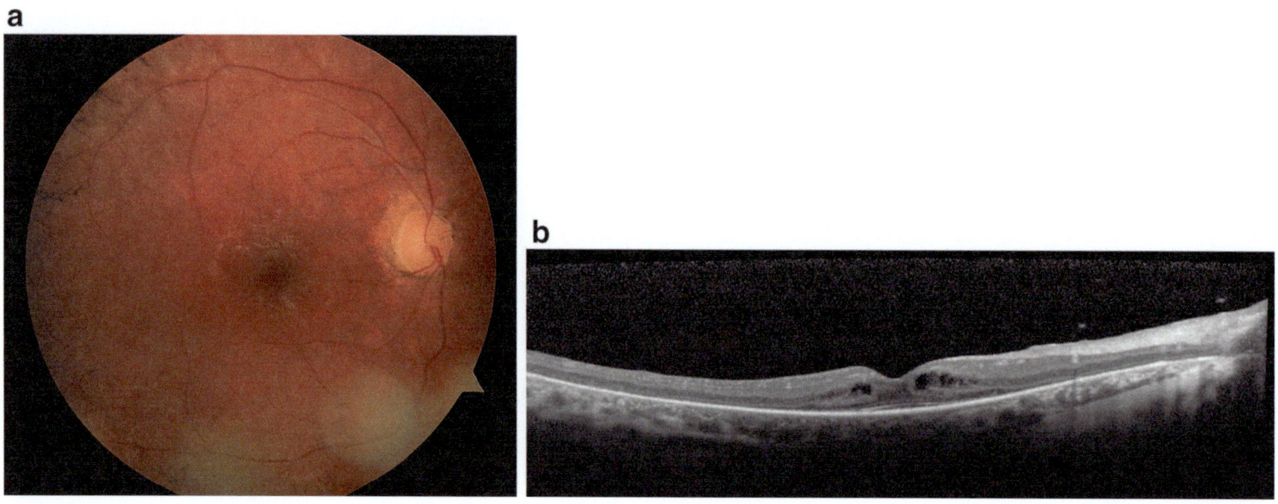

Fig. 47.2 Case summary: 26-year-old male (CEI19845) with Usher Syndrome Type 1. (**a**) Color fundus photograph of the right eye, showing patchy RPE atrophy along the arcades, with sparse bone spicule pigmentation and peripapillary atrophy. (**b**) Spectral-domain optical coherence tomography (OCT), showing extensive loss of the ellipsoid zone and outer nuclear layer (sparing the foveola), with intraretinal cystic changes (Images courtesy of Dr. Richard Weleber).

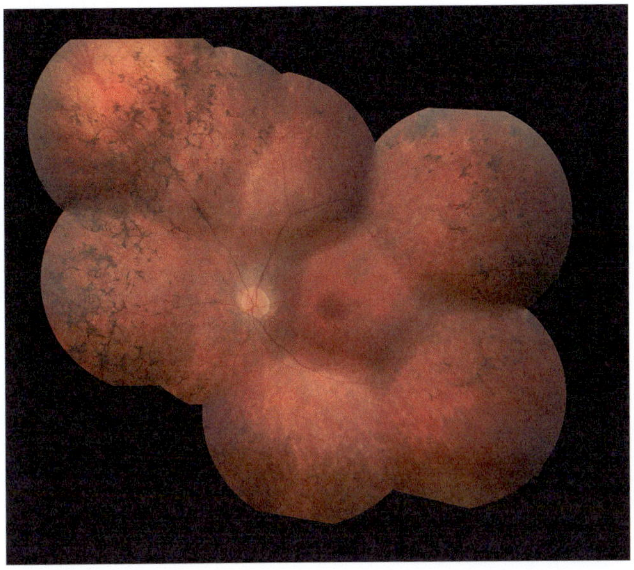

Fig. 47.3 16-year-old male (CEI26125) with Usher Syndrome Type 1. Color fundus photograph of the left eye, showing typical findings of retinitis pigmentosa, with mid-peripheral RPE atrophy and bone spicule pigment deposits.

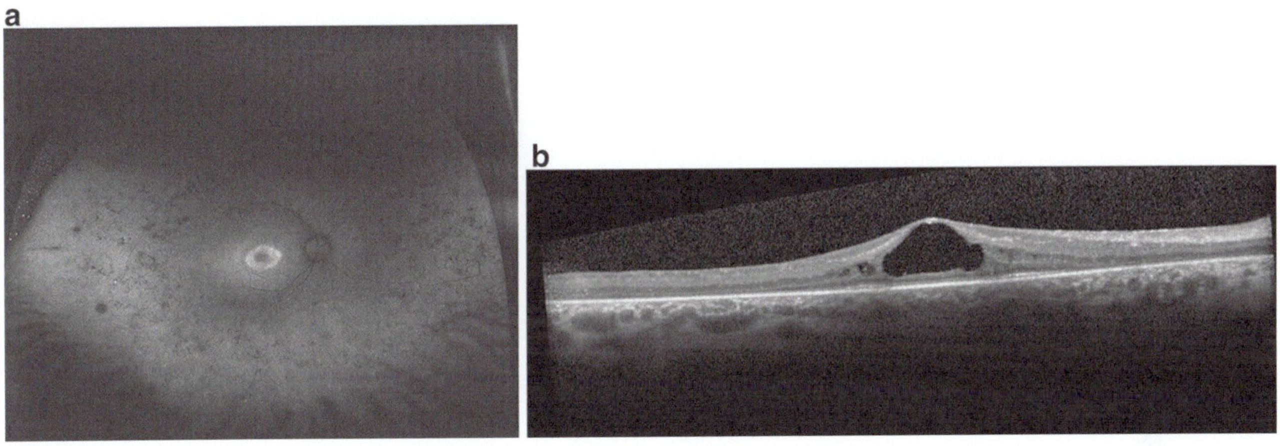

Fig. 47.4 Case summary: 17-year-old (CEI24278) with Usher Syndrome Type 1. (Images courtesy of Dr. Richard Weleber.) (**a**) Wide-field fundus autofluorescence, showing a hyperautofluorescent ring surrounding the fovea and areas of hypoautofluorescence in the mid-periphery corresponding to areas of RPE atrophy and pigment deposition. (**b**) Spectral-domain optical coherence tomography (OCT), showing extensive loss of the ellipsoid zone and outer nuclear layer (involving the foveola), with foveal intraretinal cystic changes.

References

1. Lopes VS, Gibbs D, Libby RT, Aleman TS, Welch DL, Lillo C, et al. The Usher 1B protein, MYO7A, is required for normal localization and function of the visual retinoid cycle enzyme, RPE65. Hum Mol Genet. 2011;20(13):2560–70.
2. Jacobson SG, Cideciyan AV, Gibbs D, Sumaroka A, Roman AJ, Aleman TS, et al. Retinal disease course in Usher syndrome 1B due to MYO7A mutations. Invest Ophthalmol Vis Sci. 2011;52(11):7924–36.
3. Hildebrand MS, Thorne NP, Bromhead CJ, Kahrizi K, Webster JA, Fattahi Z, et al. Variable hearing impairment in a DFNB2 family with a novel MYO7A missense mutation. Clin Genet. 2010;77(6):563–71.
4. Yoshimura H, Iwasaki S, Kanda Y, Nakanishi H, Murata T, Iwasa Y, et al. An Usher syndrome type 1 patient diagnosed before the appearance of visual symptoms by MYO7A mutation analysis. Int J Pediatr Otorhinolaryngol. 2013;77(2):298–302.
5. Liu F, Li P, Liu Y, Li W, Wong F, Du R, et al. Novel compound heterozygous mutations in MYO7A in a Chinese family with Usher syndrome type 1. Mol Vis. 2013;19:695–701.
6. Rizel L, Safieh C, Shalev SA, Mezer E, Jabaly-Habib H, Ben-Neriah Z, et al. Novel mutations of MYO7A and USH1G in Israeli Arab families with Usher syndrome type 1. Mol Vis. 2011;17:3548–55.
7. Roux AF, Faugère V, Le Guédard S, Pallares-Ruiz N, Vielle A, Chambert S, et al. Survey of the frequency of USH1 gene mutations in a cohort of Usher patients shows the importance of cadherin 23 and protocadherin 15 genes and establishes a detection rate of above 90%. J Med Genet. 2006;43(9):763–8.

48 NMNAT1

NMNAT (nicotinamide mononucleotide adenylyltransferase) is an enzyme involved in catalyzing NMN (nicotinamide mononucleotide) into NAD (nicotinamide-adenine dinucleotide). It also acts as a chaperone for neuronal maintenance and protection, particularly axonal protection [1]. The *NMNAT1* gene product protects against neuronal activity-induced degeneration in mature photoreceptors. Mutations are responsible for a severe form of Leber congenital amaurosis (LCA) [2]. The c.769G > A (p.Glu257Lys) mutation (allele frequency ≈ 0.001 [3]) is the most common and is hypothesized to be a founder mutation in those of European descent [2, 4, 5].

NMNAT1 mutations likely cause <5% of LCA [5, 6]. The inheritance pattern is autosomal recessive. Patients present in the first years of life with severe and rapidly progressive macular degeneration, causing severe central atrophy with congenital macular coloboma in the neonatal period, and with early-onset atrophy of the optic nerve. Pseudocoloboma and optic atrophy are not present at birth; they are likely due to rapid degeneration of central photoreceptors and ganglion cells due to light exposure after birth [2]. As seen in other forms of LCA, patients also demonstrate nystagmus and severe vision loss [4]. Symptoms associated with *NMNAT1* mutations tend to be earlier onset and more rapidly progressive than in other LCA patients. Homozygotes and compound heterozygotes are legally blind, with some demonstrating light perception or hand motion visual acuity [5]. Fundus exam shows macular atrophy with macular coloboma or pseudocoloboma, attenuated blood vessels, pigmentary retinal changes, and optic disc pallor (Figs. 48.1a, b) [4, 5]. ERG is typically undetectable [7].

S. Zahid et al., *Retinal Dystrophy Gene Atlas*, https://doi.org/10.1007/978-3-319-10867-4_48

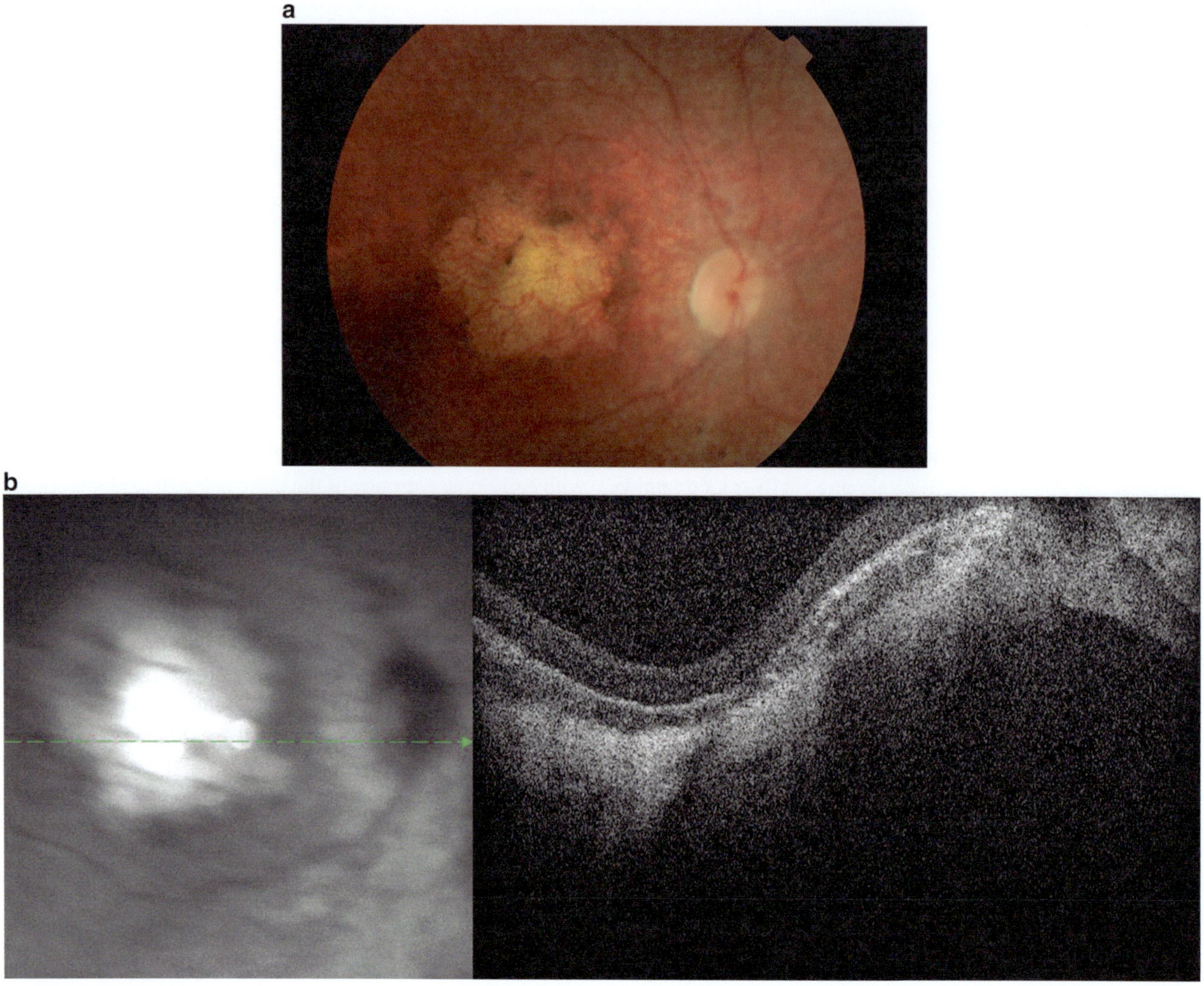

Fig. 48.1 Nine year old girl with Leber congenital amaurosis with onset at 2 months of age and light perception visual acuity. (**a**) Color fundus photograph of the right eye, showing a pale disc, attenuated vessels, peripheral RPE atrophy, and marked macular retinal/RPE/choroid atrophy. (**b**) Spectral domain-optical coherence tomography, showing a coloboma in the setting of extensive macular outer retinal atrophy.

References

1. Hartz PA. Nicotinamide nucleotide adenylyltransferase 1; NMNAT1. OMIM. 608700. 2012. Retrieved from http://www.omim.org/entry/608700?search=nmnat1&highlight=nmnat1.
2. Perrault I, Hanein S, Zanlonghi X, Serre V, Nicouleau M, Defoort-Delhemmes S, et al. Mutations in NMNAT1 cause Leber congenital amaurosis with early-onset severe macular and optic atrophy. Nat Genet. 2012;44(9):975–7.
3. Chiang PW, Wang J, Chen Y, Fu Q, Zhong J, Chen Y, et al. Exome sequencing identifies NMNAT1 mutations as a cause of Leber congenital amaurosis. Nat Genet. 2012;44(9):972–4.
4. Koenekoop RK, Wang H, Majewski J, Wang X, Lopez I, Ren H, et al. Mutations in NMNAT1 cause Leber congenital amaurosis and identify a new disease pathway for retinal degeneration. Nat Genet. 2012;44(9):1035–9.
5. Siemiatkowska AM, van den Born LI, van Genderen MM, Bertelsen M, Zobor D, Rohrschneider K, et al. Novel compound heterozygous NMNAT1 variants associated with Leber congenital amaurosis. Mol Vis. 2014;20:753–9.
6. Falk MJ, Zhang Q, Nakamaru-Ogiso E, Kannabiran C, Fonseca-Kelly Z, Chakarova C, et al. NMNAT1 mutations cause Leber congenital amaurosis. Nat Genet. 2012;44(9):1040–5.
7. Hedergott A, Volk AE, Herkenrath P, et al. Clinical and genetic findings in a family with NMNAT1-associated Leber congenital amaurosis: case report and review of literature. Graefes Arch Clin Exp Ophthalmol. 2015;253(12):2239–46.

NR2E3

49

NR2E3 encodes a nuclear receptor that plays a role in retinal photoreceptor differentiation [1]. Mutations in *NR2E3* cause autosomal recessive enhanced S cone syndrome (ESCS), Goldman-Favre Syndrome (GFS), clumped pigmentary retinal degeneration (CPRD), recessive retinitis pigmentosa, and dominant retinitis pigmentosa [2, 3].

Patients with autosomal recessive ESCS caused by *NR2E3* mutations present in the first decade with night blindness and reduced visual acuity [2]. Color vision is often defective, showing tritan sparing. Many patients are hyperopic, and cataracts have been observed; nystagmus is uncommon. The fundus is classically characterized by nummular pigment deposits at the level of the RPE along or outside the vascular arcades with RPE atrophy (Figs. 49.1a–c and 49.2a, d). However, the fundus may be normal in some young patients, and other patients may exhibit only mild focal hyperpigmentation or yellow-white dots rather than the classic nummular pigmentation [4]. Foveal schisis is commonly observed (Figs. 49.1e and 49.2c). Vitreous cells are common, and some patients have other vitreous opacities, such as haze and veils [4]. OCT may reveal foveal schisis, intraretinal cysts, increased retinal thickness early in disease, and lamellar disorganization with disease progression (Figs. 49.1e and 49.2c) [5]. Fundus autofluorescence may reveal hypoautofluorescence outside the arcades, patchy hyperautofluorescence inside the arcades, and spoke-like hyperautofluorescence at the fovea in the context of foveal schisis (Fig. 49.1d). The ERG is characterized by these pathognomonic findings: undetectable rod-only responses, similar waveforms in response to a bright flash under scotopic and photopic conditions, reduced flicker amplitude, and increased latency for the single flash photopic response [6]. These findings result from rod photoreceptor precursors being directed to a different fate, resulting in an increase in the concentration of S-cones. This phenomenon is also illustrated by increased amplitudes in response to shorter wavelength stimuli. Certain mutations have been shown to retain residual rod function and therefore may represent milder disease [7, 8]. GVF may reveal constricted peripheral fields, ring scotomata or relative central scotoma (Fig. 49.2b).

NR2E3 mutations can also cause Goldmann-Favre syndrome, which is part of a clinical spectrum of disease that includes ESCS [9]. It is also characterized by childhood onset of night blindness and reduced visual acuity. Posterior subcapsular cataracts (PSC) are commonly observed. Common funduscopic findings include progressively increasing clumped pigment deposits, peripheral or macular schisis, and liquefaction or fibrillary vitreous degeneration (Figs. 49.1 and 49.2). ERG often reveals non-recordable or severely reduced rod and cone parameters and may show enhanced S-cone function [10].

Recessive *NR2E3* mutations have also been identified in clumped pigmentary retinal degeneration (CPRD) and in RP, which may both be parts of the spectrum of ESCS. CPRD, first described by To et al., is characterized by night blindness, gradually constricting peripheral fields, and progressively increasing clumped pigment deposits in the fundus (especially in the mid-periphery) [11, 12]. Hyperopia is common in these patients. Subretinal white dots, macular holes, vessel attenuation, and atrophic scars may also be seen.

Most patients with recessive RP caused by mutations in *NR2E3* present with reduced visual acuity, hyperopia, and clumped pigmentary deposits (similar to CPRD) [13–15]. Some of these patients exhibit reduced rod parameters and supranormal dark- and light-adapted cone parameters, similar to patients with ESCS, but others have significantly reduced cone and rod parameters. Fundus features are variable, even in patients with the same mutations [13]. Findings range from flecks similar to *ABCA4*-related disease, cystoid macular edema and schisis, macular atrophy, and nummular pigmentation outside the arcades.

There is significant intra- and interfamilial phenotypic variability in disease caused by *NR2E3* mutations [13]. Escher et al. [16] reported a family with some members that had ADRP while others had ESCS [16]. There are

S. Zahid et al., *Retinal Dystrophy Gene Atlas*, https://doi.org/10.1007/978-3-319-10867-4_49

a

b

c

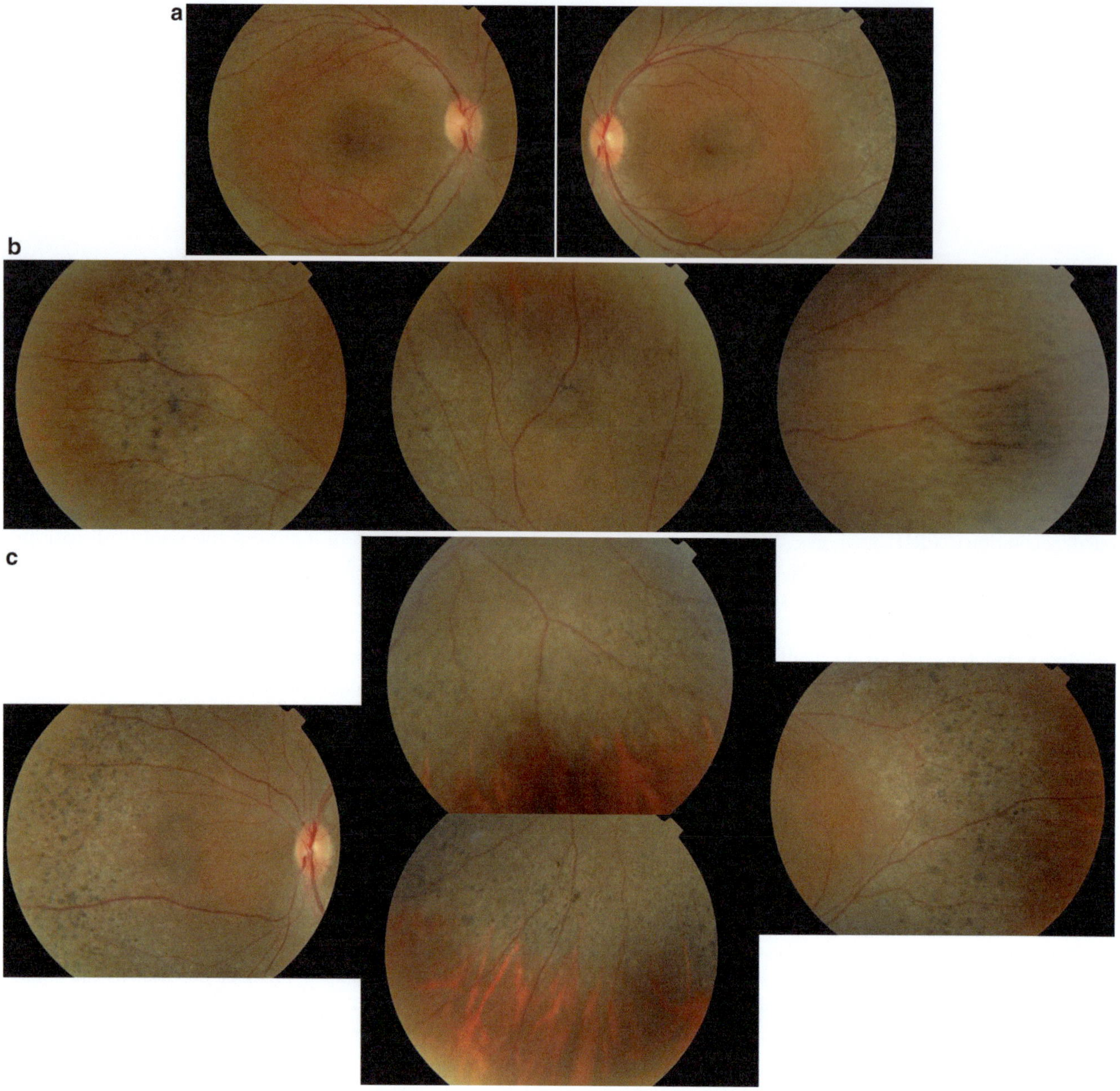

Fig. 49.1 Case summary: 34-year-old female diagnosed with RP at age 12 presented with photopsias in the right eye for 6–8 months and "dark spots in the inferior field" for 1–2 months; good general health otherwise; no other affected family members; visual acuity 20/40 OD and 20/30 OS. (**a**) Fundus photos OD and OS, showing RPE atrophy and pigment clumping outside the arcades. (**b**) Peripheral photos OD, showing peripheral RPE atrophy and pigment clumping. (**c**) Peripheral photos OS, showing peripheral RPE atrophy and pigment clumping. (**d**) FAF OD and OS, showing hyperautofluorescence in the parafovea with hypoautofluorescence outside the arcades corresponding to areas of RPE atrophy and pigment clumping. (**e**) Spectral domain OCT OD and OS, showing inner retinal schisis temporal to the fovea.

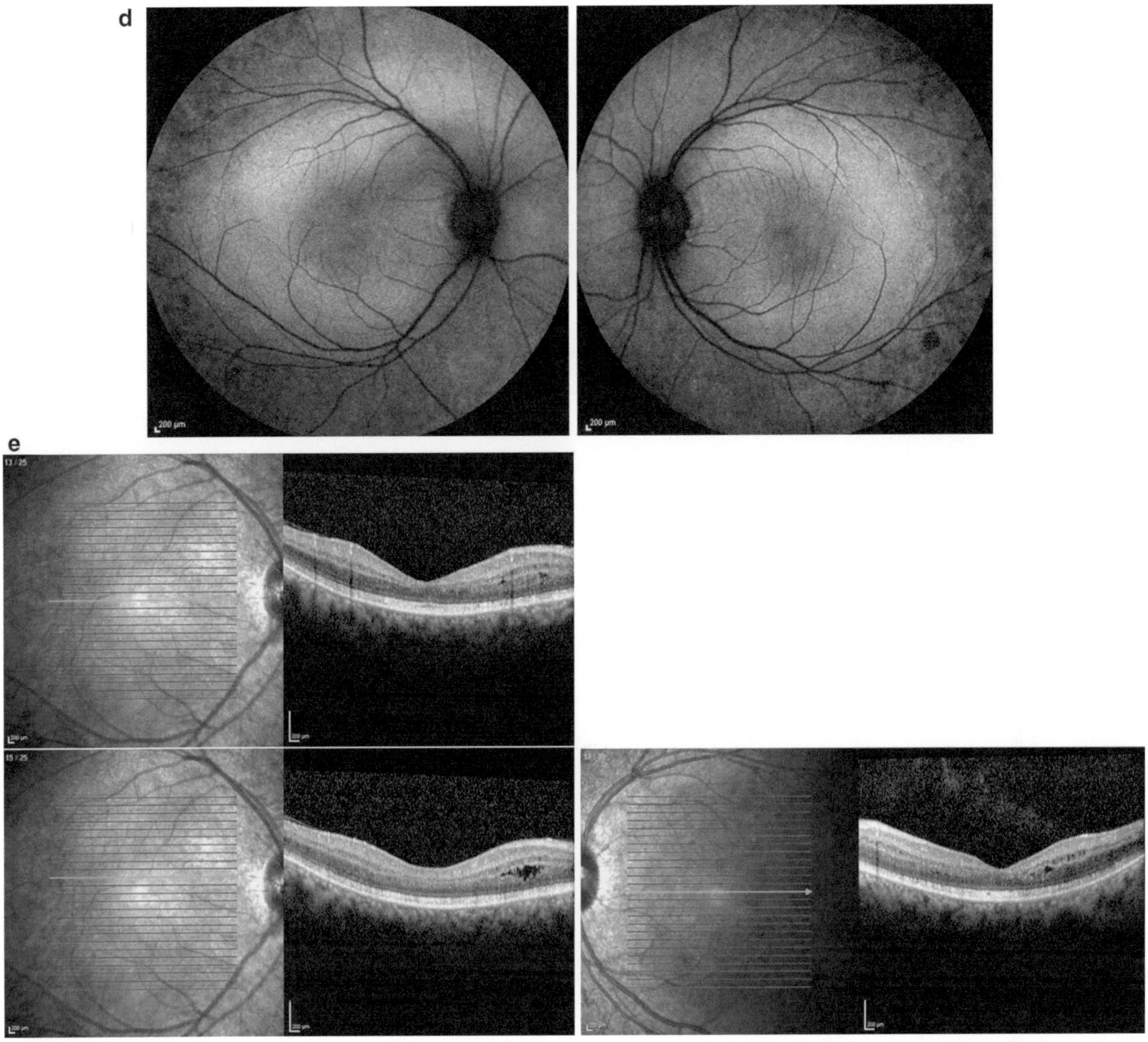

Fig. 49.1 (continued)

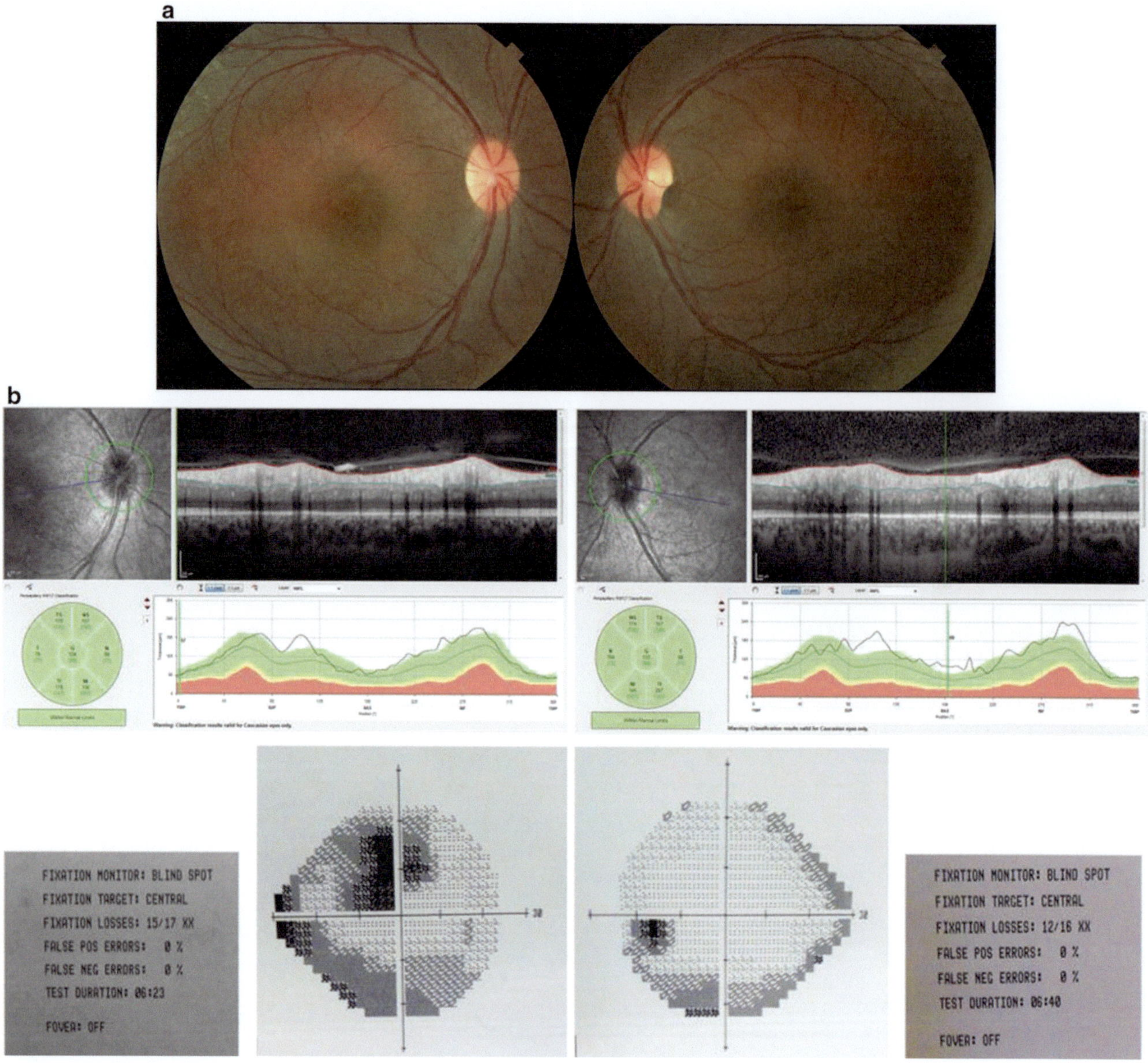

Fig. 49.2 Case: 23-year-old female with poor vision in both eyes (courtesy of Dr. Rosa Dolz-Marco, MD, PhD and Lawrence A. Yannuzzi, MD, Vitreous Retina Macula Consultants of New York). (**a**) Fundus photos OD and OS with OD showing signs of macular schisis. (**b**) Spectral domain-OCT of the nerves, showing full retinal nerve fiber layer thickness (OD and OS). Humphrey visual field testing shows reduced central sensitivities (OD greater than OS). (**c**) Spectral domain-OCT of the macula OD and OS, showing macular schisis OD greater than OS; arrows show cystic changes OS. (**d**) Wide-field fundus photos and spectral domain-OCT composite OD and OS, showing clumped pigmentary deposits and macular schisis OD greater than OS.

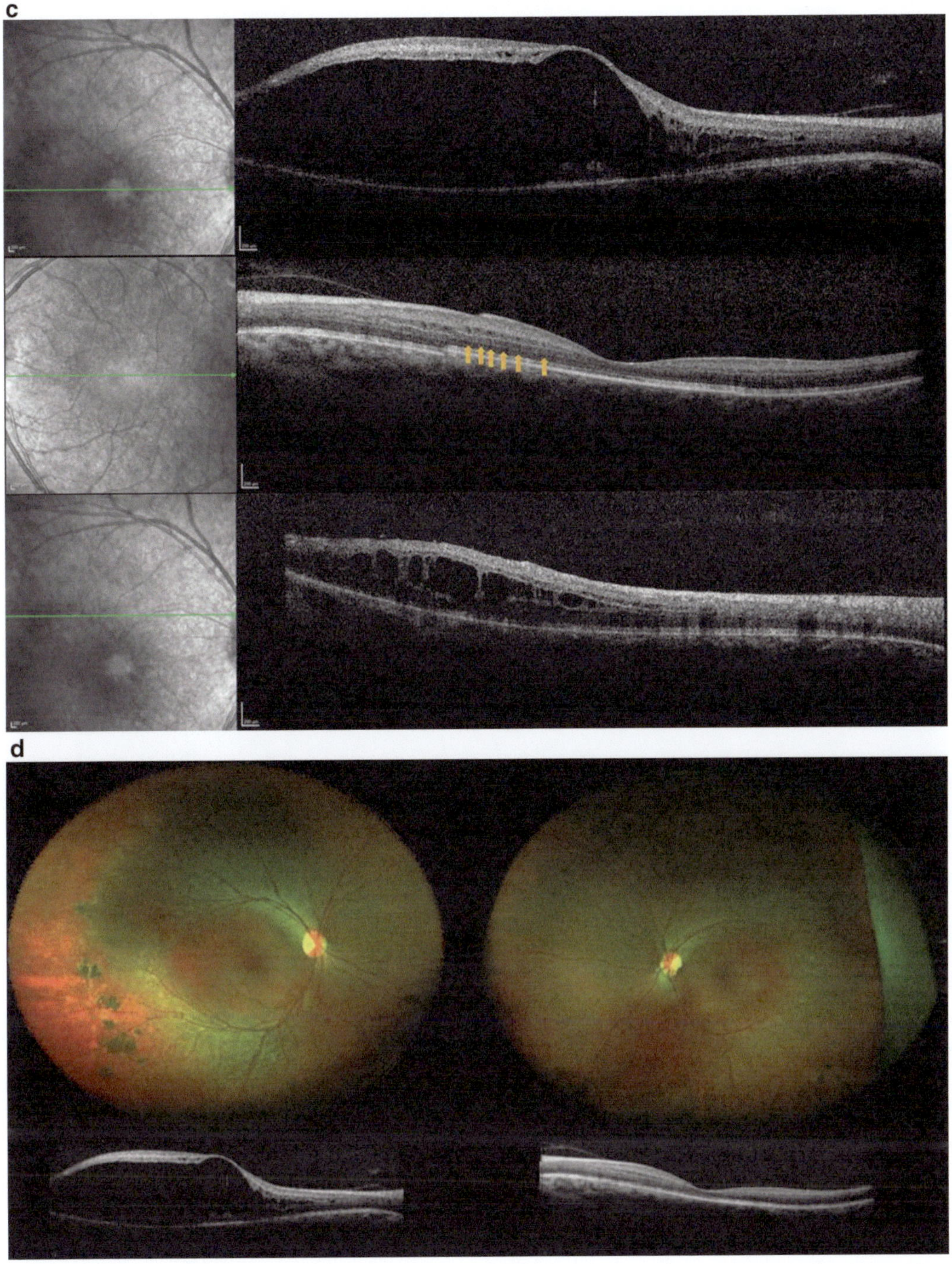

Fig. 49.2 (continued)

reports of subfoveal neovascularization and cystic maculopathy associated with *NR2E3* mutations. One study reported diffuse subretinal bleeding and fibrosis, and another reported reduced visual acuity with bilateral subretinal helicoid fibrosis without other fundus features in a consanguineous family with homozygous mutations [17, 18]. In addition, this same homozygous mutation (p. R311Q) has also been reported to result in ESCS, GFS, CPRD, and recessive RP in different patients, further emphasizing the phenotypic variability associated with mutations in this gene.

Autosomal dominant RP has also been reported to be caused by mutations in *NR2E3* [3, 19]. These patients present with night blindness and sometimes with photophobia between the first and third decades. Funduscopy may reveal pigmentary deposits in a mixed bone spicule and nummular

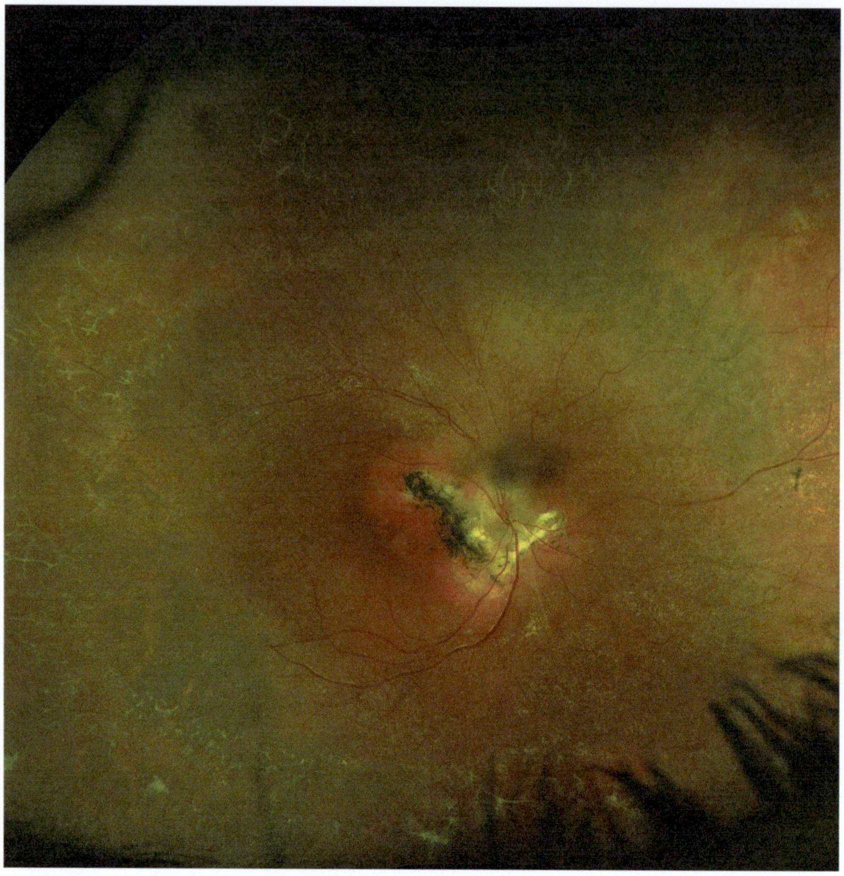

Fig. 49.3 Right eye fundus photograph of a 42 year old woman with subretinal fibrosis.

clumped pattern, optic nerve pallor, vessel attenuation, and peripheral atrophy. ERG usually reveals a rod-cone pattern of degeneration but may be non-recordable, especially in older patients. Unlike autosomal recessive mutations in *NR2E3*, S-cone function has not been reported to be increased in patients with autosomal dominant *NR2E3*-related RP. Fundus autofluorescence often reveals two rings of hyperfluorescence - a ring in the macula (which constricts with age) and another ring along the arcades, which can expand with time [20]. Escher et al. [20] report that the IS-OS line (ellipsoid zone), which reflects photoreceptor integrity, is lost within the confines of these two hyperfluorescent rings [20]. Nummular hypoautofluorescent areas have been reported around the arcades in patients without funduscopic evidence of pigmentation. GVF reveals constricted fields and peripheral loss with mid-peripheral scotomata. One study has shown that pupil responses to rod-specific stimuli may be useful to detect progression of disease [21].

References

1. Milam AH, Rose L, Cideciyan AV, Barakat MR, Tang WX, Gupta N, et al. The nuclear receptor NR2E3 plays a role in human retinal photoreceptor differentiation and degeneration. Proc Natl Acad Sci U S A. 2002;99(1):473–8.
2. Haider NB, Jacobson SG, Cideciyan AV, Swiderski R, Streb LM, Searby C, et al. Mutation of a nuclear receptor gene, NR2E3, causes enhanced S cone syndrome, a disorder of retinal cell fate. Nat Genet. 2000;24(2):127–31.
3. Coppieters F, Leroy BP, Beysen D, Hellemans J, De Bosscher K, Haegeman G, et al. Recurrent mutation in the first zinc finger of the orphan nuclear receptor NR2E3 causes autosomal dominant retinitis pigmentosa. Am J Hum Genet. 2007;81(1):147–57.
4. Audo I, Michaelides M, Robson AG, Hawlina M, Vaclavik V, Sandbach JM, et al. Phenotypic variation in enhanced S-cone syndrome. Invest Ophthalmol Vis Sci. 2008;49(5):2082–93.
5. Jacobson SG, Sumaroka A, Aleman TS, Cideciyan AV, Schwartz SB, Roman AJ, et al. Nuclear receptor NR2E3 gene mutations distort human retinal laminar architecture and cause an unusual degeneration. Hum Mol Genet. 2004;13(17):1893–902.
6. Vincent A, Robson AG, Holder GE. Pathognomonic (diagnostic) ERGs. A review and update. Retina. 2013;33(1):5–12.

7. Kinori M, Pras E, Kolker A, Ferman-Attar G, Moroz I, Moisseiev J, et al. Enhanced S-cone function with preserved rod function: a new clinical phenotype. Mol Vis. 2011;17:2241–7.
8. Kuniyoshi K, Hayashi T, Sakuramoto H, Nakao A, Sato T, Utsumi T, et al. Novel mutations in enhanced S-cone syndrome. Ophthalmology. 2013;120(2):431–431.e6.
9. Udar N, Small K, Chalukya M, Silva-Garcia R, Marmor M. Developmental or degenerative–NR2E3 gene mutations in two patients with enhanced S cone syndrome. Mol Vis. 2011;17:519–25.
10. Jacobson SG, Roman AJ, Roman MI, Gass JD, Parker JA. Relatively enhanced S cone function in the Goldmann-Favre syndrome. Am J Ophthalmol. 1991;111(4):446–53.
11. To KW, Adamian M, Jakobiec FA, Berson EL. Clinical and histopathologic findings in clumped pigmentary retinal degeneration. Arch Ophthalmol. 1996;114(8):950–5.
12. Sharon D, Sandberg MA, Caruso RC, Berson EL, Dryja TP. Shared mutations in NR2E3 in enhanced S-cone syndrome, Goldmann-Favre syndrome, and many cases of clumped pigmentary retinal degeneration. Arch Ophthalmol. 2003;121(9):1316–23.
13. Bandah D, Merin S, Ashhab M, Banin E, Sharon D. The spectrum of retinal diseases caused by NR2E3 mutations in Israeli and Palestinian patients. Arch Ophthalmol. 2009;127(3):297–302.
14. Bernal S, Solans T, Gamundi MJ, Hernan I, de Jorge L, Carballo M, et al. Analysis of the involvement of the NR2E3 gene in autosomal recessive retinal dystrophies. Clin Genet. 2008;73(4):360–6.
15. Kannabiran C, Singh H, Sahini N, Jalali S, Mohan G. Mutations in TULP1, NR2E3, and MFRP genes in Indian families with autosomal recessive retinitis pigmentosa. Mol Vis. 2012;18:1165–74.
16. Escher P, Gouras P, Roduit R, Tiab L, Bolay S, Delarive T, et al. Mutations in NR2E3 can cause dominant or recessive retinal degenerations in the same family. Hum Mutat. 2009;30(3):342–51.
17. Cassiman C, Spileers W, De Baere E, de Ravel T, Casteels I. Peculiar fundus abnormalities and pathognomonic electrophysiological findings in a 14-month-old boy with NR2E3 mutations. Ophthalmic Genet. 2013;34(1–2):105–8.
18. Khan AO, Aldahmesh MA, Al-Harthi E, Alkuraya FS. Helicoid subretinal fibrosis associated with a novel recessive NR2E3 mutation p.S44X. Arch Ophthalmol. 2010;128(3):344–8.
19. Yang Y, Zhang X, Chen LJ, Chiang SW, Tam PO, Lai TY, et al. Association of NR2E3 but not NRL mutations with retinitis pigmentosa in the Chinese population. Invest Ophthalmol Vis Sci. 2010;51(4):2229–35.
20. Escher P, Tran HV, Vaclavik V, Borruat FX, Schorderet DF, Munier FL. Double concentric autofluorescence ring in NR2E3-p.G56R-linked autosomal dominant retinitis pigmentosa. Invest Ophthalmol Vis Sci. 2012;53(8):4754–64.
21. Kawasaki A, Crippa SV, Kardon R, Leon L, Hamel C. Characterization of pupil responses to blue and red light stimuli in autosomal dominant retinitis pigmentosa due to NR2E3 mutation. Invest Ophthalmol Vis Sci. 2012;53(9):5562–9.

50 NRL

NRL encodes the transcription factor neural retina leucine zipper, which is involved in regulating the expression of rod-specific genes. It is essential for rod photoreceptor differentiation during retinal development. Mutations in *NRL* are associated with retinitis pigmentosa and clumped pigmentary retinal degeneration [1–3].

NRL-related retinitis pigmentosa most commonly follows an autosomal dominant pattern of inheritance, with autosomal recessive disease less commonly described. Patients experience night blindness initially, with an onset between early childhood and the second decade of life, with significant peripheral visual field constriction by their third to fourth decades of life [1–3]. Fundoscopy reveals typical signs of RP (Figs. 50.1a and 50.2a). Peripapillary atrophy may also be observed in both younger and older patients [1]. Fundus autofluorescence imaging may identify a perifoveal ring of increased autofluoresence at an early stage in young patients (Figs. 50.1b, c and 50.2b) [1]. Spectral domain-optical coherence tomography (SD-OCT) is useful to demonstrate the extent of photoreceptor loss in the macula and may show foveal-sparing early in the disease course (Figs. 50.1d and 50.2c). Full-field electroretinograms (ERG) may reveal non-recordable scotopic responses, but well-preserved photopic responses in younger patients. Older patients may have both non-recordable scotopic and photopic ERGs [1–3].

S. Zahid et al., *Retinal Dystrophy Gene Atlas*, https://doi.org/10.1007/978-3-319-10867-4_50

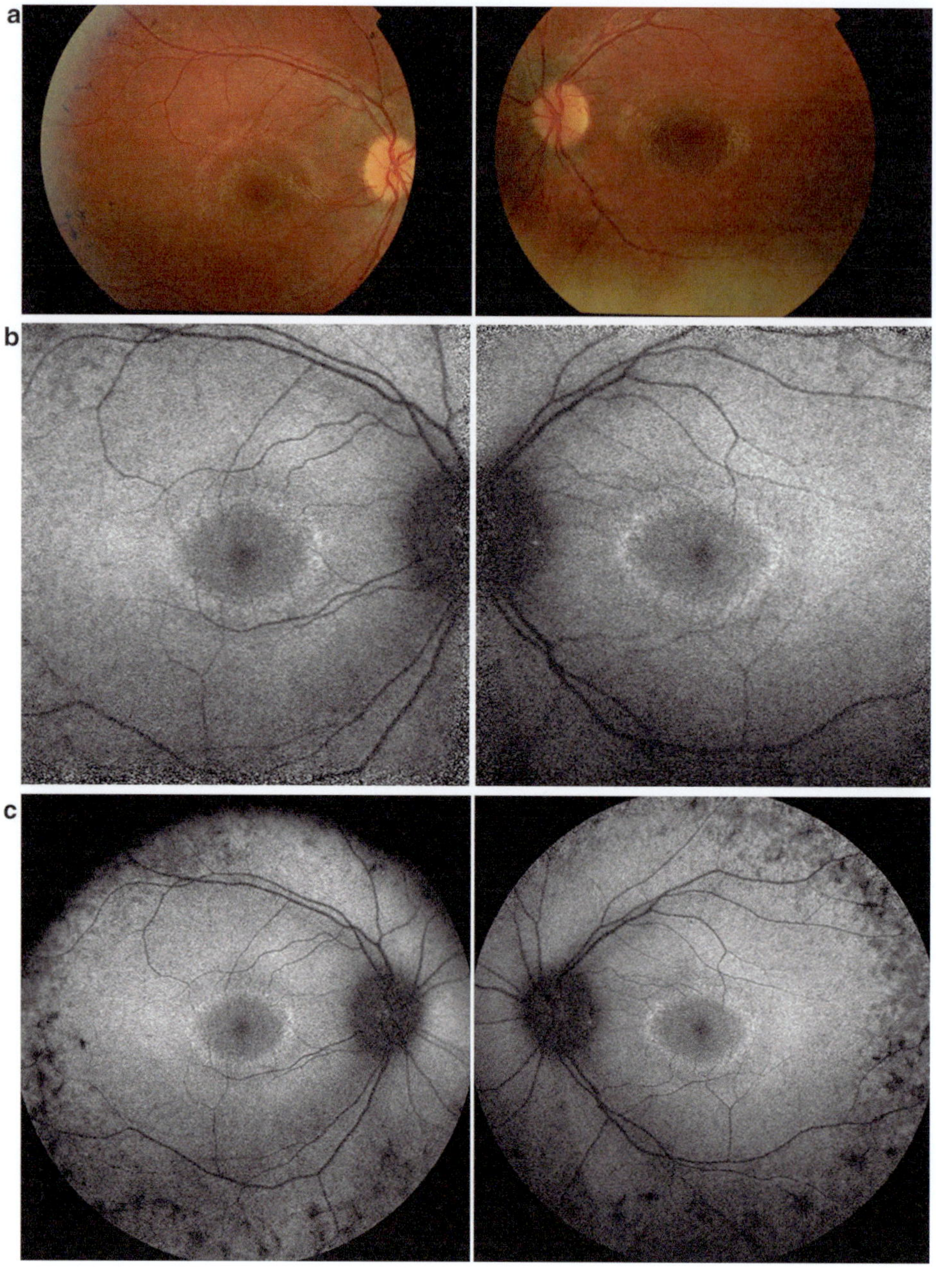

Fig. 50.1 Case Summary: Male patient with a mutation in *NRL*. (**a**) Color fundus photos of the right and left eyes at age 12, showing an unremarkable macular appearance with peripheral pigment deposits visible outside the arcades (OD > OS). (**b**) Macular fundus autofluorescence of the right and left eyes at age 13, showing a macular ring of hyperautofluorescence. (**c**) Wide-field fundus autofluorescence of the right and left eyes at age 13, showing the macular rings of hyperautofluorescence as well as hypoautofluorescence outside the arcades, corresponding to areas of atrophy and pigment deposition. (**d**) Spectral domain-optical coherence tomography (SD-OCT) of the macula in the right and left eyes, showing outer nuclear layer and ellipsoid zone (EZ) loss outside the foveal center, with a faint epiretinal membrane.

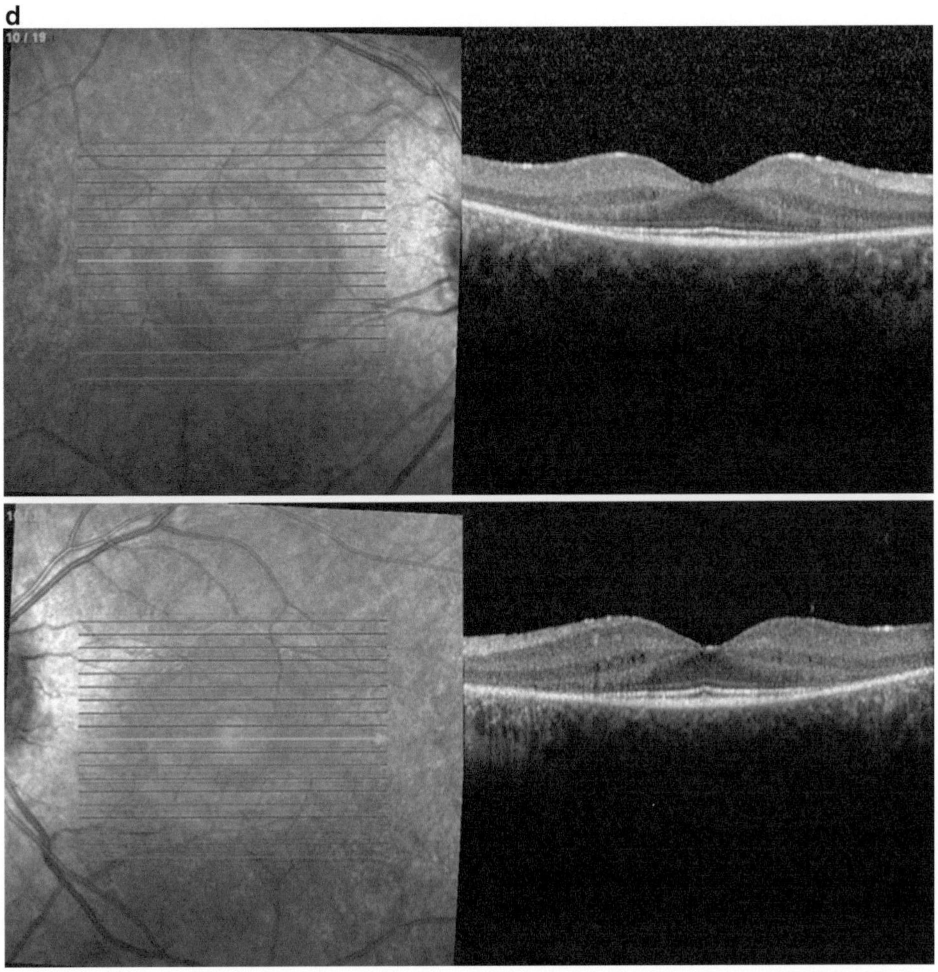

Fig. 50.1 (continued)

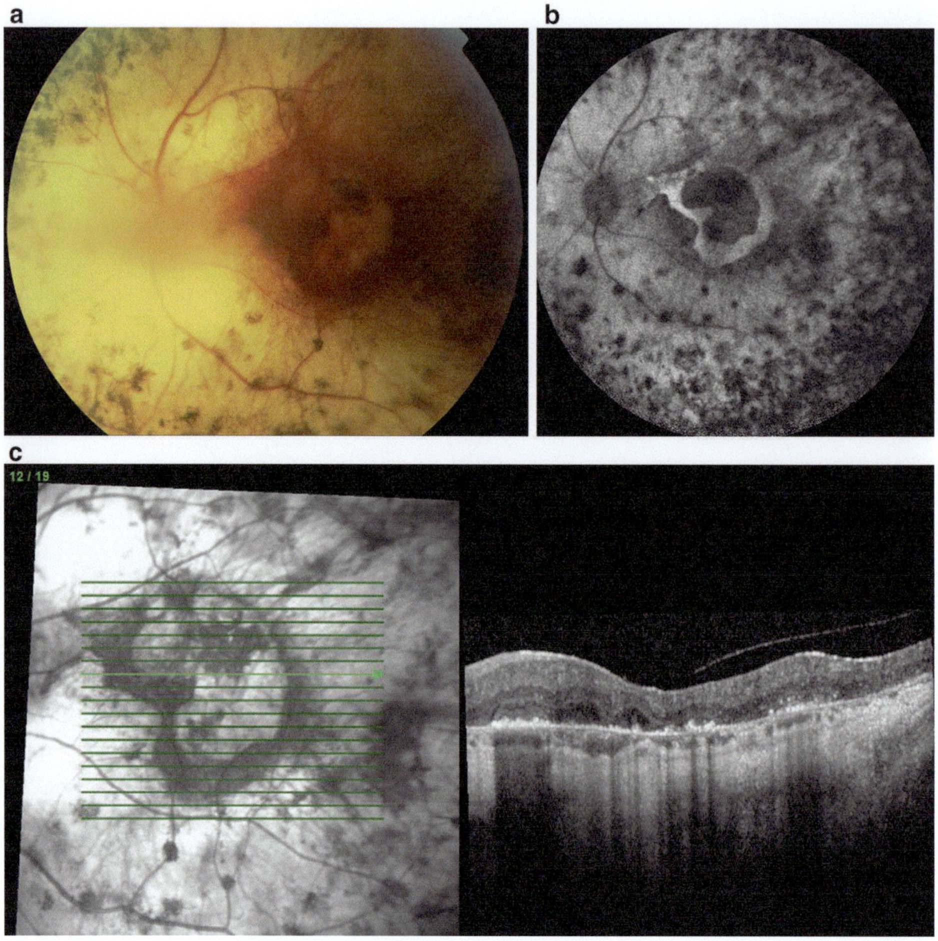

Fig. 50.2 Case Summary: (**a**) Color fundus photo left eye at age 63 (media opacity over optic nerve suspected to be secondary to cataract), showing extensive macular atrophy with pigment deposition as well as peripheral chorioretinal atrophy with dense pigmentation outside the arcades. There appears to be a residual area of parafoveal retinal pigment epithelium (RPE) surrounding the central atrophy. (**b**) Fundus autofluorescence of the right eye at age 70, showing macular and peripheral hypoautofluorescence corresponding to areas of atrophy and pigmentation. The residual RPE in the parafovea exhibits abnormal hyperautofluorescence. (**c**) Spectral domain-OCT at age 70, showing extensive loss of the EZ in the macula with a residual (abnormal-appearing) scattered RPE band corresponding to hyperautofluorescent areas in the macula shown in Fig. 50.2b.

References

1. Bessant DA, Holder GE, Fitzke FW, Payne AM, Bhattacharya SS, Bird AC. Phenotype of retinitis pigmentosa associated with the Ser50Thr mutation in the NRL gene. Arch Ophthalmol. 2003;121(6):793–802.
2. Chen LJ, Lai TY, Tam PO, Chiang SW, Zhang X, Lam S, et al. Compound heterozygosity of two novel truncation mutations in RP1 causing autosomal recessive retinitis pigmentosa. Invest Ophthalmol Vis Sci. 2010;51(4):2236–42.
3. DeAngelis MM, Grimsby JL, Sandberg MA, Berson EL, Dryja TP. Novel mutations in the NRL gene and associated clinical findings in patients with dominant retinitis pigmentosa. Arch Ophthalmol. 2002;120(3):369–75.

51 NYX

Mutations in *NYX*, which encodes nyctalopin, causes 45% of X-linked congenital stationary night blindness [1]. Males with CSNB caused by mutations in *NYX* often present in the first decade with reduced visual acuity (20/30–20/200), night blindness in up to 97.2% of patients, myopia (average refraction −9.19 diopters in one study, more myopic than *CACNA1F* patients), usually normal color vision, nystagmus (40%) and strabismus (29.4%) [2, 3]. The fundus usually appears normal on fundoscopy (Figs. 51.1a and 51.2a), fundus autofluorescence (Figs. 51.1b and 51.2b), and optical coherence tomography (Fig. 51.2c), but patients with high myopia may exhibit myopic degeneration. Full-field ERG reveals severely decreased responses to dim scotopic flashes; a characteristic negative ERG on maximum scotopic stimulation testing, in which the b-wave to a-wave ratio is less than 1; and squaring of the photopic a-wave due to loss of the second oscillatory potential. These changes are thought to reflect an ON-pathway [2]. At high flicker frequencies, the photopic flicker amplitudes were attenuated in one study [4]. One study has shown that patients with *NYX* mutations exhibit less phenotypic variability with respect to visual acuity, refractive error, and scotopic b/a wave ratio than patients with mutations in *CACNA1F* [2, 3]. Female carriers of *NYX* mutations tend to be asymptomatic and exhibit normal funduscopic and electrophysiologic examinations.

Studies by Zhang et al. [5] and Yip et al. [6] have reported high myopia without features of CSNB in some patients with mutations in *NYX*.

S. Zahid et al., *Retinal Dystrophy Gene Atlas*, https://doi.org/10.1007/978-3-319-10867-4_51

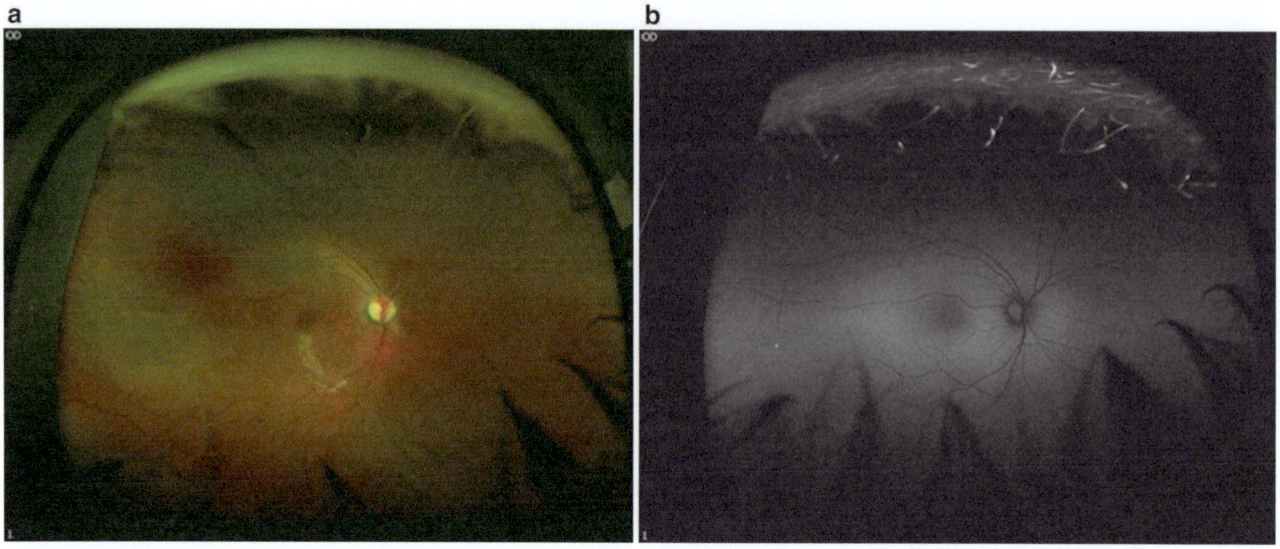

Fig. 51.1 Case Summary: 6-year-old male with CSNB with a mutation in *NYX*. (**a**) Wide-field color fundus photograph of the right eye, showing an essentially unremarkable right fundus. (**b**) Wide-field fundus autofluorescence, showing a normal pattern of autofluorescence.

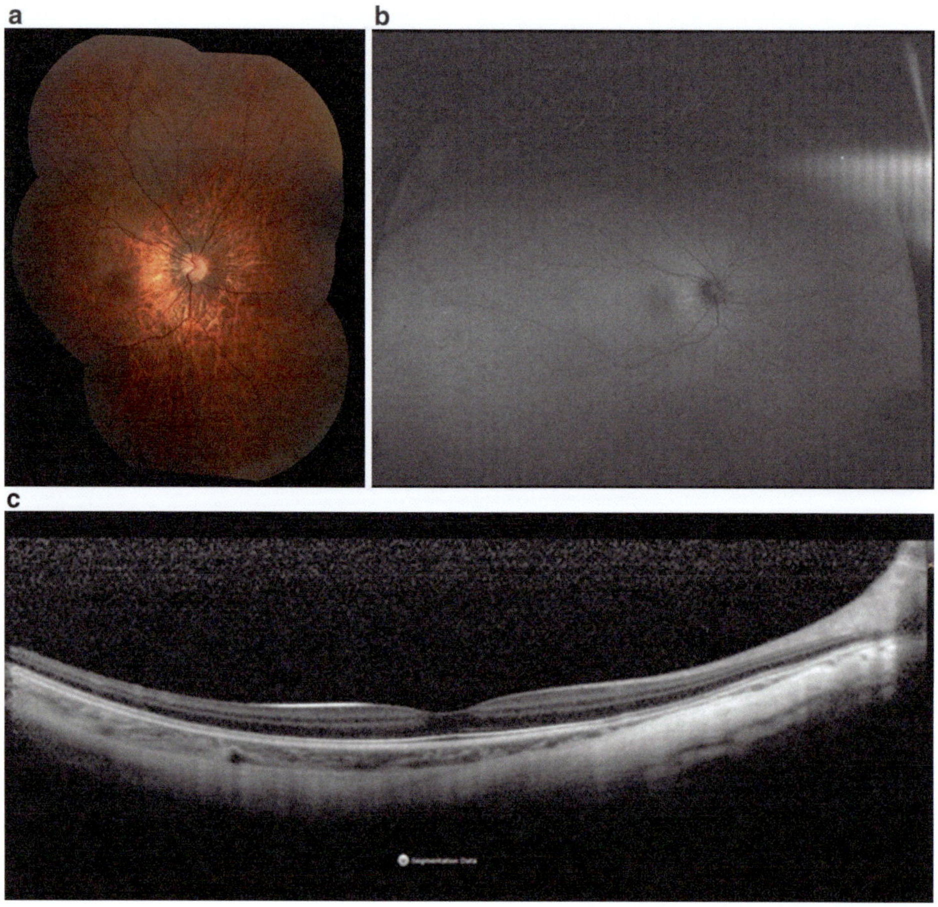

Fig. 51.2 Case Summary: 11-year-old male (CEI28443) with complete CSNB with a mutation in *NYX*. (**a**) Montage color fundus photograph of the right eye, showing an essentially unremarkable fundus. (**b**) Wide-field fundus autofluorescence, showing a normal pattern of autofluorescence except for patchy hyperautofluorescence around the optic nerve. (**c**) Spectral domain optical coherence tomography, showing good preservation of the retinal layers.

References

1. Boycott KM, Sauvé Y, MacDonald IM. X-Linked congenital stationary night blindness. 2008 [Updated 2012]. In: Pagon RA, Adam MP, Ardinger HH, et al., editors. GeneReviews® [Internet]. Seattle: University of Washington; 1993–2017. https://www.ncbi.nlm.nih.gov/books/NBK1245/. Accessed 25 Jan 2017.
2. Lodha N, Loucks CM, Beaulieu C, Parboosingh JS, Bech-Hansen NT. Congenital stationary night blindness: mutation update and clinical variability. Adv Exp Med Biol. 2012;723:371–9.
3. Bijveld MM, Florijn RJ, Bergen AA, van den Born LI, Kamermans M, Prick L, et al. Genotype and phenotype of 101 dutch patients with congenital stationary night blindness. Ophthalmology. 2013;120(10):2072–81.
4. McAnany JJ, Alexander KR, Kumar NM, Ying H, Anastasakis A, Fishman GA. Electroretinographic findings in a patient with congenital stationary night blindness due to a novel NYX mutation. Ophthalmic Genet. 2013;34(3):167–73.
5. Zhang Q, Xiao X, Li S, Jia X, Yang Z, Huang S, et al. Mutations in NYX of individuals with high myopia, but without night blindness. Mol Vis. 2007;13:330–6.
6. Yip SP, Li CC, Yiu WC, Hung WH, Lam WW, Lai MC, et al. A novel missense mutation in the NYX gene associated with high myopia. Ophthalmic Physiol Opt. 2013;33(3):346–53.

52 OAT

OAT is a nuclear gene that encodes a mitochondrial enzyme that acts as an ornithine aminotransferase. Mutations in *OAT* are associated with gyrate atrophy of the choroid and retina, which follows an autosomal recessive pattern of inheritance [1–5]. Patients typically present with nyctalopia and/or loss of peripheral vision in their second decade of life, though some patients may present with progressive myopia or poor central vision. Patients may also manifest early cataracts (typically in the second decade of life) [2, 3, 6, 7]. Visual acuities vary within age groups, ranging from 20/40 to light perception, and decline with age [1].

Patients with gyrate atrophy typically have higher plasma ornithine levels (usually 10–20 times higher than normal) [8, 9]. Fundoscopy reveals scalloped retinal pigment epithelium (RPE) and circular chorioretinal atrophic areas in the periphery (Fig. 52.1a). Optic disc atropy, macular changes, and arteriolar attenuation may also be observed. The macula and central vision are typically preserved until the fourth and fifth decades of life. Fundus autofluorescence (FAF) imaging reveals characteristic areas of hypoautofluorescence corresponding to areas of atrophy; a hyperautofluorescent region may surround these areas. Some patients may exhibit a hyperautofluorecent ring in an otherwise normal parafovea, while others may reveal speckled hyperautofluorescence in areas of the macula with normal retinal cross-sectional architecture [5, 10]. Spectral-domain optical coherence tomography (SD-OCT) may reveal cystoid spaces in the inner nuclear layer and exhibit hyper-reflective deposits in the ganglion cell layer (Fig. 52.1b) [2, 5]. Areas of preserved ellipsoid zone (EZ) have been noted to correspond to areas of normal or hyperautofluorescent areas on FAF imaging, similar to other retinal dystrophies [2]. As would be expected, the areas corresponding to hypoautofluorescent atrophy on FAF exhibit thinning and loss of outer retinal layers [2, 5]. Thickening of the foveola may be observed in younger patients, while older patients may exhibit outer retinal tubulation, which is characterized by tubular hyporeflective spaces surrounded by hyperreflective borders [2, 3]. There are varying degrees of retinal atrophy in areas of peripheral chorioretinal degeneration, or, at a minimum, interruption of the ellipsoid zone [2]. Cystoid macular edema has also been reported in some patients [2, 3]. Full-field electroretinography (ERG) recordings are variable but typically show both abnormal cone and rod responses, which can sometimes be completely extinguished [1, 10].

Microperimetry reveals that areas with maintained retinal architecture and normal autofluorescence may exhibit reduced sensitivity, while areas corresponding to atrophy show no response to bright stimuli [2]. Patients with gyrate atrophy may be treated with a low arginine protein diet to slow progression of disease [10–13]. There is a subset of patients that may respond to pyridoxine (vitamin B6), which is a cofactor for the OAT enzyme. These patients exhibit reduced plasma ornithine levels and slower progression of disease with daily pyridoxine supplementation [14, 15].

S. Zahid et al., *Retinal Dystrophy Gene Atlas*, https://doi.org/10.1007/978-3-319-10867-4_52

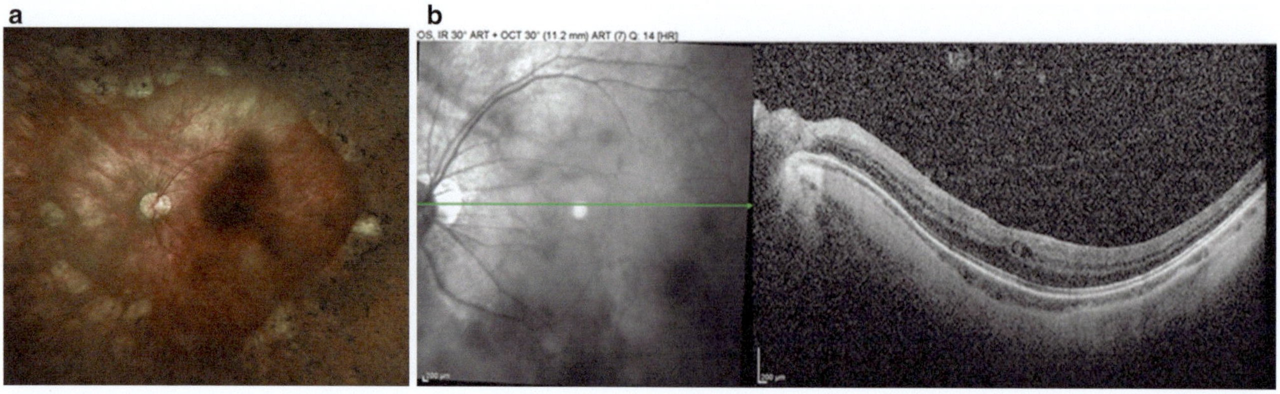

Fig. 52.1 Case Summary: 30-year-old woman with gyrate atrophy, diagnosed based on elevated ornithine levels, OCT performed at age 34. (**a**) Wide-field color fundus photograph of the left eye, showing scalloped chorioretinal atrophy with pigment deposition and retinal vessel attenuation. (**b**) Spectral domain optical coherence tomography of the left eye, showing intraretinal cystic changes with overall maintenance of the ellipsoid zone in the macula.

References

1. Peltola KE, Nanto-Salonen K, Heinonen OJ, Jääskeläinen S, Heinänen K, Simell O, et al. Ophthalmologic heterogeneity in subjects with gyrate atrophy of choroid and retina harboring the L402P mutation of ornithine aminotransferase. Ophthalmology. 2001;108(4):721–9.
2. Sergouniotis PI, Davidson AE, Lenassi E, Devery SR, Moore AT, Webster AR. Retinal structure, function, and molecular pathologic features in gyrate atrophy. Ophthalmology. 2012;119(3):596–605.
3. Oliveira TL, Andrade RE, Muccioli C, Sallum J, Belfort R Jr. Cystoid macular edema in gyrate atrophy of the choroid and retina: a fluorescein angiography and optical coherence tomography evaluation. Am J Ophthalmol. 2005;140(1):147–9.
4. Doimo M, Desbats MA, Baldoin MC, Lenzini E, Basso G, Murphy E, et al. Functional analysis of missense mutations of OAT, causing gyrate atrophy of choroid and retina. Hum Mutat. 2013;34(1):229–36.
5. Renner AB, Walter A, Fiebig BS, Jagle H. Gyrate atrophy: clinical and genetic findings in a female without arginine-restricted diet during her first 39 years of life and report of a new OAT gene mutation. Doc Ophthalmol. 2012;125(1):81–9.
6. Buyuktortop N, Alp MN, Sivri S, Coskun T, Kural G. Gyrate atrophy of the choroid and retina: a case report. Turk J Pediatr. 2011;53(1):94–6.
7. Bangal S, Bhandari A, Dhaytadak P, Gogri P. Gyrate atrophy of choroid and retina with myopia, cataract and systemic proximal myopathy: a rare case report from rural India. Australas Med J. 2012;5(12):639–42.
8. Khan MY, Ibraheim AS, Firoozmand S. Gyrate atrophy of the choroid and retina with hyperornithinaemia, cystinuria and lysinuria. Eye. 1994;8(Pt 3):284–7.
9. Simell O, Takki K. Raised plasma-ornithine and gyrate atrophy of the choroid and retina. Lancet. 1973;1(7811):1031–3.
10. Katagiri S, Gekka T, Hayashi T, et al. OAT mutations and clinical features in two Japanese brothers with gyrate atrophy of the choroid and retina. Doc Ophthalmol. 2014;128(2):137–48.
11. Wang T, Steel G, Milam AH, Valle D. Correction of ornithine accumulation prevents retinal degeneration in a mouse model of gyrate atrophy of the choroid and retina. Proc Natl Acad Sci U S A. 2000;97(3):1224–9.
12. Kim SJ, Lim DH, Kim JH, Kang SW. Gyrate atrophy of the choroid and retina diagnosed by ornithine-delta-aminotransferase gene analysis: a case report. Korean J Ophthalmol. 2013;27(5):388–91.
13. Kaiser-Kupfer MI, Caruso RC, Valle D. Gyrate atrophy of the choroid and retina: further experience with long-term reduction of ornithine levels in children. Arch Ophthalmol. 2002;120(2):146–53.
14. Mashima YG, Weleber RG, Kennaway NG, Inana G. Genotype-phenotype correlation of a pyridoxine-responsive form of gyrate atrophy. Ophthalmic Genet. 1999;20(4):219–24.
15. Ohkubo Y, Ueta A, Ito T, Sumi S, Yamada M, Ozawa K, et al. Vitamin B6-responsive ornithine aminotransferase deficiency with a novel mutation G237D. Tohoku J Exp Med. 2005;205(4):335–42.

OPN1LW and OPN1MW

53

OPN1LW and *OPN1MW* lie side by side on the X-chromosome and encode the long-wavelength (red) and middle-wavelength (green) cone opsins, respectively. Mutations in these genes cause a wide array of X-linked conditions ranging from red-green dyschromatopsia, blue cone monochromacy (BCM), cone/cone-rod dystrophy, and high myopia.

BCM is caused by mutations involving both *OPN1LW* and *OPN1MW* (sometimes from unequal crossing over that results in a single mutated hybrid gene) or in the locus control region lying upstream of these genes [1–5]. Patients typically present within the first decade with photophobia, pendular nystagmus, and poor visual acuity (typically between 20/60 and 20/400) [3, 6, 7]. Patients may exhibit central scotomas and eccentric fixation. Patients also typically exhibit severe color vision defects, observed with various types of testing (i.e. Mollon-Rifflen [RF] Minimal and Hardy-Rand-Rittler [HRR] pseudoisochromatic Plates), showing poor discrimination along the protan and deutan axes but maintained discrimination of tritan axes [3]. Myopia is very common in patients with BCM [3, 8]. Fundus examinations in younger patients are often unremarkable or show mild macular retinal pigment epithelium (RPE) changes, while older patients may exhibit macular atrophy, which may be better visualized with fundus autofluorescence (FAF) imaging (Figs. 53.1 and 53.2a) [3, 9, 10]. Spectral domain optical coherence tomography may reveal reduced foveal thicknesses and varied disruption of the ellipsoid band around the foveal center (Fig. 53.2b) [10–12]. Patients crossing-over mutations may exhibit a wider area of ellipsoid band loss than those with missense mutations [12]. Adaptive optics may be useful in further evaluating the degree of foveal cone photoreceptor loss in areas of ellipsoid disruption [10, 12]. Electroretinograms (ERG) usually show normal rod responses but severely reduced photopic parameters. ERG testing using monochromatic stimuli may reveal absent green and red responses and normal responses to blue light [11].

Certain mutations have also been reported to cause X-linked cone/cone-rod dystrophy [2, 5, 13–16]. These patients also tend to present with poor visual acuity within the first decade; myopia is common (not high myopia), while nystagmus is uncommon [13]. One study reported that these patients may present in the second or third decades and retain better visual acuity [2] than those with BCM. Similar to those BCM, most of these patients retain discrimination along the tritan axis, with abnormalities in the protan and deutan axes [13]. Fundus findings range from mild RPE pigment changes at an early age to macular atrophy in older patients. FAF may be normal in young patients or exhibit a parafoveal ring of hyperautofluorescence; there is hypoautofluorescence in areas of atrophy [13]. ERG usually reveals abnormal photopic parameters with normal scotopic parameters [2, 5, 13]. Some patients may exhibit a cone-rod dystrophy phenotype with progressive deterioration in both photopic and scotopic ERG parameters [2].

Some patients exhibit a phenotype described as X-linked myopia with cone dysfunction [14]. These patients exhibit moderate-to-high myopia, reduced visual acuity, and protanopia. The fundoscopic exam is usually normal except for myopic changes in some patients. The full-field ERG reveals abnormal cone function that does not deteriorate with time [14].

Female carriers are typically clinically unaffected, but some may exhibit evidence of cone dysfunction with ERG testing [13] There has been a report of BCM in a female resulting from an abnormal X-inactivation pattern [11].

S. Zahid et al., *Retinal Dystrophy Gene Atlas*, https://doi.org/10.1007/978-3-319-10867-4_53

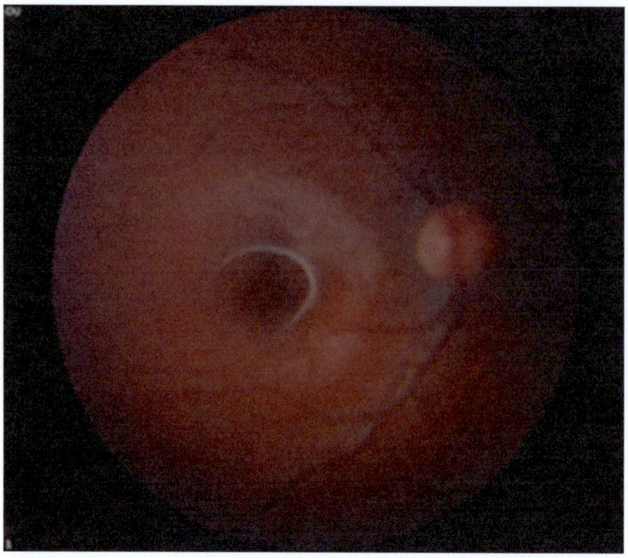

Fig. 53.1 Case Summary: 3-year-old male with BCM. Color fundus photograph of the right eye, showing a normal fundus.

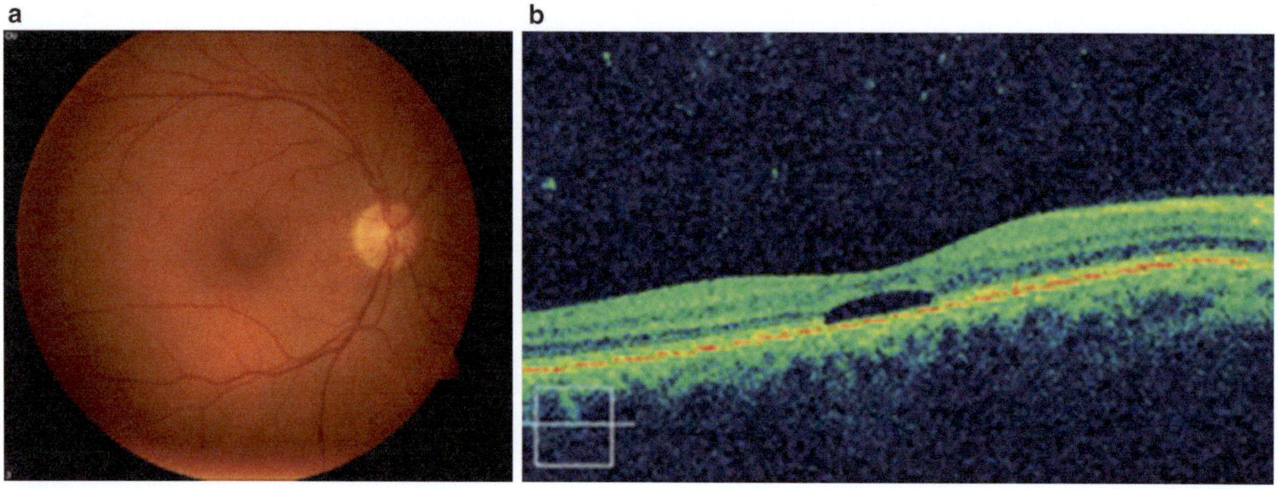

Fig. 53.2 Case summary: 49-year-old man with BCM. (**a**) Color fundus photograph of the right eye, showing loss of the foveal reflex and foveal atrophy. (**b**) Spectral domain optical coherence tomography, showing foveal ellipsoid zone loss with cavitation.

References

1. Kazmi MA, Sakmar TP, Ostrer H. Mutation of a conserved cysteine in the X-linked cone opsins causes color vision deficiencies by disrupting protein folding and stability. Invest Ophthalmol Vis Sci. 1997;38(6):1074–81.
2. Carroll J, Rossi EA, Porter J, Neitz J, Roorda A, Williams DR, et al. Deletion of the X-linked opsin gene array locus control region (LCR) results in disruption of the cone mosaic. Vis Res. 2010;50(19):1989–99.
3. Michaelides M, Johnson S, Simunovic MP, Bradshaw K, Holder G, Mollon JD, et al. Blue cone monochromatism: a phenotype and genotype assessment with evidence of progressive loss of cone function in older individuals. Eye. 2005;19(1):2–10.
4. Wang Y, Macke JP, Merbs SL, Zack DJ, Klaunberg B, Bennett J, et al. A locus control region adjacent to the human red and green visual pigment genes. Neuron. 1992;9(3):429–40.
5. Mizrahi-Meissonnier L, Merin S, Banin E, Sharon D. Variable retinal phenotypes caused by mutations in the X-linked photopigment gene array. Invest Ophthalmol Vis Sci. 2010;51(8):3884–92.
6. Ladekjaer-Mikkelsen AS, Rosenberg T, Jorgensen AL. A new mechanism in blue cone monochromatism. Hum Genet. 1996;98(4):403–8.
7. Kellner U, Wissinger B, Tippmann S, Kohl S, Kraus H, Foerster MH. Blue cone monochromatism: clinical findings in patients with mutations in the red/green opsin gene cluster. Graefes Arch Clin Exp Ophthalmol. 2004;242(9):729–35.
8. Weiss AH, Biersdorf WR. Blue cone monochromatism. J Pediatr Ophthalmol Strabismus. 1989;26(5):218–23.
9. Ayyagari R, Kakuk LE, Coats CL, Bingham EL, Toda Y, Felius J, et al. Bilateral macular atrophy in blue cone monochromacy (BCM) with loss of the locus control region (LCR) and part of the red pigment gene. Mol Vis. 1999;5:13.
10. Cideciyan AV, Hufnagel RB, Carroll J, Sumaroka A, Luo X, Schwartz SB, et al. Human cone visual pigment deletions spare sufficient photoreceptors to warrant gene therapy. Hum Gene Ther. 2013;24(12):993–1006.
11. Frederiksen AL, Duno M, Welinder LG. Blue cone monochromatism in a female due to skewed X-inactivation. Ophthalmic Genet. 2013;34(1–2):101–4.
12. Carroll J, Dubra A, Gardner JC, Mizrahi-Meissonnier L, Cooper RF, Dubis AM, et al. The effect of cone opsin mutations on retinal structure and the integrity of the photoreceptor mosaic. Invest Ophthalmol Vis Sci. 2012;53(13):8006–15.
13. Gardner JC, Webb TR, Kanuga N, Robson AG, Holder GE, Stockman A, et al. X-linked cone dystrophy caused by mutation of the red and green cone opsins. Am J Hum Genet. 2010;87(1):26–39.
14. Michaelides M, Johnson S, Bradshaw K, Holder GE, Simunovic MP, Mollon JD, et al. X-linked cone dysfunction syndrome with myopia and protanopia. Ophthalmology. 2005;112(8):1448–54.
15. Kellner U, Sadowski B, Zrenner E, Foerster MH. Selective cone dystrophy with protan genotype. Invest Ophthalmol Vis Sci. 1995;36(12):2381–7.
16. Reichel E, Bruce AM, Sandberg MA, Berson EL. An electroretinographic and molecular genetic study of X-linked cone degeneration. Am J Ophthalmol. 1989;108(5):540–7.

54 PDE6A

PDE6A encodes the alpha-subunit of the cGMP phosphodiesterase in rod photoreceptor cells that transmits visual signals during phototransduction. Mutations in *PDE6A* cause 2–5% of autosomal recessive retinitis pigmentosa (rod-cone dystrophy) [1–5]. Increased intracellular calcium and apoptosis resulting from reduced cGMP phosphodiesterase activity is thought to be a possible mechanism for rod photoreceptor cell loss [6].

These patients typically present with nyctalopia and peripheral field loss in early childhood. Visual acuity is usually maintained until later in the disease course. Fundus findings demonstrate typical signs of RP, including optic disc pallor, retinal vascular attenuation, and classic bone-spicule deposits in the mid-peripheral retina, which may be extensive (Fig. 54.1a) [4]. The full-field electroretinogram reveals a rod-cone pattern of degeneration; scotopic responses are often non-recordable. Tsang et al. [4] reported that vitreomacular traction is seen in some patients, and this may be best visualized on optical coherence tomography (Fig. 54.1c); fundus autofluorescence may reveal a hyperautofluorescent ring in the macula (Fig. 54.1b), in which the microperimetric thresholds are elevated. Bilateral cystoid macular edema has also been reported [4].

S. Zahid et al., *Retinal Dystrophy Gene Atlas*, https://doi.org/10.1007/978-3-319-10867-4_54

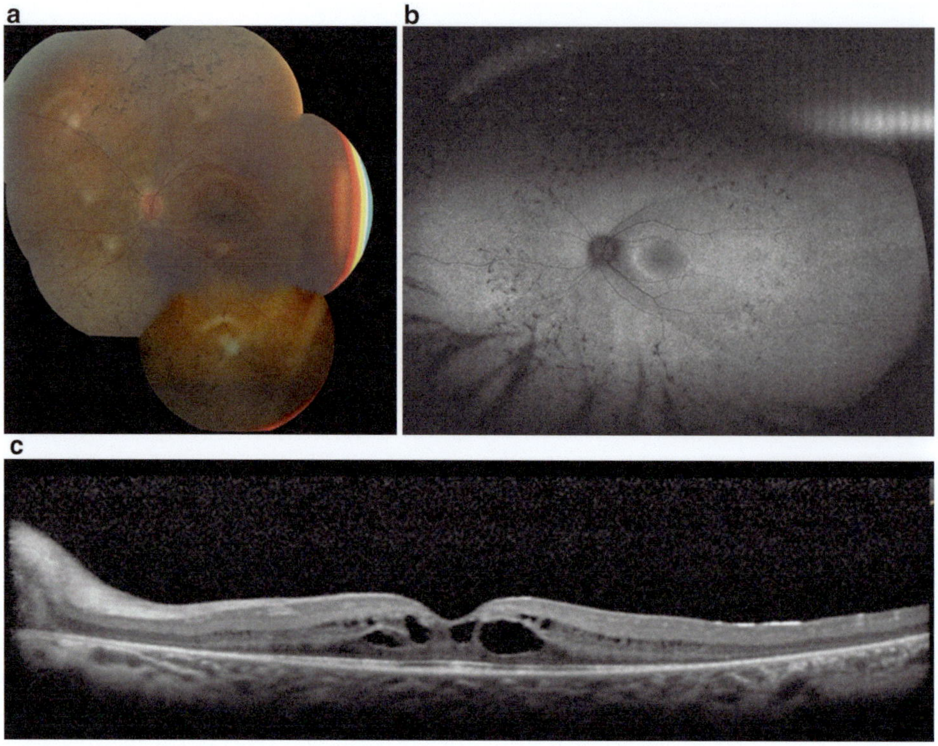

Fig. 54.1 Case Summary: 15-year-old female with retinitis pigmentosa (simplex) (CEI26433) with mutations in *PDE6A*. (**a**) Montage color fundus photograph of the left eye, showing bone spicule pigmentation and RPE atrophy in the mid-peripheral retina. (**b**) Wide-field fundus autofluorescence of the left eye, showing hypoautofluorescence associated with bone spicule pigmentation, with surrounding foci of hyperautofluorescence. There is also a hyperautofluorescent ring in the macula. (**c**) Spectral domain optical coherence tomography of the left eye, showing extrafoveal loss of the ellipsoid zone and outer nuclear layer, cystoid changes at the fovea, as well as a faint temporal epiretinal membrane.

References

1. Huang SH, Pittler SJ, Huang X, Oliveira L, Berson EL, Dryja TP. Autosomal recessive retinitis pigmentosa caused by mutations in the alpha subunit of rod cGMP phosphodiesterase. Nat Genet. 1995;11(4):468–71.
2. Corton M, Blanco MJ, Torres M, Sanchez-Salorio M, Carracedo A, Brion M. Identification of a novel mutation in the human PDE6A gene in autosomal recessive retinitis pigmentosa: homology with the nmf28/nmf28 mice model. Clin Genet. 2010;78(5):495–8.
3. Dryja TP, Rucinski DE, Chen SH, Berson EL. Frequency of mutations in the gene encoding the alpha subunit of rod cGMP-phosphodiesterase in autosomal recessive retinitis pigmentosa. Invest Ophthalmol Vis Sci. 1999;40(8):1859–65.
4. Tsang SH, Tsui I, Chou CL, Zernant J, Haamer E, Iranmanesh R, et al. A novel mutation and phenotypes in phosphodiesterase 6 deficiency. Am J Ophthalmol. 2008;146(5):780–8.
5. Riazuddin SA, Zulfiqar F, Zhang Q, Yao W, Li S, Jiao X, et al. Mutations in the gene encoding the alpha-subunit of rod phosphodiesterase in consanguineous Pakistani families. Mol Vis. 2006;12:1283–91.
6. Ferrari S, Di Iorio E, Barbaro V, Ponzin D, Sorrentino FS, Parmeggiani F. Retinitis pigmentosa: genes and disease mechanisms. Curr Genomics. 2011;12(4):238–49.

55 PDE6B

PDE6B encodes the beta-subunit of the cGMP phosphodiesterase in rod photoreceptor cells that plays a key role during phototransduction. Mutations in *PDE6B* cause 2–5% of autosomal recessive retinitis pigmentosa (rod-cone dystrophy) [1] and rarely autosomal dominant congenital stationary night blindness (CSNB) [2].

Patients with recessive mutations in *PDE6B* report nyctalopia and peripheral field loss starting in early childhood [1, 3, 4]. Visual acuity is generally maintained (better than 20/40) until later in the disease course. Fundus findings are typical for retinitis pigmentosa, including optic disc pallor, retinal vascular attenuation, and bone-spicule deposits in the mid-peripheral retina, which progresses to peripheral atrophy that may ultimately involve the macula (Fig. 55.1); some patients may exhibit cystoid macular edema. The full-field electroretinogram (ERG) reveals a rod-cone pattern of degeneration; scotopic responses are often non-recordable [4]. Dark adaptation thresholds are elevated, and Goldmann visual field testing reveals constriction starting in the mid-peripheral fields followed by extension to the periphery and finally constriction centrally. Spectral domain-optical coherence tomography may demonstrate outer retinal atrophy with ellipsoid zone loss, faint epiretinal membrane, and inner retinal cystic changes (Fig. 55.2a, b). Fundus autofluorescence reveals areas of hypoautofluorescence corresponding to areas of retinal pigment epithelium atrophy; some patients may exhibit a ring of hyperautofluorescence surrounding the fovea (Fig. 55.2c, d) [4]. Microperimetry shows reduced sensitivities in areas of hypoautofluorescence [4].

Certain mutations in *PDE6B* can cause dominant CSNB [2, 5]. These patients typically experience stable night blindness but maintain good central visual acuity and color vision. Funduscopy usually reveals a normal fundus, and testing reveals elevated dark adaptation thresholds, reduced to absent dark-adapted a- and b-waves, and normal photopic responses. A negative ERG, in which the b-wave to a-wave ratio is less than 1 for the scotopic b-wave under dark-adapted maximum stimulus conditions, may be observed in patients with dominant CSNB associated with mutations in *PDE6B* [5].

S. Zahid et al., *Retinal Dystrophy Gene Atlas*, https://doi.org/10.1007/978-3-319-10867-4_55

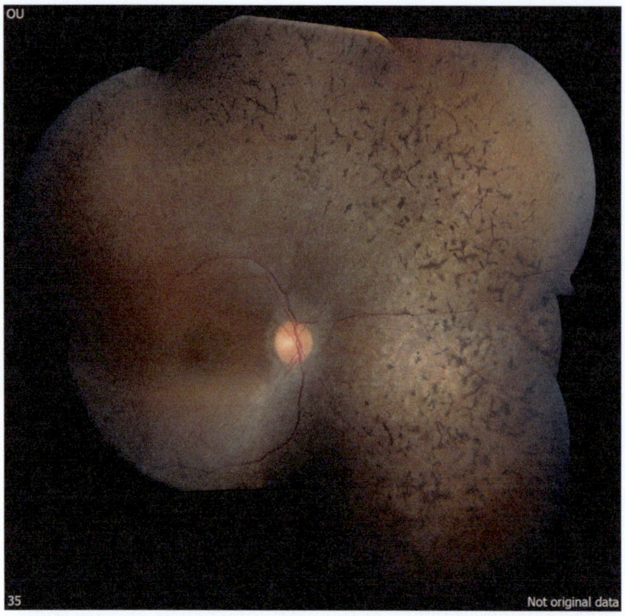

Fig. 55.1 Color fundus photograph of the right eye, showing mid-peripheral bone-spicule pigmentation and peripheral retinal atrophy. Case Summary: Twenty-eight year old woman with rod-cone dystrophy.

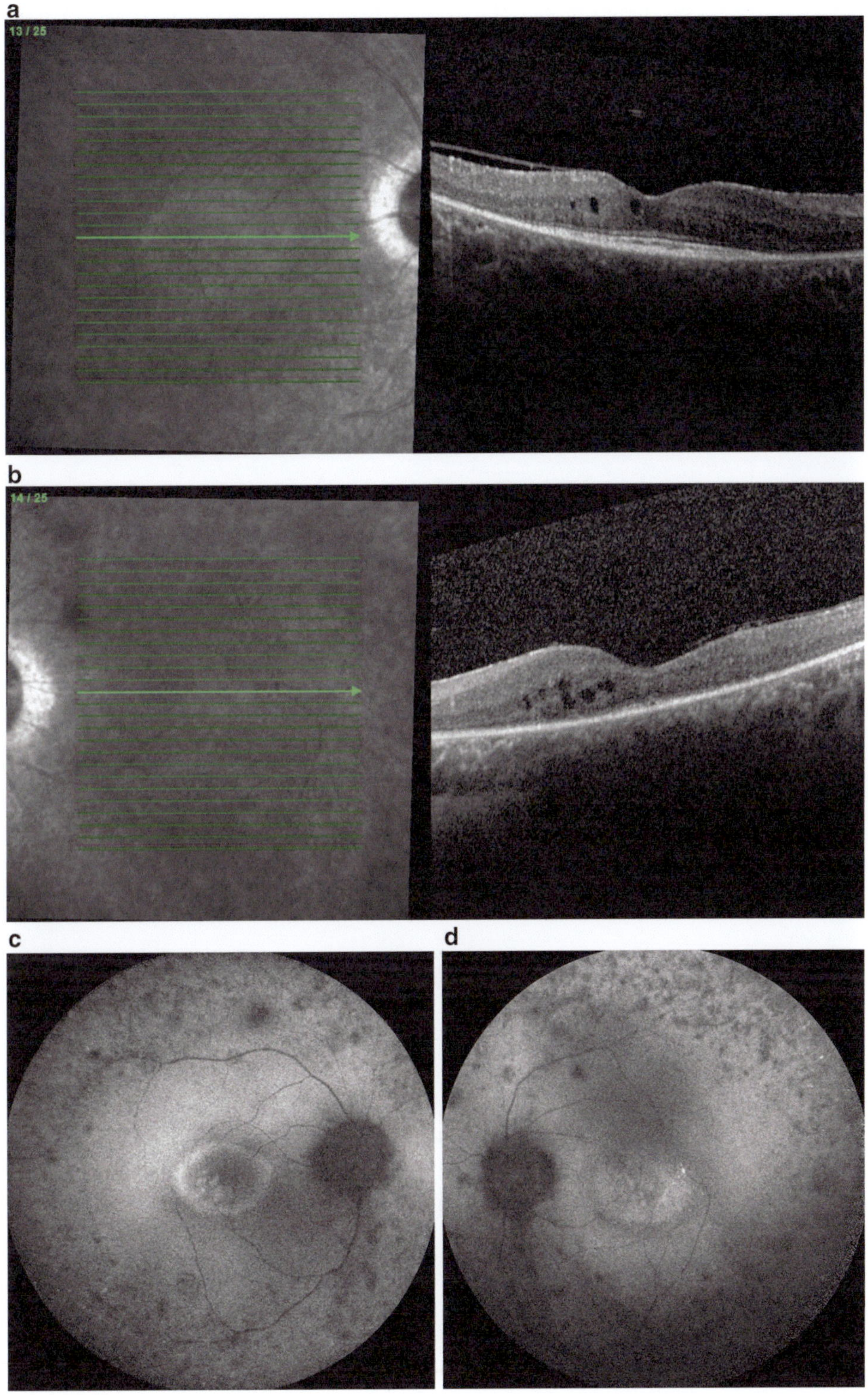

Fig. 55.2 Case Summary: 33-year-old female with cystoid macular edema. (**a**) Spectral domain-optical coherence tomography of the right eye, showing outer retinal atrophy with ellipsoid zone (EZ) loss outside the fovea, with a faint epiretinal membrane and inner retinal cystic changes. (**b**) Spectral domain-OCT of the left eye, showing EZ loss involving the fovea, with a trace ERM and inner retinal cystic changes. (**c**) Fundus autofluorescence, showing a ring of hyperautofluorescence surrounding the fovea and patchy hypoautofluoresence outside the arcades in the right eye. (**d**) Fundus autofluorescence, showing macular hyperautofluorescence and patchy hypoautofluorescence outside the arcades in the left eye.

References

1. McLaughlin ME, Sandberg MA, Berson EL, Dryja TP. Recessive mutations in the gene encoding the beta-subunit of rod phosphodiesterase in patients with retinitis pigmentosa. Nat Genet. 1993;4(2):130–4.
2. Gal A, Orth U, Baehr W, Schwinger E, Rosenberg T. Heterozygous missense mutation in the rod cGMP phosphodiesterase beta-subunit gene in autosomal dominant stationary night blindness. Nat Genet. 1994;7(4):551.
3. Ali S, Riazuddin SA, Shahzadi A, Nasir IA, Khan SN, Husnain T, et al. Mutations in the beta-subunit of rod phosphodiesterase identified in consanguineous Pakistani families with autosomal recessive retinitis pigmentosa. Mol Vis. 2011;17:1373–80.
4. Tsang SH, Tsui I, Chou CL, Zernant J, Haamer E, Iranmanesh R, et al. A novel mutation and phenotypes in phosphodiesterase 6 deficiency. Am J Ophthalmol. 2008;146(5):780–8.
5. Tsang SH, Woodruff ML, Jun L, Mahajan V, Yamashita CK, Pedersen R, et al. Transgenic mice carrying the H258N mutation in the gene encoding the beta-subunit of phosphodiesterase-6 (PDE6B) provide a model for human congenital stationary night blindness. Hum Mutat. 2007;28(3):243–54.

56 PDE6C

PDE6C encodes cone cGMP-specific 3′,5′-cyclic phosphodiesterase subunit alpha (cGMP phosphodiesterase 6C), which is an enzyme expressed in cone photoreceptors. Autosomal recessive mutations in *PDE6C* cause cone-specific disorders ranging from achromatopsia to cone dystrophy [1, 2].

Patients can present within the first decade with poor visual acuity, photophobia, abnormal color vision, and nystagmus; most tend to be myopic. Fundoscopy may be unremarkable or reveal mild macular pigment changes with an absent foveal reflex in the context of a normal peripheral retina; some patients may exhibit atrophy at the macula (Fig. 56.1a) [1, 2]. The electroretinogram (ERG) is notable for abnormal cone function with normal rod function, although reduced rod parameters have been reported in some patients [1–4]. Cone function worsens with age in many patients until responses are extinguished, but some patients may exhibit a non-recordable cone ERG within the first decade of life. Goldmann visual field testing and microperimetry reveal central scotomas [1, 3]. Fundus autofluorescence may show abnormal foveal autofluorescence, ranging from hyperautofluorescence to hypoautofluorescence in cases with foveal atrophy (Fig. 56.1b). Spectral domain optical coherence tomography typically reveals a loss of the photoreceptor layer at the fovea that appears as a cavitation (or empty optical cavity) at the foveola with loss of the ellipsoid zone (Fig. 56.1c) [2, 3, 5]. While mutations in *PDE6C* cause a spectrum of disease from progressive cone dystrophy to achromatopsia, the final phenotype may be determined by the type and nature of inherited disease-causing mutations and the degree to which enzyme activity is affected [5].

S. Zahid et al., *Retinal Dystrophy Gene Atlas*, https://doi.org/10.1007/978-3-319-10867-4_56

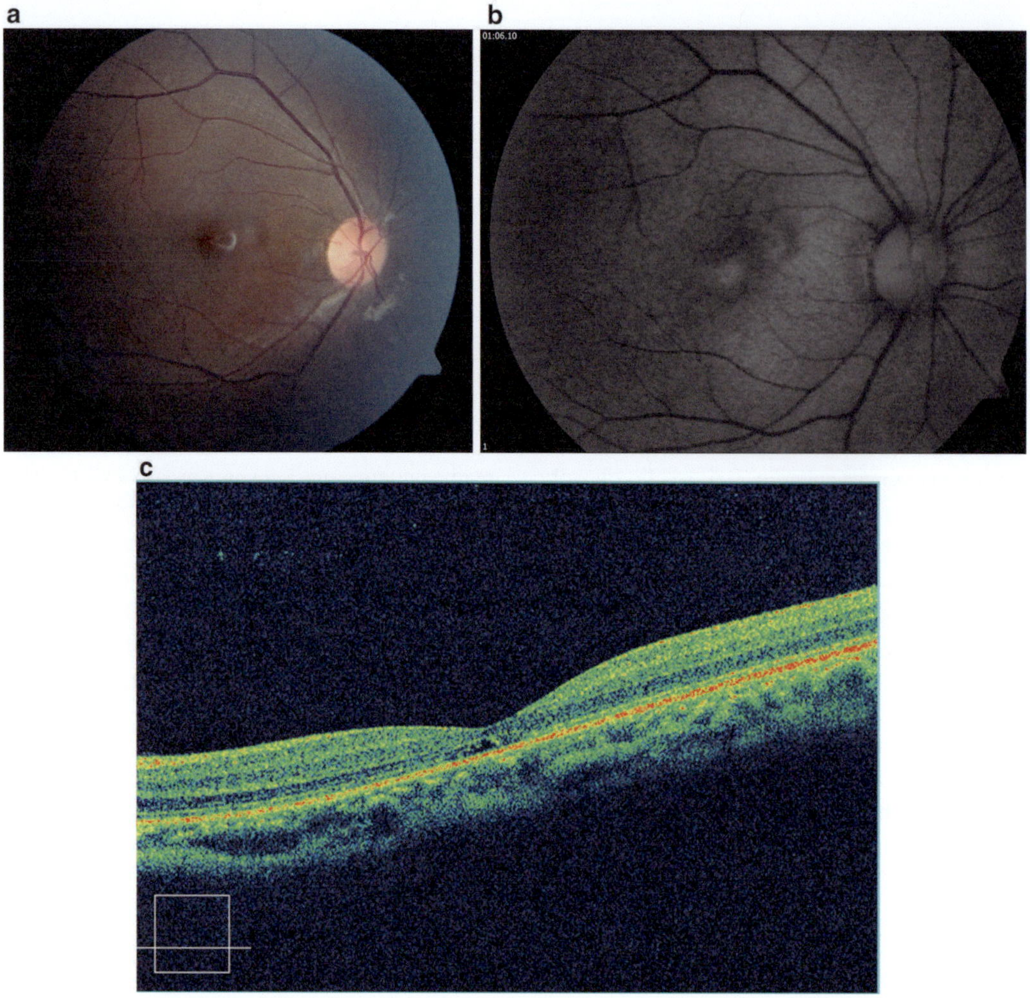

Fig. 56.1 Case summary: 10-year-old girl with achromatopsia. (**a**) Color fundus photograph of the right eye, showing an abnormal foveal reflex at age 10 years. (**b**) Fundus autoflourescence of the right eye, showing abnormal areas of hyperautofluorescence at and surrounding the fovea at age 12 years. (**c**) Spectral-domain optical coherence tomography, showing outer retinal foveal atrophy with ellipsoid zone loss and cavitation in the context of a broadened foveal pit at age 10.

References

1. Chang B, Grau T, Dangel S, Hurd R, Jurklies B, Sener EC, et al. A homologous genetic basis of the murine cpfl1 mutant and human achromatopsia linked to mutations in the PDE6C gene. Proc Natl Acad Sci U S A. 2009;106(46):19581–6.
2. Thiadens AA, den Hollander AI, Roosing S, Nabuurs SB, Zekveld-Vroon RC, Collin RW, et al. Homozygosity mapping reveals PDE6C mutations in patients with early-onset cone photoreceptor disorders. Am J Hum Genet. 2009;85(2):240–7.
3. Sundaram V, Wilde C, Aboshiha J, Cowing J, Han C, Langlo CS, et al. Retinal structure and function in achromatopsia: implications for gene therapy. Ophthalmology. 2014;121(1):234–45.
4. Huang L, Zhang Q, Li S, Guan L, Xiao X, Zhang J, et al. Exome sequencing of 47 chinese families with cone-rod dystrophy: mutations in 25 known causative genes. PLoS One. 2013;8(6):e65546.
5. Grau T, Artemyev NO, Rosenberg T, Dollfus H, Haugen OH, Cumhur Sener E, et al. Decreased catalytic activity and altered activation properties of PDE6C mutants associated with autosomal recessive achromatopsia. Hum Mol Genet. 2011;20(4):719–30.

57 PDE6G

PDE6G encodes the gamma-subunit of the cGMP phosphodiesterase in rod photoreceptor cells that plays a key role during phototransduction. Mutations in *PDE6G* are a rare cause of autosomal recessive retinitis pigmentosa (RP; rod-cone dystrophy) and autosomal dominant congenital stationary night blindness [1, 2]. Due to the rarity of mutations in this gene, limited information is available on the phenotype. Compared to other forms of RP, it exhibits an earlier onset of photoreceptor dysfunction on electroretinography (ERG); however, best corrected visual acuity was relatively good (as high as 20/40 at age 10–16). Patients present with the typical features of RP, including night blindness, reduced peripheral vision, and preserved central visual acuity. Funduscopic findings demonstrate retinal pigment epithelium (RPE) atrophy and bone-spicule pigment deposits starting in the mid-periphery and spreading to the periphery, retinal vascular attenuation, and optic disc pallor. Macular atrophy and cystoid macular edema may also develop in some patients. Full-field ERG is usually non-recordable at an early age (as early as 4 years). Visual field testing usually reveals a central island of remaining vision (<5–10°) from 10–16 years of age. [1].

References

1. Dvir L, Srour G, Abu-Ras R, Miller B, Shalev SA, Ben-Yosef T. Autosomal-recessive early-onset retinitis pigmentosa caused by a mutation in PDE6G, the gene encoding the gamma subunit of rod cGMP phosphodiesterase. Am J Hum Genet. 2010;87(2):258–64.
2. Muradov KG, Granovsky AE, Artemyev NO. Mutation in rod PDE6 linked to congenital stationary night blindness impairs the enzyme inhibition by its gamma-subunit. Biochemistry. 2003;42(11):3305–10.

S. Zahid et al., *Retinal Dystrophy Gene Atlas*, https://doi.org/10.1007/978-3-319-10867-4_57

58 *PHYH*

PHYH (also called PAHX) encodes the peroxisomal protein phytanoyl-CoA hydroxylase, which is involved in the peroxisomal α-oxidation of phytanic acid. Mutations in *PHYH* cause adult Refsum disease, which is an autosomal-recessive peroxisomal disorder resulting from serum and tissue accumulation of phytanic acid. The disease has numerous features, including retinitis pigmentosa (RP) as well as peripheral polyneuropathy, anosmia, hearing loss, cardiomyopathy, cerebellar ataxia, and elevated protein levels in the cerebrospinal fluid [1, 2]. It is as yet unclear how elevated levels of phytanic acid result in disease.

All cases of adult Refsum disease exhibit retinitis pigmentosa, and most patients report ophthalmic symptoms long before other systemic issues [3]. There is typically an onset of night blindness and visual field constriction from early childhood to the second decade of life [2, 4, 5]. Visual acuities may be normal early in the disease course to very severely affected (hand movement vision) in older patients [2]. Concentric narrowing of the visual field is also common, as with other types of rod-cone dystrophy. However, progressive visual field and acuity deterioration occur over several decades after the initial onset of night blindness [2, 4]. Some patients may exhibit earlier macular atrophy, resulting in loss of visual acuity at a younger age [6]. Electroretinography (ERG) usually reveals significantly reduced or nonrecordable rod and cone responses, although it is reasonable to expect a rod-cone pattern of degeneration in patients [1]. Dietary restriction of phytanic acid levels (to less than 10 mg/day) has been shown to successfully improve ichthyosis and neurologic symptoms such as ataxia and peripheral neuropathy, but it is unknown whether this affects the progression of retinal disease [4–7].

References

1. Fertl E, Foldy D, Vass K, Auff E, Vass C, Molzer B, et al. Refsum's disease in an Arabian family. J Neurol Neurosurg Psychiatry. 2001;70(4):564–5.
2. Wanders RJA, Waterham HR, Leroy BP. Refsum Disease. In: Pagon RA, Adam MP, Ardinger HH, Wallace SE, Amemiya A, Bean LJH, et al., editors. GeneReviews(R). Seattle: University of Washington; 2006. (Updated 2015).
3. Claridge KG, Gibberd FB, Sidey MC. Refsum disease: the presentation and ophthalmic aspects of Refsum disease in a series of 23 patients. Eye (Lond). 1992;6(Pt 4):371–5.
4. Horn MA, van den Brink DM, Wanders RJ, Duran M, Poll-The BT, Tallaksen CM, et al. Phenotype of adult Refsum disease due to a defect in peroxin 7. Neurology. 2007;68(9):698–700.
5. Kohlschutter A, Santer R, Lukacs Z, Altenburg C, Kemper MJ, Rüther K. A child with night blindness: preventing serious symptoms of Refsum disease. J Child Neurol. 2012;27(5):654–6.
6. Traboulsi EI. Genetic diseases of the eye. 2nd ed. Oxford: Oxford University Press; 2012.
7. Klockgether T. Handbook of ataxia disorders. New York: Marcel Dekker; 2000.

S. Zahid et al., *Retinal Dystrophy Gene Atlas*, https://doi.org/10.1007/978-3-319-10867-4_58

59 PRCD

PRCD encodes progressive rod-cone degeneration protein, whose function is poorly defined, but which is known to be a membrane protein expressed in photoreceptors [1]. Autosomal recessive mutations in *PRCD* cause retinitis pigmentosa (rod-cone dystrophy) [2, 3]. A founder mutation has been identified in the Muslim Arab population in Israel [3]. Symptoms include nyctalopia and reduced visual acuity within the first decade, with most patients exhibiting very poor visual acuity by the second decade. Myopia and posterior subcapsular cataracts are common findings [3, 4]. Fundus findings include classic RP features, such as bone-spicule pigment deposits, optic nerve pallor, and arteriolar attenuation (Fig. 59.1a, b). Many patients also exhibit abnormal findings at the macula, such as macular puckering, central atrophy, or a bull's eye maculopathy [2–4]. The full-field ERG has been reported to be non-recordable in all published patients, including a child only 6 years of age [2–4]. Goldmann visual field testing tends to reveal peripheral field loss [2]. Spectral domain OCT reveals reduced foveal thickness, with shortened outer segments and loss of the ONL and RPE [4].

S. Zahid et al., *Retinal Dystrophy Gene Atlas*, https://doi.org/10.1007/978-3-319-10867-4_59

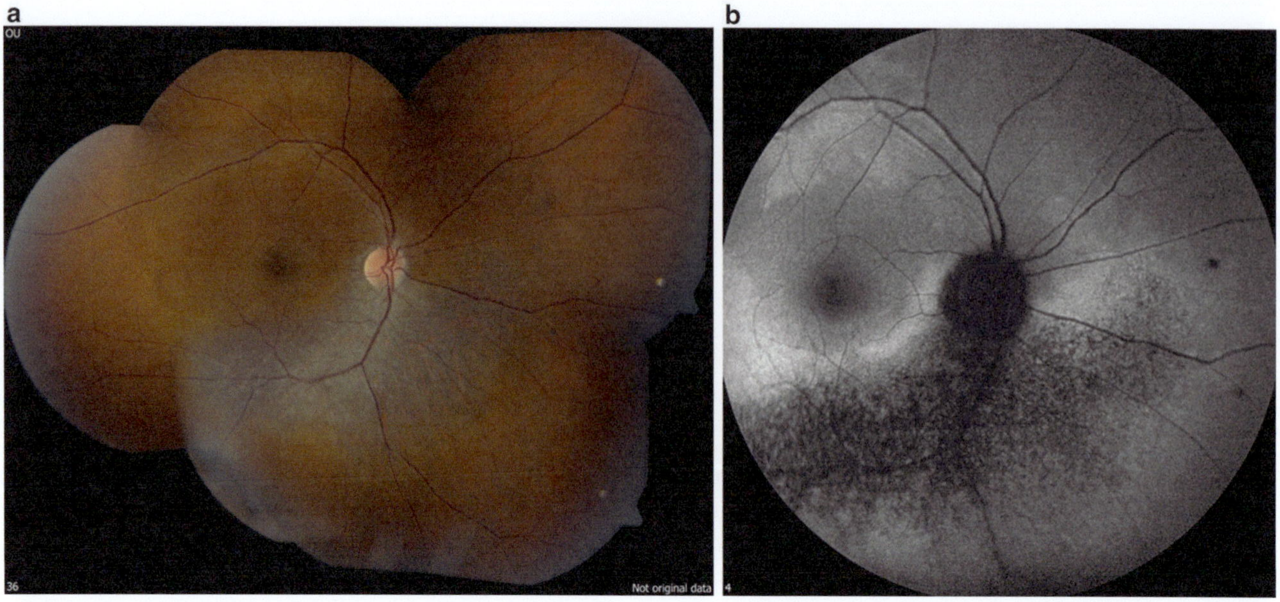

Fig. 59.1 Case summary: 45-year-old woman with pericentral retinitis pigmentosa. (**a**) Color fundus photograph of the right eye, showing pericentral pigment deposits and retinal pigment epithelium (RPE) atrophy along the inferior arcades with an otherwise unremarkable fundus. (**b**) Fundus autofluorescence, showing hypoautofluorescence along the inferior arcades in areas of RPE atrophy with surrounding areas of hyperautofluorescence and with hyperautofluorescence along the arcades.

References

1. Skiba NP, Spencer WJ, Salinas RY, Lieu EC, Thompson JW, Arshavsky VY. Proteomic identification of unique photoreceptor disc components reveals the presence of PRCD, a protein linked to retinal degeneration. J Proteome Res. 2013;12(6):3010–8.
2. Zangerl B, Goldstein O, Philp AR, Lindauer SJ, Pearce-Kelling SE, Mullins RF, et al. Identical mutation in a novel retinal gene causes progressive rod-cone degeneration in dogs and retinitis pigmentosa in humans. Genomics. 2006;88(5):551–63.
3. Nevet MJ, Shalev SA, Zlotogora J, Mazzawi N, Ben-Yosef T. Identification of a prevalent founder mutation in an Israeli Muslim Arab village confirms the role of PRCD in the aetiology of retinitis pigmentosa in humans. J Med Genet. 2010;47(8):533–7.
4. Pach J, Kohl S, Gekeler F, Zobor D. Identification of a novel mutation in the PRCD gene causing autosomal recessive retinitis pigmentosa in a Turkish family. Mol Vis. 2013;19:1350–5.

60 *PROM1*

PROM1 encodes prominin-1, a membrane protein involved in disk morphogenesis. Mutations in *PROM1* cause autosomal dominant macular dystrophy, autosomal recessive or dominant retinitis pigmentosa (RP), or recessive cone-rod dystrophy [1–3].

Patients with macular dystrophy may present in their teens to thirties and with reduced visual acuity, photophobia, and abnormal color vision [4]. Funduscopic findings are characterized by bilateral macular degeneration and may include retinal pigment epithelium (RPE) changes, bull's-eye maculopathy with atrophy, or flecks (Fig. 60.1a). Fluorescein angiography usually shows hyperfluorescent macular lesions with window defects; a dark choroid has been reported in one patient but is not necessarily pathognomonic for this mutation. FAF may reveal a hyperautofluorescent perifoveal ring (Fig. 60.1b). In cases of isolated macular involvement, the full-field electroretinogram (ERG) is normal, while rod-cone or cone-rod pattern dysfunction suggests more widespread retinal involvement. Goldmann visual field (GVF) usually shows central scotomata. Optical coherence tomography (OCT) may reveal macular atrophy with retinal thinning such as a loss of the ellipsoid zone, reflecting lack of photoreceptor integrity (Fig. 60.1c); retinal tissue in the more peripheral macula may be less affected [4].

PROM1 mutations have also been shown to cause dominant RP. The initial symptom is usually reduced central vision, with night blindness becoming more noticeable with time. Age of onset may be variable, between the teens to the 50s. Unlike many other forms of RP, funduscopy commonly reveals a bull's eye maculopathy, with variable other features of RP, including attenuated vessels, optic disc pallor, peripheral pigment, and macular atrophy. Fluorescein angiography has never been noted to exhibit a dark choroid. ERG reveals rod-cone dysfunction. OCT may reveal reduced retinal thickness, macular atrophy, or loss of photoreceptor outer segments.

Recessive RP may also be caused by *PROM1* mutations [5]. The presenting symptoms are usually night blindness and reduced acuity, which begin in early childhood. Visual acuity reduces rapidly to significantly worse than 20/200 before age 20. Nystagmus may be observed, but photophobia and keratoconus are uncommon. Fundus findings include disc pallor, progressive macular atrophy beginning with pigment clumping (often exhibiting a bull's-eye lesion), vascular attenuation, and bone-spicule pigment deposits in the mid-periphery. ERG reveals rod-cone dysfunction and is often non-recordable by the third decade. Polydactyly has been reported in one patient [5].

Recessive cone-rod dystrophy has also been reported to be caused by mutations in *PROM1* [2]. Patients present in early childhood with reduced visual acuity (may progress to counting fingers before age 20), photosensitivity, and color vision defects; night vision is affected later in life. High myopia and nystagmus are commonly observed. Fundus findings are usually limited to the macula, including bull's-eye maculopathy, with rare deposits in the periphery (Fig. 60.2). ERG is characterized by cone dysfunction with progressively deteriorating rod function over time.

S. Zahid et al., *Retinal Dystrophy Gene Atlas*, https://doi.org/10.1007/978-3-319-10867-4_60

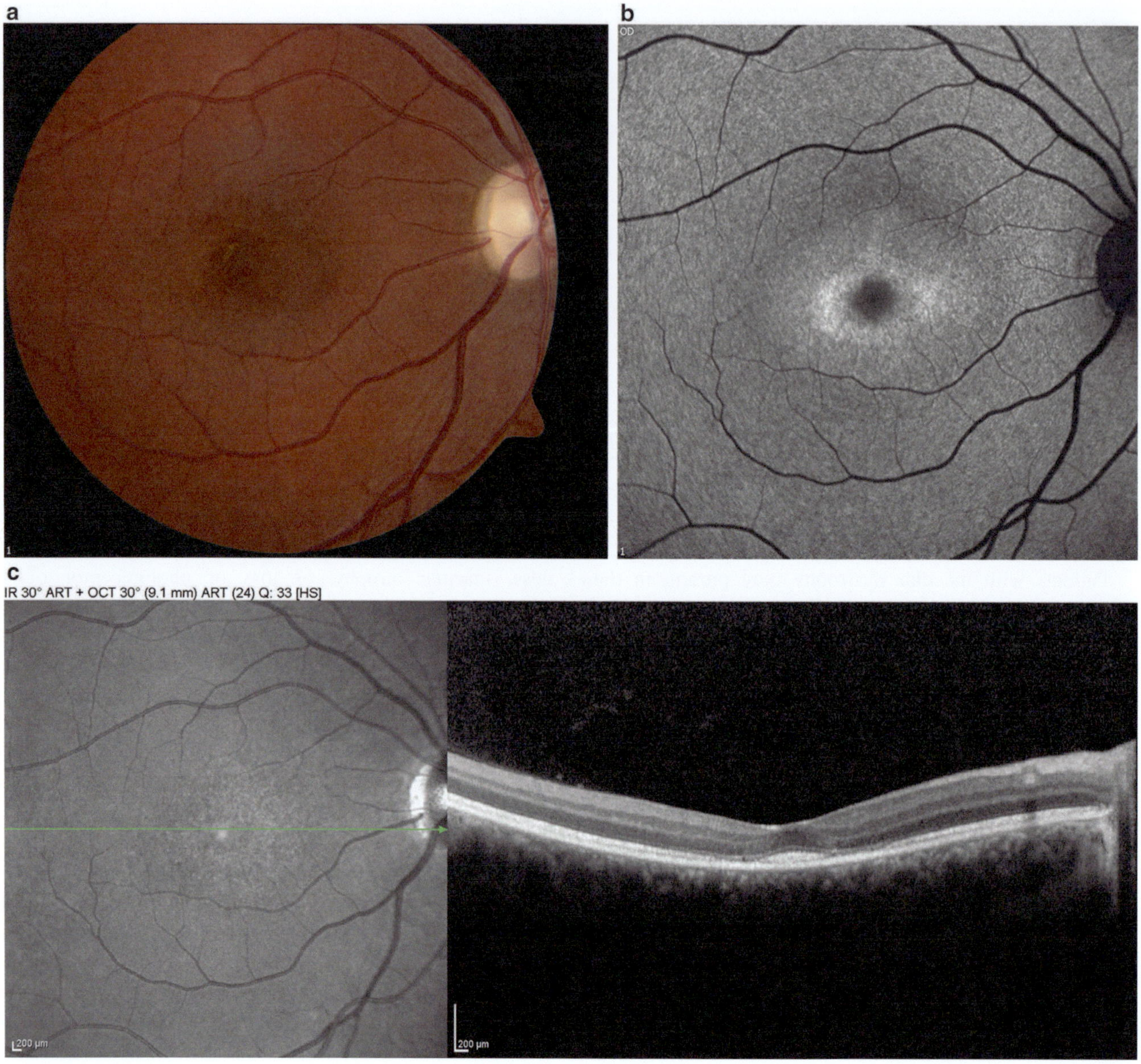

Fig. 60.1 Case summary: 25-year-old woman with dominant macular dystrophy. (**a**) Color fundus photograph of the right eye, showing faint RPE abnormalities in the macula. (**b**) Fundus autofluorescence of the right eye, showing a ring of hyperautofluorescence surrounding the fovea. (**c**) Spectral domain optical coherence tomography, showing a broadened foveal pit and focal disruption of the ellipsoid zone surrounding the foveola, with an anatomically intact underlying RPE.

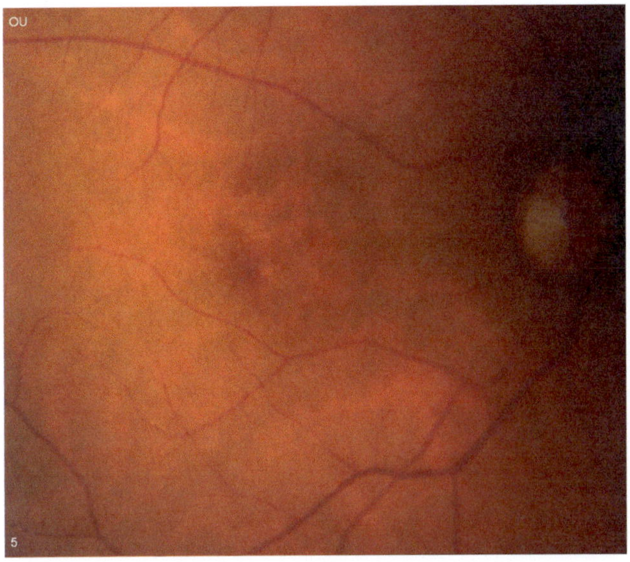

Fig. 60.2 Color fundus photograph of the right eye from a 51-year-old woman with cone-rod dystrophy, showing macular atrophy and retinal pigment epithelium abnormality.

References

1. Zhang Q, Zulfiqar F, Xiao X, Riazuddin SA, Ahmad Z, Caruso R, et al. Severe retinitis pigmentosa mapped to 4p15 and associated with a novel mutation in the PROM1 gene. Hum Genet. 2007;122(3–4):293–9.
2. Pras E, Abu A, Rotenstreich Y, Avni I, Reish O, Morad Y, et al. Cone-rod dystrophy and a frameshift mutation in the PROM1 gene. Mol Vis. 2009;15:1709–16.
3. Yang Z, Chen Y, Lillo C, Chien J, Yu Z, Michaelides M, et al. Mutant prominin 1 found in patients with macular degeneration disrupts photoreceptor disk morphogenesis in mice. J Clin Invest. 2008;118(8):2908–16.
4. Michaelides M, Gaillard MC, Escher P, Tiab L, Bedell M, Borruat FX, et al. The PROM1 mutation p.R373C causes an autosomal dominant bull's eye maculopathy associated with rod, rod-cone, and macular dystrophy. Invest Ophthalmol Vis Sci. 2010;51(9):4771–80.
5. Maw MA, Corbeil D, Koch J, Hellwig A, Wilson-Wheeler JC, Bridges RJ, et al. A frameshift mutation in prominin (mouse)-like 1 causes human retinal degeneration. Hum Mol Genet. 2000;9(1):27–34.

PRPF3

61

PRPF3 encodes U4/U6 small nuclear ribonucleoprotein Prp3, a nuclear protein that plays a role in mRNA splicing. It is highly expressed in the retina, among many other tissues; mutations affect its interaction with the U4/U6 snRNP complex of the spliceosome [1]. Mutations in *PRPF3* cause about one percent of autosomal dominant retinitis pigmentosa (rod-cone dystrophy) [2–6]. It is not well understood how mutations in the components of the spliceosome result in a phenotype that affects only the retina [7].

Patients usually present with night blindness in childhood (first and second decades), then progressively lose peripheral fields into their thirties and forties, and usually exhibit a non-recordable electroretinogram (ERG) by the fourth decade [8–10]. Some studies, however, have reported a later onset of night blindness, as late as age 40 [4, 6]. Patients with an earlier onset of nyctalopia (within the first decade) tend to lose visual acuity more rapidly than those who experience nyctalopia in the second and third decades [6]. Most patients are myopic; nystagmus and color vision abnormalities are uncommon. Some patients develop photophobia later in the disease course [10].

Fundus findings feature classic features of rod-cone dystrophy, such as retinal vascular attenuation, optic disc pallor, retinal pigment epithelium (RPE) mottling, and bone spicule pigment deposits in the mid-periphery and peripheral retina that progresses to atrophy later in the disease course. Younger patients may exhibit a normal fundus [6]. FAF reveals hypoautofluorescence in the peripheral and mid-peripheral retina due to atrophy; some patients may exhibit granular hyperautofluorescence at the macula [8]. A hyperautofluorescent ring in the macula is common, the inner ring of which may correlate with the extent of the remaining visual field detected with the I-4e or I-3e isopters [6]. This ring may be present early in the disease course in the context of a relatively normal fundus, before any symptoms manifest. The full-field ERG is often non-recordable by the fourth decade of life, and Goldmann Visual Field (GVF) reveals visual field constriction in a rod-cone pattern. When the full-field ERG is recordable (usually earlier in life), it exhibits a rod-cone pattern of degeneration. Dark-adaptation thresholds are elevated, as would be expected for a rod-cone dystrophy. Cystoid macular edema (CME) is uncommonly observed with mutations in *PRPF3*. Phenotypic variability, even in patients within the same family, is common, and there may be differences in visual acuity, field size, and ERG findings in patients harboring the same mutations [6].

References

1. Gonzalez-Santos JM, Cao H, Duan RC, Hu J. Mutation in the splicing factor Hprp3p linked to retinitis pigmentosa impairs interactions within the U4/U6 snRNP complex. Hum Mol Genet. 2008;17(2):225–39.
2. Chakarova CF, Hims MM, Bolz H, Abu-Safieh L, Patel RJ, Papaioannou MG, et al. Mutations in HPRP3, a third member of pre-mRNA splicing factor genes, implicated in autosomal dominant retinitis pigmentosa. Hum Mol Genet. 2002;11(1):87–92.
3. Gamundi MJ, Hernan I, Muntanyola M, Maseras M, López-Romero P, Alvarez R, et al. Transcriptional expression of cis-acting and trans-acting splicing mutations cause autosomal dominant retinitis pigmentosa. Hum Mutat. 2008;29(6):869–78.
4. Martinez-Gimeno M, Gamundi MJ, Hernan I, Maseras M, Millá E, Ayuso C, et al. Mutations in the pre-mRNA splicing-factor genes PRPF3, PRPF8, and PRPF31 in Spanish families with autosomal dominant retinitis pigmentosa. Invest Ophthalmol Vis Sci. 2003;44(5):2171–7.
5. Sullivan LS, Bowne SJ, Birch DG, Hughbanks-Wheaton D, Heckenlively JR, Lewis RA, et al. Prevalence of disease-causing mutations in families with autosomal dominant retinitis pigmentosa: a screen of known genes in 200 families. Invest Ophthalmol Vis Sci. 2006;47(7):3052–64.
6. Vaclavik V, Gaillard MC, Tiab L, Schorderet DF, Munier FL. Variable phenotypic expressivity in a Swiss family with autosomal dominant retinitis pigmentosa due to a T494M mutation in the PRPF3 gene. Mol Vis. 2010;16:467–75.
7. Liu MM, Zack DJ. Alternative splicing and retinal degeneration. Clin Genet. 2013;84(2):142–9.
8. Wada Y, Itabashi T, Sato H, Tamai M. Clinical features of a Japanese family with autosomal dominant retinitis pigmentosa

S. Zahid et al., *Retinal Dystrophy Gene Atlas*, https://doi.org/10.1007/978-3-319-10867-4_61

associated with a Thr494Met mutation in the HPRP3 gene. Graefes Arch Clin Exp Ophthalmol. 2004;242(11):956–61.
9. Inglehearn CF, Tarttelin EE, Keen TJ, Bhattacharya SS, Moore AT, Taylor R, et al. A new dominant retinitis pigmentosa family mapping to the RP18 locus on chromosome 1q11-21. J Med Genet. 1998;35(9):788–9.
10. Xu SY, Schwartz M, Rosenberg T, Gal A. A ninth locus (RP18) for autosomal dominant retinitis pigmentosa maps in the pericentromeric region of chromosome 1. Hum Mol Genet. 1996;5(8):1193–7.

62 PRPF31

PRPF31 encodes U4/U6 small nuclear ribonucleoprotein Prp31, which is involved in mRNA splicing. Mutations in *PRPF31* cause 8–9% of autosomal dominant retinitis pigmentosa (adRP) (rod-cone dystrophy) [1–4].

Patients with adRP caused by *PRPF31* mutations present in the first-to-third decades with nyctalopia and reduced peripheral fields but generally maintain visual acuity until late in the disease course. *PRPF31* has incomplete penetrance, as many patients carrying the disease allele do not manifest signs of disease [3–6]. There is also a great deal of variable expressivity in *PRPF31*-related disease: even patients who carry the same mutations may exhibit variable phenotypes and disease severity [2]. There is evidence that this may be caused by haploinsufficiency (reduced levels of wild-type Prp31) and has led to a model of pathogenesis in which higher levels of normal protein are protective against disease [7, 8]. Co-occurrence of disease-causing alleles of *PRPF31* and *RHO* in a family has been reported [9].

Fundus findings are typical for RP, including peripheral bone spicule deposits and pigment mottling, optic disc pallor, and attenuated retinal vessels. As with other forms of RP, patients often develop CME and posterior sub-capsular cataracts [2, 10, 11]. OCT may reveal normal retinal lamination or exhibit CME, ERMs, or foveal thinning. FAF may reveal hypoautofluorescence outside the arcades with patchy loss of signal in the macula; there may be a perifoveal ring of hyperautofluorescence, or, rarely, hyperfluorescence at the fovea. Full-field ERG and GVF reveal a rod-cone pattern of degeneration, while multifocal ERG shows preservation of responses at the central hexagons (Figs. 62.1 and 62.2).

S. Zahid et al., *Retinal Dystrophy Gene Atlas*, https://doi.org/10.1007/978-3-319-10867-4_62

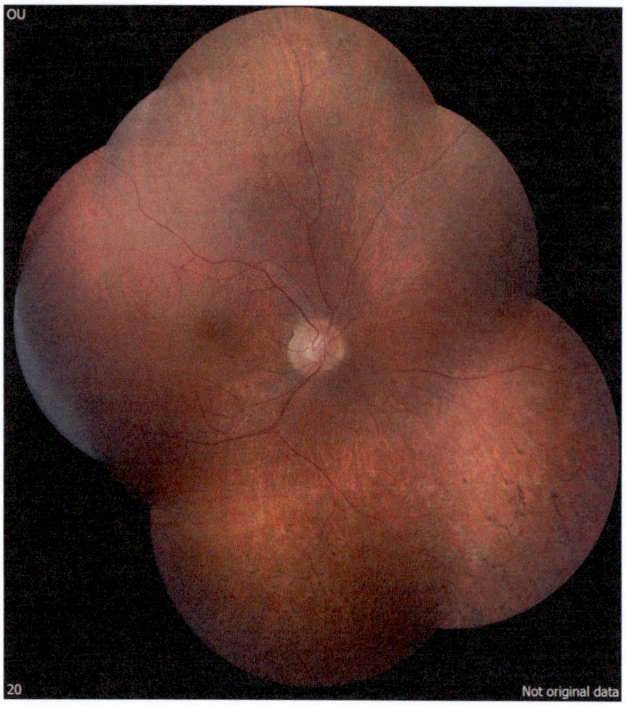

Fig. 62.1 Color fundus photograph from a 22-year-old man, showing attenuated retinal vasculature and midperipheral bone spicule pigment deposits.

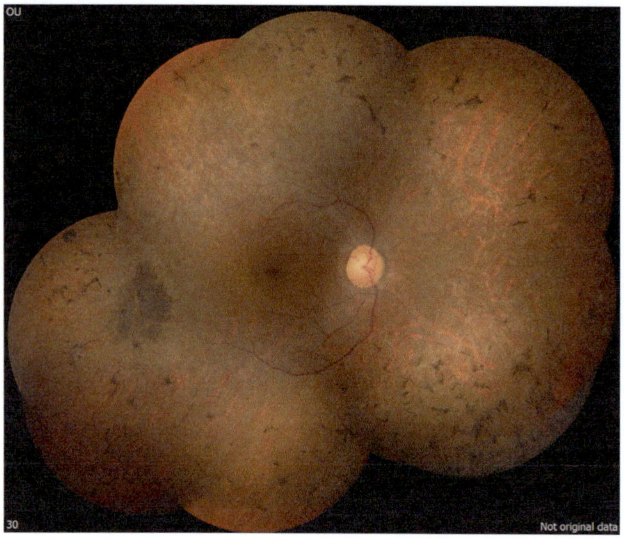

Fig. 62.2 Color fundus photograph from the 44-year-old mother of the patient in Fig. 62.1, showing attenuated retinal vasculature and more extensive midperipheral bone spicule pigment deposits.

References

1. Vithana EN, Abu-Safieh L, Allen MJ, Carey A, Papaioannou M, Chakarova C, et al. A human homolog of yeast pre-mRNA splicing gene, PRP31, underlies autosomal dominant retinitis pigmentosa on chromosome 19q13.4 (RP11). Mol Cell. 2001;8(2):375–81.
2. Waseem NH, Vaclavik V, Webster A, Jenkins SA, Bird AC, Bhattacharya SS. Mutations in the gene coding for the pre-mRNA splicing factor, PRPF31, in patients with autosomal dominant retinitis pigmentosa. Invest Ophthalmol Vis Sci. 2007;48(3):1330–4.
3. Al-Maghtheh M, Vithana E, Tarttelin E, Jay M, Evans K, Moore T, et al. Evidence for a major retinitis pigmentosa locus on 19q13.4 (RP11) and association with a unique bimodal expressivity phenotype. Am J Hum Genet. 1996;59(4):864–71.
4. Daiger SP, Bowne SJ, Sullivan LS, Blanton SH, Weinstock GM, Koboldt DC, et al. Application of next-generation sequencing to identify genes and mutations causing autosomal dominant retinitis pigmentosa (adRP). Adv Exp Med Biol. 2014;801:123–9.
5. Rio Frio T, McGee TL, Wade NM, Iseli C, Beckmann JS, Berson EL, et al. A single-base substitution within an intronic repetitive element causes dominant retinitis pigmentosa with reduced penetrance. Hum Mutat. 2009;30(9):1340–7.
6. Berson EL, Gouras P, Gunkel RD, Myrianthopoulos NC. Dominant retinitis pigmentosa with reduced penetrance. Arch Ophthalmol. 1969;81(2):226–34.
7. Rio Frio T, Wade NM, Ransijn A, Berson EL, Beckmann JS, Rivolta C. Premature termination codons in PRPF31 cause retinitis pigmentosa via haploinsufficiency due to nonsense-mediated mRNA decay. J Clin Invest. 2008;118(4):1519–31.
8. Rivolta C, McGee TL, Rio Frio T, Jensen RV, Berson EL, Dryja TP. Variation in retinitis pigmentosa-11 (PRPF31 or RP11) gene expression between symptomatic and asymptomatic patients with dominant RP11 mutations. Hum Mutat. 2006;27(7):644–53.
9. Lim KP, Yip SP, Cheung SC, Leung KW, Lam ST, To CH. Novel PRPF31 and PRPH2 mutations and co-occurrence of PRPF31 and RHO mutations in Chinese patients with retinitis pigmentosa. Arch Ophthalmol. 2009;127(6):784–90.
10. Utz VM, Beight CD, Marino MJ, Hagstrom SA, Traboulsi EI. Autosomal dominant retinitis pigmentosa secondary to pre-mRNA splicing-factor gene PRPF31 (RP11): review of disease mechanism and report of a family with a novel 3-base pair insertion. Ophthalmic Genet. 2013;34(4):183–8.
11. Audo I, Bujakowska K, Mohand-Said S, Lancelot ME, Moskova-Doumanova V, Waseem NH, et al. Prevalence and novelty of PRPF31 mutations in French autosomal dominant rod-cone dystrophy patients and a review of published reports. BMC Med Genet. 2010;11:145.

63 PRPF8

PRPF8 encodes pre-mRNA-processing-splicing factor 8, which interacts with the 5′ and 3′ ends of pre-mRNA molecules and plays a role in the assembly of spliceosome components onto pre-mRNA molecules. Mutations in *PRPF8* cause about 2–3% of autosomal dominant retinitis pigmentosa (rod-cone dystrophy) [1–10].

Patients present within the first-to-second decades of life with nyctalopia, usually followed by peripheral field loss. However, there is often significant phenotypic variability, even in family members carrying the same mutation [3–5]. For example, patients with the p.H2309P mutation were shown to exhibit an earlier age of onset (age of 6.6 years) than patients with the p.H2309R(10.7 years) and p. R2310K(22 years) mutations [3]. Visual acuity may be maintained until later in the disease course (e.g., in a family described in Walia et al, some members of the family retained visual better than 20/30 into their 40s while a few members had acuities as poor as 20/400 in their 20s [5]), though some patients may experience reductions in visual acuity as early as the second decade [4, 7]. Some mutations (p.R2310K) may exhibit a milder phenotype, with patients presenting as late as their forties and exhibiting better visual acuity over time [3].

As is typical for RP, patients may develop early-onset posterior subcapsular cataracts (Towns et al. reported 17 of 75 patients with cataracts [3], while Maubaret et al. [4] reported bilateral PCS cataracts in nearly half of their patients). Fundus findings usually feature diffuse bone-spicule pigment deposits and retinal vessel attenuation and may also show optic disc pallor with or without optic nerve drusen (Fig. 63.1a) [3, 5]. Like other forms of RP, cystoid macular edema (CME) is common (11 of 17 patients per Towns et al. [3]). Some patients may exhibit macular pigment clumping and RPE atrophy [3, 4]. FAF reveals areas of hypoautofluorescent RPE atrophy, usually beyond the arcades, while some patients may exhibit a hyperautofluorescent perifoveal ring in the macula (Fig. 63.1b) [4, 6]. Full-field ERG is often non-recordable; when detectable, it exhibits a rod-cone pattern of degeneration [6]. Dark adaptation thresholds are elevated. GVF testing exhibits a rod-cone pattern of field loss that ultimately leaves behind a central island of vision. OCT may reveal CME, thinning, and atrophy at the macula (Fig. 63.1c), or loss of the outer retinal layers at the fovea; the outer retinal layers and architecture are usually maintained within the confines of the macular hyperautofluorescent ring on FAF imaging [3, 4]. There is often significant phenotypic variability, even in family members carrying the same mutation [3–5]. Maubaret et al. [4] reported one patient who developed a monocular Coats-like retinal telangiectasia that caused vitreous hemorrhage in his mid-thirties; they also reported one mutation-carrying patient who reported only mild symptoms and did not manifest any clinical signs of disease.

S. Zahid et al., *Retinal Dystrophy Gene Atlas*, https://doi.org/10.1007/978-3-319-10867-4_63

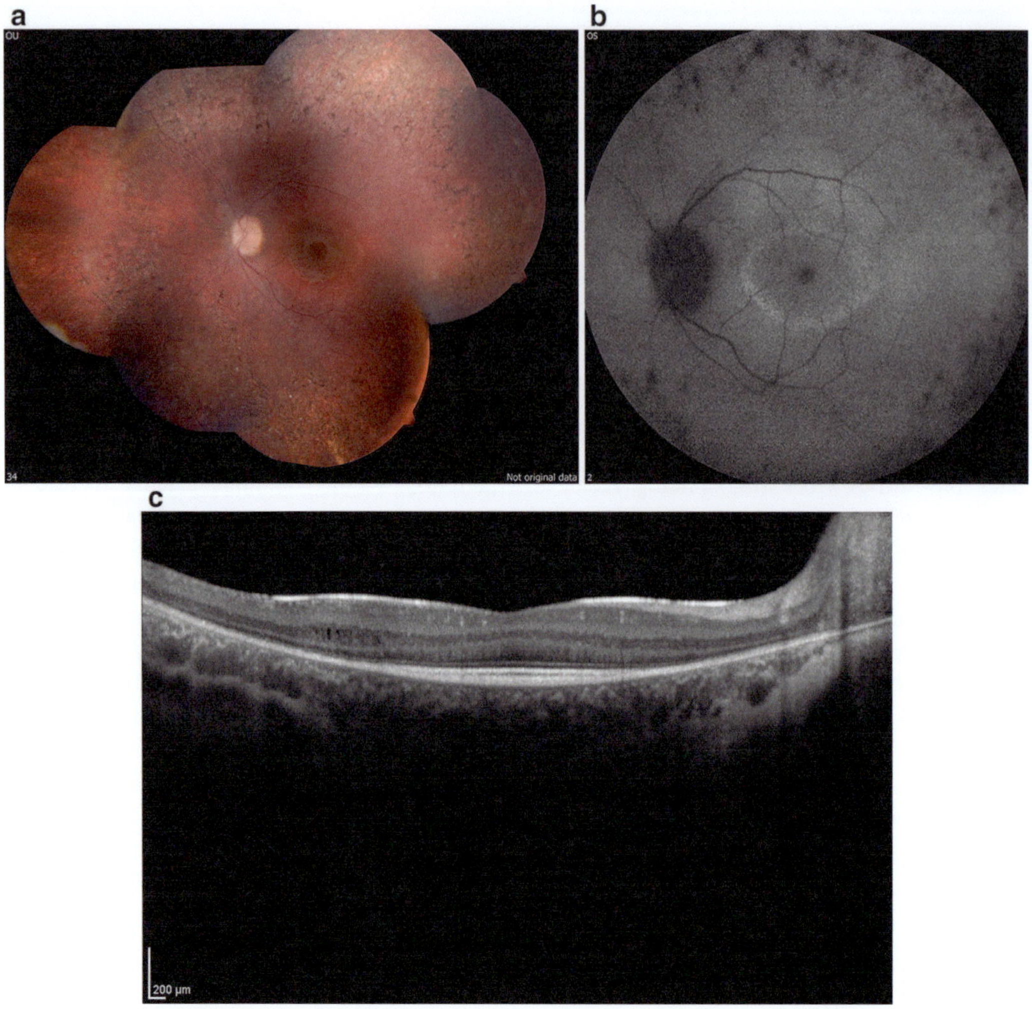

Fig. 63.1 Case summary: 10-year-old boy with retinitis pigmentosa (rod-cone dystrophy). (**a**) Color fundus photograph of the left eye, showing peripheral RPE atrophy with bone spicule pigment deposits and retinal vascular attenuation. (**b**) Fundus autofluorescence, showing a ring of hyperautofluorescence in the parafovea with midperipheral hypoautofluorescence corresponding to RPE loss and bone-spicule deposits. (**c**) Spectral domain optical coherence tomography, showing extensive loss of the ellipsoid zone and outer nuclear layer outside the central fovea, with a mild epiretinal membrane and with mild cystoid macular edema visible in the inner nuclear layer.

References

1. McKie AB, McHale JC, Keen TJ, Tarttelin EE, Goliath R, van Lith-Verhoeven JJ, et al. Mutations in the pre-mRNA splicing factor gene PRPC8 in autosomal dominant retinitis pigmentosa (RP13). Hum Mol Genet. 2001;10(15):1555–62.
2. Greenberg J, Goliath R, Beighton P, Ramesar R. A new locus for autosomal dominant retinitis pigmentosa on the short arm of chromosome 17. Hum Mol Genet. 1994;3(6):915–8.
3. Towns KV, Kipioti A, Long V, McKibbin M, Maubaret C, Vaclavik V, et al. Prognosis for splicing factor PRPF8 retinitis pigmentosa, novel mutations and correlation between human and yeast phenotypes. Hum Mutat. 2010;31(5):E1361–76.
4. Maubaret CG, Vaclavik V, Mukhopadhyay R, Waseem NH, Churchill A, Holder GE, et al. Autosomal dominant retinitis pigmentosa with intrafamilial variability and incomplete penetrance in two families carrying mutations in PRPF8. Invest Ophthalmol Vis Sci. 2011;52(13):9304–9.
5. Walia S, Fishman GA, Zernant-Rajang J, Raime K, Allikmets R. Phenotypic expression of a PRPF8 gene mutation in a Large African American family. Arch Ophthalmol. 2008;126(8):1127–32.
6. Testa F, Ziviello C, Rinaldi M, Rossi S, Di Iorio V, Interlandi E, et al. Clinical phenotype of an Italian family with a new mutation in the PRPF8 gene. Eur J Ophthalmol. 2006;16(5):779–81.
7. Martinez-Gimeno M, Gamundi MJ, Hernan I, Maseras M, Millá E, Ayuso C, et al. Mutations in the pre-mRNA splicing-factor genes PRPF3, PRPF8, and PRPF31 in Spanish families with autosomal dominant retinitis pigmentosa. Invest Ophthalmol Vis Sci. 2003;44(5):2171–7.
8. Sullivan LS, Bowne SJ, Birch DG, Hughbanks-Wheaton D, Heckenlively JR, Lewis RA, et al. Prevalence of disease-causing mutations in families with autosomal dominant retinitis pigmentosa: a screen of known genes in 200 families. Invest Ophthalmol Vis Sci. 2006;47(7):3052–64.
9. van Lith-Verhoeven JJ, van der Velde-Visser SD, Sohocki MM, Deutman AF, Brink HM, Cremers FP, et al. Clinical characterization, linkage analysis, and PRPC8 mutation analysis of a family with autosomal dominant retinitis pigmentosa type 13 (RP13). Ophthalmic Genet. 2002;23(1):1–12.
10. Daiger SP, Bowne SJ, Sullivan LS, Blanton SH, Weinstock GM, Koboldt DC, et al. Application of next-generation sequencing to identify genes and mutations causing autosomal dominant retinitis pigmentosa (adRP). Adv Exp Med Biol. 2014;801:123–9.

64 PRPH2 (RDS)

PRPH2 encodes a membrane protein involved in photoreceptor disc morphogenesis. There is significant inter- and intrafamilial phenotypic variability with *PRPH2* mutations dystrophy [1–4]. For example, mutations in this gene have been associated with dominant retinitis pigmentosa (including retinitis punctata albescens), pattern macular dystrophy, central areolar choroidal dystrophy (CACD), or cone-rod dystrophy [5–7].

Seven-and-a-half percent of dominant RP may be caused by *PRPH2* mutations, and there is significant phenotypic variability [8–11]. Patients present with abnormal night vision and progressively constricting peripheral vision in the third to fifth decades, though some mutations may present in the first to third decades [12]. Visual acuity is usually maintained until the fifth decade. The fundus typically resembles classical RP and features bone spicule pigment deposits, peripheral atrophy, disc pallor, and vascular attenuation. ERG and GVF reveal a rod-cone pattern of degeneration. Dark adaptation thresholds are elevated, and color vision is usually normal. Some studies have reported patients with dominant RP who exhibit a maculopathy, which may range from a bull's-eye lesion to atrophy [4, 13–15]. This subset of patients may exhibit extinguished electroretingram (ERG) parameters as early as the second decade (Fig. 64.1).

PRPH2 mutations have also been associated with a phenotype resembling retinitis punctata albescens (RPA), which is characterized by distinctive white round deposits present diffusely throughout the retina, with progressive vessel attenuation (Figs. 64.2a–c and 64.3a, b) [16, 17]. Kajiwara et al found their patients to have a predominant rod photoreceptor degeneration [18].

PRPH2 mutations can also cause macular pattern dystrophies, which are a diverse group of diseases characterized by deposits, pigment, and/or atrophy in the macula [19–22]. *PRPH2* mutations have been associated with adult-onset foveomacular vitelliform dystrophy (AOFVD), butterfly-shaped pattern dystrophy, and multifocal pattern dystrophy resembling *ABCA4*-related disease [23–25]. Onset of disease is variable, but many patients are asymptomatic until their 50s [5]. Central vision is lost gradually with time; many patients (up to 50%) exhibit severe vision loss because of atrophy or choroidal neovascularization [5, 20]. Fluorescein angiography can be helpful in distinguishing between different types of pattern dystrophy [26]. Importantly, a dark choroid may not be not observed with pattern dystrophies associated with *PRPH2* mutations [26]. AOFVD typically illustrates bilateral round yellow-white subretinal lesions with central pigmentation in the macula (Figs. 64.4, 64.5, 64.6, and 64.7). These appear bright on fundus autofluorescence (FAF) due to lipofuscin accumulation and dark on fluorescein angiography (FA) (surrounded by a bright ring) [23]. Optical coherence tomography (OCT) can be useful in delineating the lesion. AOFVD may be confused with Best vitelliform macular dystrophy but may be distinguished by a normal electro-oculogram (EOG) [23]. AOFVD typically exhibits a normal full-field ERG. In butterfly-shaped pattern dystrophy, the fundus is characterized by a spoked "butterfly-shaped" pigment deposit at the center of the macula, surrounded by depigmentation (Figs. 64.6 and 64.7) [20]. The lesion may have regions of low and high autofluorescence on FAF, while FA reveals hypofluorescence in areas with pigment deposits and elevated signal in areas with depigmentation and atrophy. Full-field ERG is usually normal, but, unlike AOFVD, color vision and the EOG are abnormal. Multifocal pattern dystrophy (MPD) resembles *ABCA4*-related disease in many ways [26, 27]. The flecks seen in MPD greatly resemble the yellow flecks in the macula and beyond the arcades frequently seen in *ABCA4*-related disease (Fig. 64.1a, b). Differences include a later onset of disease and a dominant inheritance pattern. The appearance of the macula ranges from pigmentary abnormalities and deposits to atrophy; some patients may exhibit AOFVD or butterfly lesions early in the disease course. As with *ABCA4*-related disease, flecks are hyperautofluorescent on FAF and FA (Fig. 64.1b). A dark choroid is usually not observed, but Kim et al. [28] reported one case of MPD with a dark choroid and CNV. Patients may develop atrophy at the macula, which may result in more diffuse posterior pole atrophy. MPD patients may experience night blindness, but central vision deficits

S. Zahid et al., *Retinal Dystrophy Gene Atlas*, https://doi.org/10.1007/978-3-319-10867-4_64

may also be present; they typically exhibit progressively deteriorating retinal function on GVF and ERG (either mixed, rod-cone or cone-rod), which is unique among pattern dystrophies [29]. As with MPD patients exhibiting vitelliform or butterfly lesions early in the disease, some patients may progress from one class of pattern dystrophy to another class; there are also reports of interocular phenotypic asymmetry.

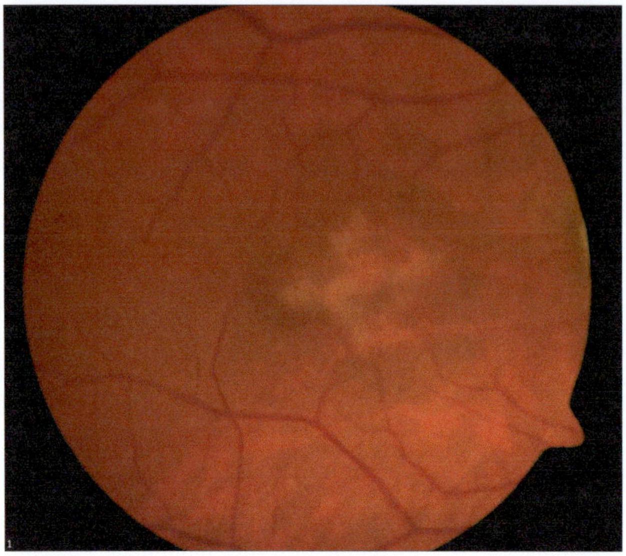

Fig. 64.1 Color fundus photograph of the right eye from a 51-year-old female with a pattern dystrophy, showing a butterfly pattern.

PRPH2 mutations also cause CACD, in which patients present in their 30s to 40s (later with some mutations) with reduced visual acuity, metamorphopsia, or photophobia [30]. Some mutations (e.g. p.Arg172Trp) are associated with significant phenotypic variability, with variable penetrance and expressivity (with reports of cone-rod dystrophy, ADRP, and CACD observed within the same family), while others exhibit a more consistent phenotype [3, 4]. The p.Arg172Trp mutation may exhibit a worse visual prognosis than other mutations [2]. Funduscopic findings range from subtle pigmentary changes early in life to areas of well-defined atrophy (broken into stages I–IV) that eventually include the fovea and optic disc in the late stages. Bull's-eye maculopathy has also been reported with CACD. As with other macular degenerative diseases, FAF and FA are useful to define the extent of retinal atrophy. FAF ranges from patchy increases in autofluorescence to hypoautofluorescent confluent areas reflecting atrophy that may resemble the late atrophic stages of dry AMD. ERG may be normal or may exhibit a cone or cone-rod pattern of degeneration in the late stages of disease. Given that this is a disease affecting the macula, multifocal and pattern ERG are frequently abnormal.

Mutation in *PRPH2* may also cause an autosomal dominant maculopathy that is similar to age-related macular degeneration (AMD) (named "AMD-like late-onset maculopathy") [31]. Patients present during the fifth decade with reduced visual acuity and may exhibit features of dry AMD

a b

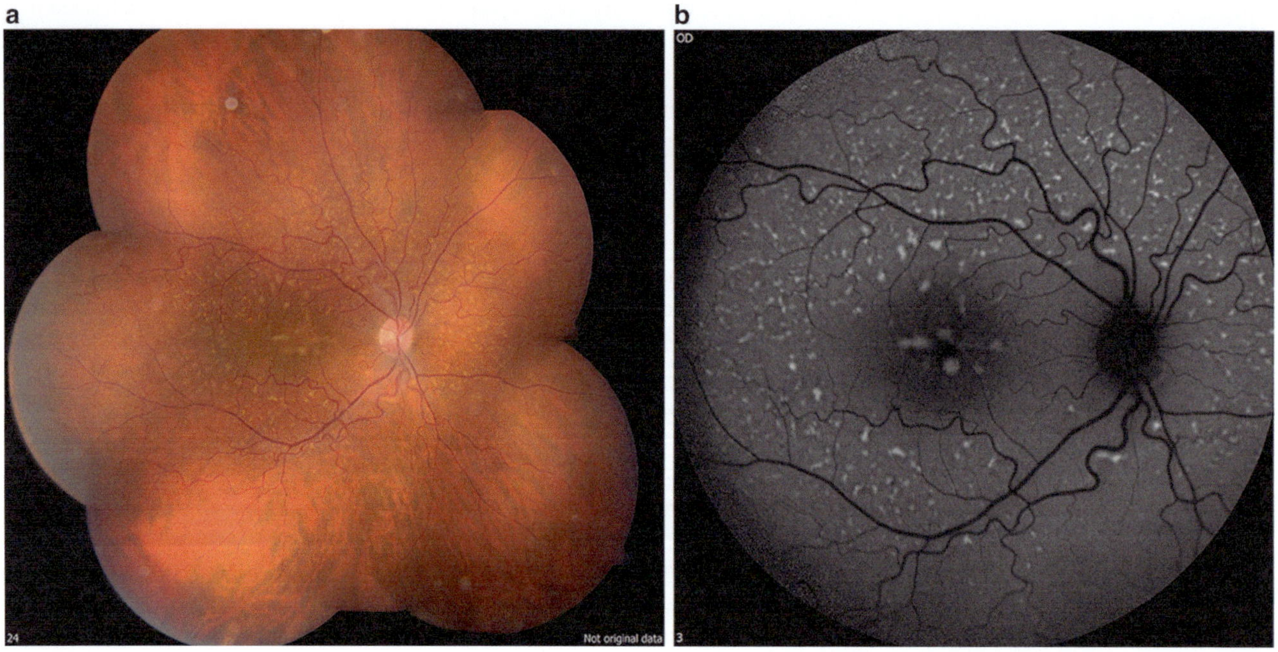

Fig. 64.2 Case summary: 37-year-old man with a multifocal pattern dystrophy. (**a**) Montage color fundus photo of the right eye, showing a multifocal pattern dystrophy resembling the pisciform flecks of Stargardt disease in the macula and along the vascular arcades. (**b**) Fundus autofluorescence of the right eye, showing hyperautofluorescence in the areas with fleck-like deposits.

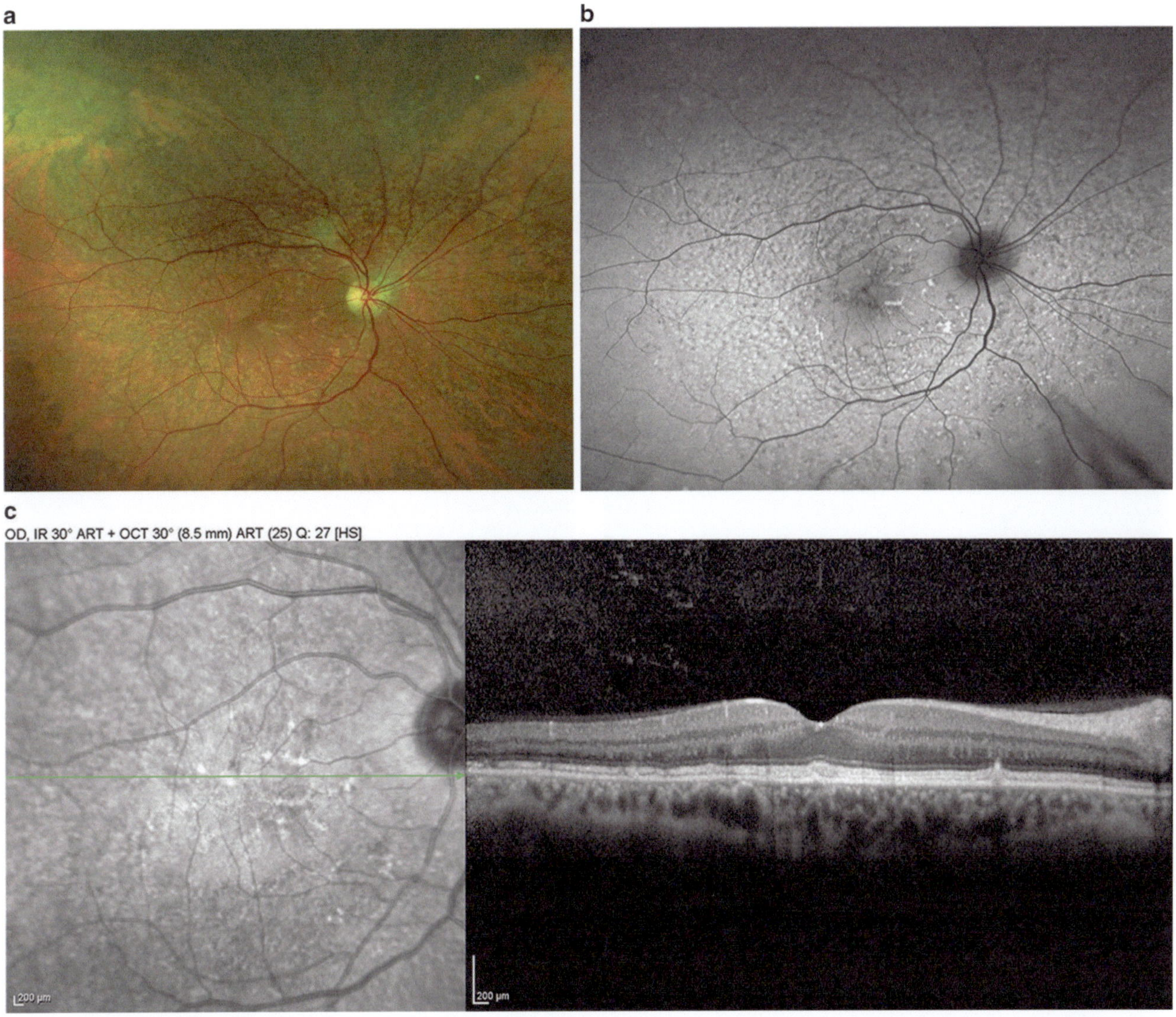

Fig. 64.3 Case summary: 51-year-old man with retinitis punctata albescens (RPA). (**a**) Color fundus photograph of the right eye showing diffuse white round deposits in the fundus. (**b**) Fundus autofluorescence of the right eye showing areas of hypo- and hyperautofluorescence associated with the white deposits. (**c**) Spectral-domain optical coherence tomography of the right eye, showing an overall maintained retinal architecture without ellipsoid loss, with deposits localized to the subretinal space.

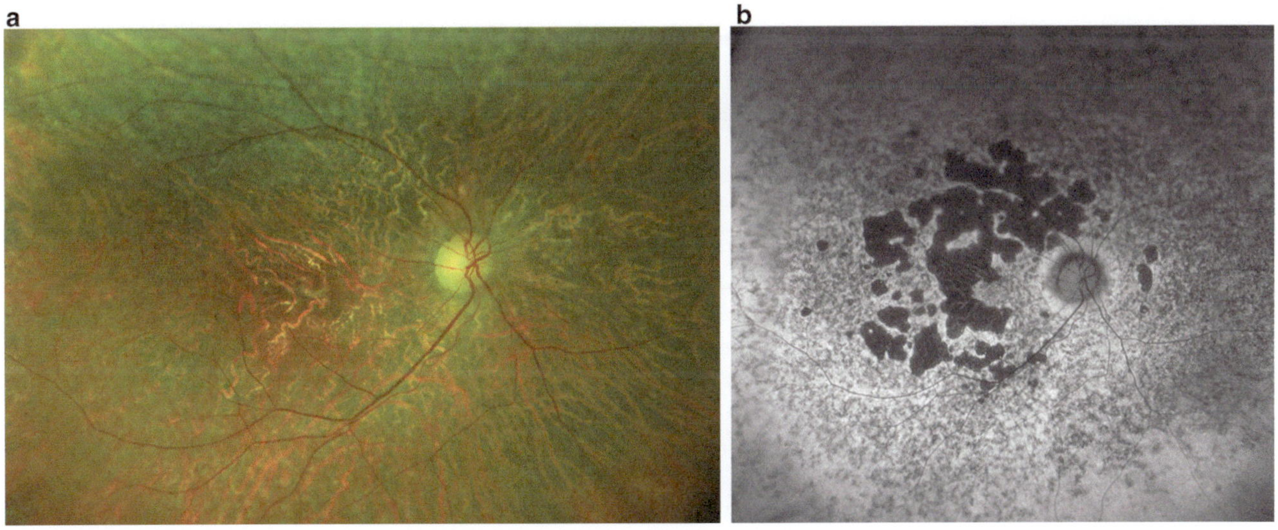

Fig. 64.4 Case summary: 74-year-old mother of the patient in Fig. 64.1 with advanced RPA. (**a**) Color fundus photograph of the right eye, showing RPE atrophy in the macula with white deposits visible throughout the posterior pole. (**b**) Fundus autofluorescence of the right eye, showing areas of hypo- and hyperautofluorescence associated with the white deposits as well as hypoautofluorescence in the macula corresponding to the areas of atrophy.

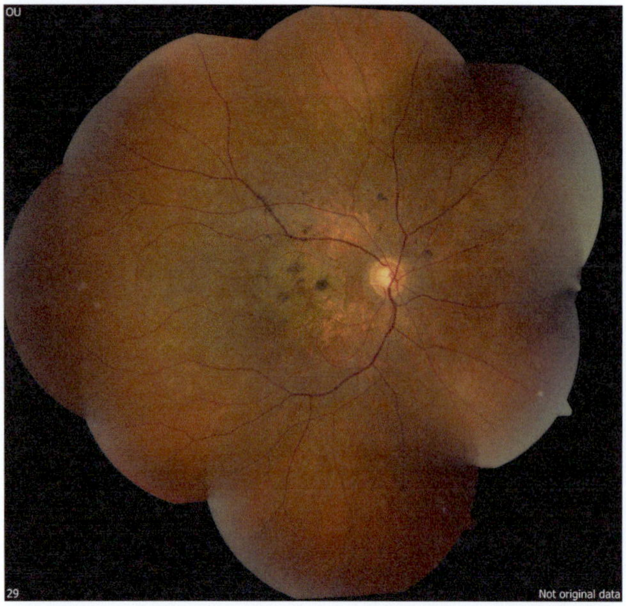

Fig. 64.5 Color fundus photograph of the right eye from a 62-year-old man with pattern dystrophy, showing the late stage of a butterfly pattern and macular atrophy with hyperpigmented spots.

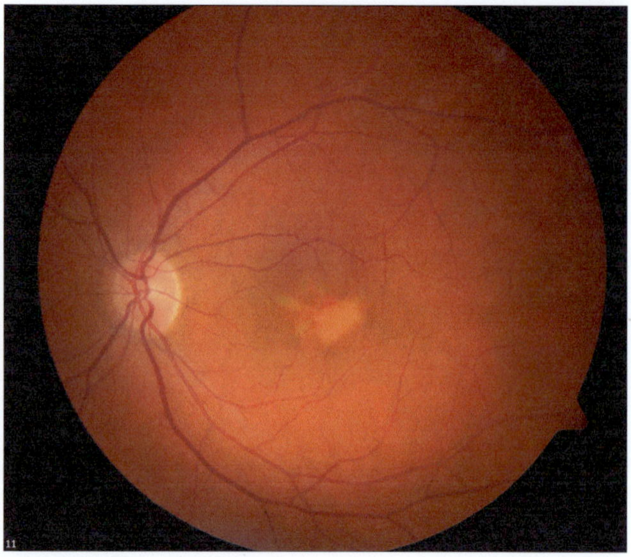

Fig. 64.6 Color fundus photograph of the left eye of a 51-year-old woman with a pattern dystrophy.

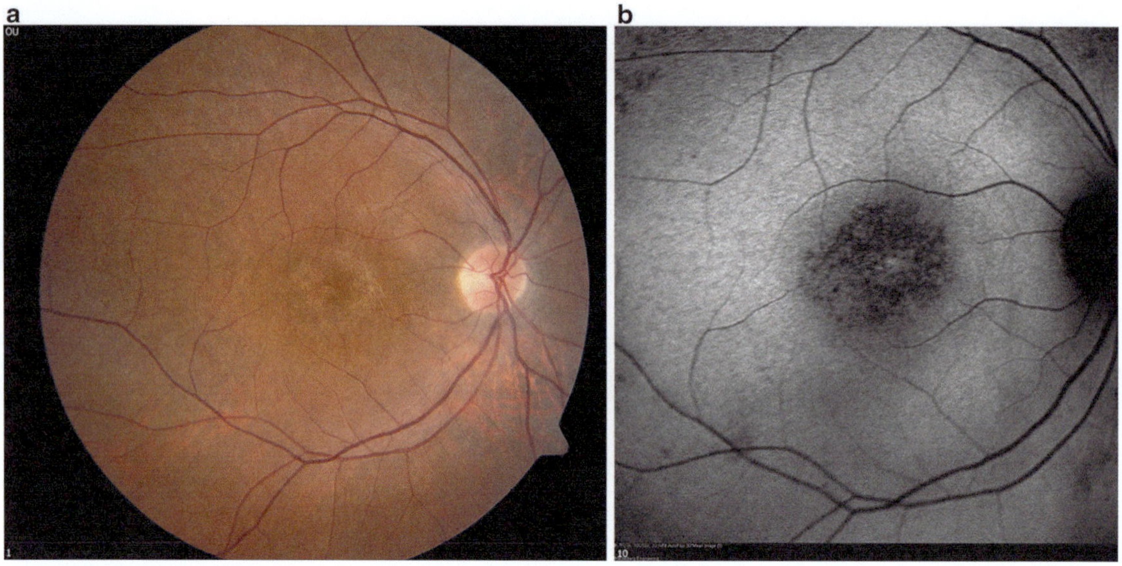

Fig. 64.7 Case summary: 37-year-old man with cone-rod dystrophy. (**a**) Color fundus photograph of the right eye, showing a macular bull's eye lesion and patchy RPE pigmentary changes within the arcades. (**b**) Fundus autofluorescence of the right eye, showing hypoautofluorescence at the macula in the areas with atrophy.

(drusen, geographic atrophy, etc.) or wet AMD (CNV, hemorrhage). FAF may be useful to detect the extent of atrophy; FA is useful to reveal the exudative changes of wet AMD associated with *PRPH2* mutations.

Dominant cone-rod dystrophy has also been shown to be caused by mutations in *PRPH2* [32]. Patients present in their 20s to 40s with reduced visual acuity with or without nyctalopia, abnormal color vision, and photophobia; peripheral vision is lost gradually later in the disease course. As with many other cone-rod dystrophies, the fundus is characterized by changes at the macula that range from mild pigmentary changes, to bull's eye maculopathy, to atrophy (Fig. 64.5a). FAF may range from patchy increases in hyperautofluorescence early in the disease to areas of hypoautofluorescence later in the disease course (Fig. 64.5b). Full-field ERG reveals a cone-rod pattern of degeneration [29]. Similar to CACD and pattern dystrophies, the pattern ERG is abnormal.

References

1. Renner AB, Fiebig BS, Weber BH, Wissinger B, Andreasson S, Gal A, et al. Phenotypic variability and long-term follow-up of patients with known and novel PRPH2/RDS gene mutations. Am J Ophthalmol. 2009;147(3):518–30. e511
2. Anand S, Sheridan E, Cassidy F, Inglehearn C, Williams G, Springell K, et al. Macular dystrophy associated with the Arg172Trp substitution in peripherin/RDS: genotype-phenotype correlation. Retina. 2009;29(5):682–8.
3. Wells J, Wroblewski J, Keen J, Inglehearn C, Jubb C, Eckstein A, et al. Mutations in the human retinal degeneration slow (RDS) gene can cause either retinitis pigmentosa or macular dystrophy. Nat Genet. 1993;3(3):213–8.
4. Nakazawa M, Kikawa E, Kamio K, Chida Y, Shiono T, Tamai M. Ocular findings in patients with autosomal dominant retinitis pigmentosa and transversion mutation in codon 244 (Asn244Lys) of the peripherin/RDS gene. Arch Ophthalmol. 1994;112(12):1567–73.
5. Boon CJ, den Hollander AI, Hoyng CB, Cremers FP, Klevering BJ, Keunen JE. The spectrum of retinal dystrophies caused by mutations in the peripherin/RDS gene. Prog Retin Eye Res. 2008;27(2):213–35.
6. Keen TJ, Inglehearn CF. Mutations and polymorphisms in the human peripherin-RDS gene and their involvement in inherited retinal degeneration. Hum Mutat. 1996;8(4):297–303.
7. Kohl S, Christ-Adler M, Apfelstedt-Sylla E, Kellner U, Eckstein A, Zrenner E, et al. RDS/peripherin gene mutations are frequent causes of central retinal dystrophies. J Med Genet. 1997;34(8):620–6.
8. Daiger SP, Bowne SJ, Sullivan LS, Blanton SH, Weinstock GM, Koboldt DC, et al. Application of next-generation sequencing to identify genes and mutations causing autosomal dominant retinitis pigmentosa (adRP). Adv Exp Med Biol. 2014;801:123–9.
9. Kalyanasundaram TS, Black GC, O'Sullivan J, Bishop PN. A novel peripherin/RDS mutation resulting in a retinal dystrophy with phenotypic variation. Eye (Lond). 2009;23(1):237–9.
10. Farrar GJ, Kenna P, Jordan SA, Kumar-Singh R, Humphries MM, Sharp EM, et al. A three-base-pair deletion in the peripherin-RDS gene in one form of retinitis pigmentosa. Nature. 1991;354(6353):478–80.
11. Gruning G, Millan JM, Meins M, Beneyto M, Caballero M, Apfelstedt-Sylla E, et al. Mutations in the human peripherin/RDS gene associated with autosomal dominant retinitis pigmentosa. Hum Mutat. 1994;3(3):321–3.
12. Bareil C, Delague V, Arnaud B, Demaille J, Hamel C, Claustres M. W179R: a novel missense mutation in the peripherin/RDS gene in a family with autosomal dominant retinitis pigmentosa. Hum Mutat. 2000;15(6):583–4.
13. Richards SC, Creel DJ. Pattern dystrophy and retinitis pigmentosa caused by a peripherin/RDS mutation. Retina. 1995;15(1):68–72.
14. Bareil C, Hamel C, Arnaud B, Demaille J, Claustres M. A complex allele (1064delTC and IVS2 + 22ins7) in the peripherin/RDS gene in retinitis pigmentosa with macular dystrophy. Ophthalmic Genet. 1997;18(3):129–38.
15. Kikawa E, Nakazawa M, Chida Y, Shiono T, Tamai M. A novel mutation (Asn244Lys) in the peripherin/RDS gene causing autosomal dominant retinitis pigmentosa associated with bull's-eye maculopathy detected by nonradioisotopic SSCP. Genomics. 1994;20(1):137–9.
16. Apfelstedt-Sylla E, Theischen M, Ruther K, Wedemann H, Gal A, Zrenner E. Extensive intrafamilial and interfamilial phenotypic variation among patients with autosomal dominant retinal dystrophy and mutations in the human RDS/peripherin gene. Br J Ophthalmol. 1995;79(1):28–34.
17. Jacobson SG, Cideciyan AV, Kemp CM, Sheffield VC, Stone EM. Photoreceptor function in heterozygotes with insertion or deletion mutations in the RDS gene. Invest Ophthalmol Vis Sci. 1996;37(8):1662–74.
18. Kajiwara K, Sandberg MA, Berson EL, Dryja TP. A null mutation in the human peripherin/RDS gene in a family with autosomal dominant retinitis punctata albescens. Nat Genet. 1993;3(3):208–12.
19. Grover S, Fishman GA, Stone EM. Atypical presentation of pattern dystrophy in two families with peripherin/RDS mutations. Ophthalmology. 2002;109(6):1110–7.
20. Zhang K, Garibaldi DC, Li Y, Green WR, Zack DJ. Butterfly-shaped pattern dystrophy: a genetic, clinical, and histopathological report. Arch Ophthalmol. 2002;120(4):485–90.
21. Francis PJ, Schultz DW, Gregory AM, Schain MB, Barra R, Majewski J, et al. Genetic and phenotypic heterogeneity in pattern dystrophy. Br J Ophthalmol. 2005;89(9):1115–9.
22. Michaelides M, Hunt DM, Moore AT. The genetics of inherited macular dystrophies. J Med Genet. 2003;40(9):641–50.
23. Renner AB, Tillack H, Kraus H, Kohl S, Wissinger B, Mohr N, et al. Morphology and functional characteristics in adult vitelliform macular dystrophy. Retina. 2004;24(6):929–39.
24. Nichols BE, Drack AV, Vandenburgh K, Kimura AE, Sheffield VC, Stone EM. A 2 base pair deletion in the RDS gene associated with butterfly-shaped pigment dystrophy of the fovea. Hum Mol Genet. 1993;2(5):601–3.
25. Felbor U, Schilling H, Weber BH. Adult vitelliform macular dystrophy is frequently associated with mutations in the peripherin/RDS gene. Hum Mutat. 1997;10(4):301–9.
26. Boon CJ, van Schooneveld MJ, den Hollander AI, van Lith-Verhoeven JJ, Zonneveld-Vrieling MN, Theelen T, et al. Mutations in the peripherin/RDS gene are an important cause of multifocal pattern dystrophy simulating STGD1/fundus flavimaculatus. Br J Ophthalmol. 2007;91(11):1504–11.
27. Weigell-Weber M, Kryenbuhl C, Buchi ER, Spiegel R. Genetic heterogeneity in autosomal dominant pattern dystrophy of the retina. Mol Vis. 1996;2:6.
28. Kim RY, Dollfus H, Keen TJ, Fitzke FW, Arden GB, Bhattacharya SS, et al. Autosomal dominant pattern dystrophy of the retina associated with a 4-base pair insertion at codon 140 in the peripherin/RDS gene. Arch Ophthalmol. 1995;113:451–5.
29. Cideciyan AV. In vivo assessment of photoreceptor function in human diseases caused by photoreceptor-specific gene mutations. Methods Enzymol. 2000;316:611–26.
30. Boon CJ, Klevering BJ, Cremers FP, Zonneveld-Vrieling MN, Theelen T, Den Hollander AI, et al. Central areolar choroidal dystrophy. Ophthalmology. 2009;116(4):771–82, 782 e771.
31. Khani SC, Karoukis AJ, Young JE, Ambasudhan R, Burch T, Stockton R, et al. Late-onset autosomal dominant macular dystrophy with choroidal neovascularization and nonexudative maculopathy associated with mutation in the RDS gene. Invest Ophthalmol Vis Sci. 2003;44(8):3570–7.
32. Nakazawa M, Kikawa E, Chida Y, Wada Y, Shiono T, Tamai M. Autosomal dominant cone-rod dystrophy associated with mutations in codon 244 (Asn244His) and codon 184 (Tyr184Ser) of the peripherin/RDS gene. Arch Ophthalmol. 1996;114(1):72–8.
33. Michaelides M, Holder GE, Bradshaw K, Hunt DM, Moore AT. Cone-rod dystrophy, intrafamilial variability, and incomplete penetrance associated with the R172W mutation in the peripherin/RDS gene. Ophthalmology. 2005;112(9):1592–8.

65 RDH12

RDH12 encodes retinol dehydrogenase, which reduces 9-cis and all-*trans*-retinol in the retina. Mutations in *RDH12* may cause a spectrum of disease, ranging from autosomal recessive Leber congenital amaurosis (LCA), which classically begins within the first year of life, to early-onset retinitis pigmentosa (rod-cone dystrophy), which starts within the first decade [1–5]. Given the phenotypic overlap between autosomal recessive LCA and early-onset rod-cone dystrophy, it may be more useful to see these diseases as part of the same spectrum of differential disease severity. There has also been a report of autosomal dominant retinitis pigmentosa associated with a mutation in *RDH12* [6].

Homozygous or compound heterozygous mutations in *RDH12* cause about 4% of LCA, in which patients present with poor vision within the first year of life [1, 6]. Visual acuity is reduced at an early age, and some patients may exhibit nyctalopia, pendular nystagmus, early-onset posterior subcapsular cataracts, and/or color vision abnormalities. Walia et al. reported that these patients exhibit visual acuities ranging from 20/63 to 20/200 (average 20/125) [7]. These patients exhibit extensive mid-peripheral bone spicule pigment deposits, RPE atrophy, waxy pallor of the optic disc, and retinal vessel attenuation (Fig. 65.1a). Some patients may have a "beaten bronze" appearance of the fundus or macular atrophy (Figs. 65.2a, 65.3a, and 65.4a) [6]. The ERG has been reported to become nonrecordable at as early as 4 years of age in one study and reveals severe pan-retinal dysfunction in both rods and cones when recordable [8]. GVF may reveal defects ranging from no residual visual field, only temporal islands remaining, or a central scotoma with scattered surrounding scotomata. A monocular Coats-like reaction has been reported in some patients [1, 9].

Some patients may present within the first decade with a clinical picture resembling early onset RP [2, 6, 10]. These patients experience nyctalopia (19% overall) [10] and visual field constriction (22% overall) [10] at an early age, which progress with time. Visual acuity in these patients is typically better than patients with the LCA phenotype described above and may exhibit mild improvement before deteriorating further [2, 10]. Walia et al. [7] reported the median VA in these patients to be 20/80 (at a mean age of 18), with 87.5% of patients having acuities better than 20/200. Fundus findings feature peripheral pigment deposits that eventually progress to a large area of macular atrophy later in the disease process. Cystoid macular edema (CME) and optic atrophy have been reported [11]. Some patients may exhibit para-arteriolar sparing of the retinal pigment epithelium [10]. FAF reveals hypoautofluorescence in areas of atrophy, such as the macula, but may also exhibit foveal hyperautofluorescence in some patients; the intervening areas between atrophic regions and the peripapillary region may also exhibit hyperautofluorescence (Figs. 65.2b, 65.3b, and 65.4b) [10]. Optical coherence tomography is helpful to visualize the extent of photoreceptor and retinal pigment epithelium loss (Fig. 65.2c and 65.3c). Full-field ERG shows severely reduced values in both rod and cone parameters when recordable [9]. GVF usually reveals bilateral constriction of peripheral fields [9], but some patients may show central scotomas or undetectable fields [8].

Autosomal dominant retinitis pigmentosa has also been reported with a mutation in *RDH12* [12]. Patients in this family presented at an average age of 28, ranging from 12 to 43 years. Visual acuity was maintained into the eighth decade. Fundus findings featured classical RP, with diffuse peripheral to mid-peripheral bone spicule deposits and RPE atrophy, vessel attenuation, and macular sparing.

S. Zahid et al., *Retinal Dystrophy Gene Atlas*, https://doi.org/10.1007/978-3-319-10867-4_65

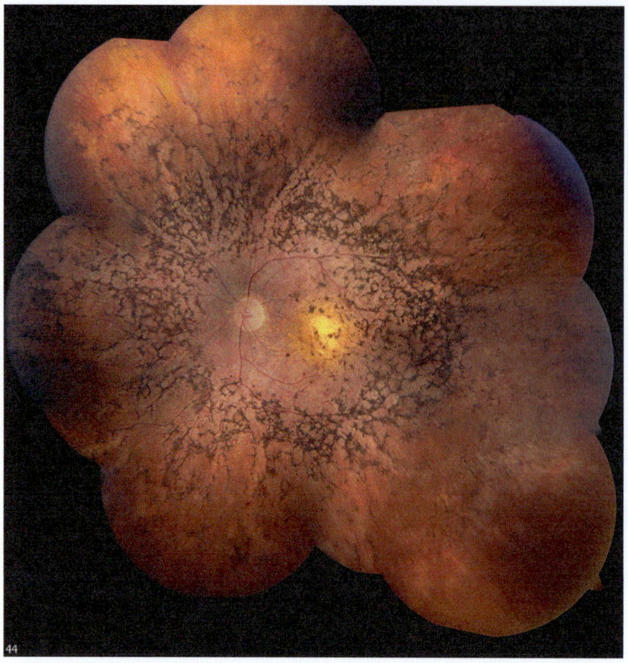

Fig. 65.1 Color fundus photograph of the left eye from a 28-year old woman with a history of juvenile-onset RP, demonstrating optic disc pallor, vessel attenuation, macular atrophy, and peripheral pigment deposition (densest in the mid-periphery outside the arcades).

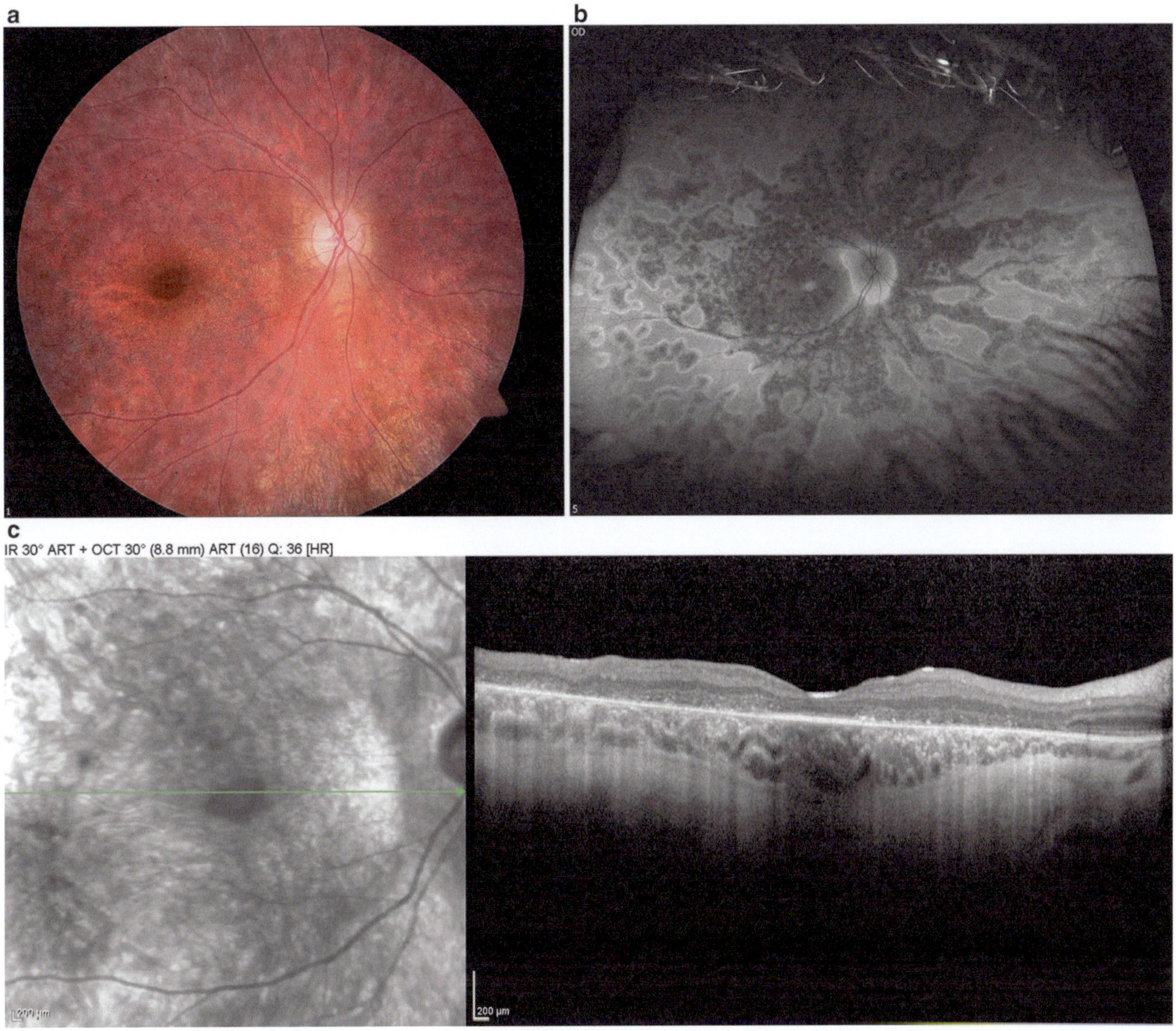

Fig. 65.2 Case summary: 11-year-old male with Leber congenital amaurosis (**a**) Color fundus photograph of the right eye, showing retinal pigment epithelium atrophy in the macula and outside the arcades and beaten bronze appearance of the macula. (**b**) Fundus autofluorescence, showing radial hypoautofluorescent regions in areas of RPE atrophy, each with a surrounding band of hyperautofluorescence. There is also foveal hyperfluorescence, as well as hyperfluorescence in the residual RPE around the optic nerve head. (**c**) Spectral domain-optical coherence tomography (SD-OCT), showing extensive loss of the ellipsoid zone (EZ) and the outer nuclear layer (ONL) band, as well as a faint epiretinal membrane, with hyperreflective deposits above the RPE.

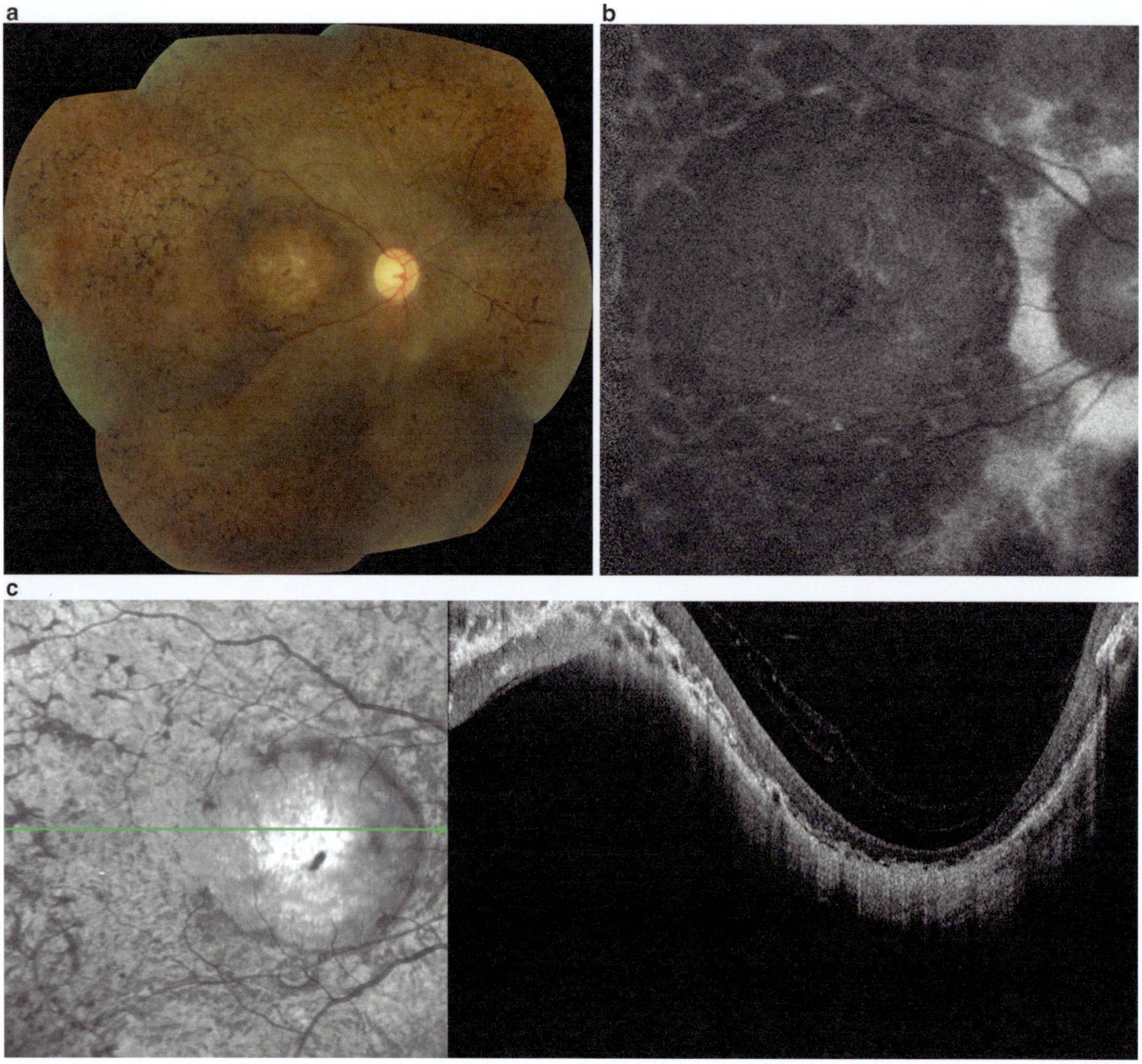

Fig. 65.3 Case summary: 27-year-old with LCA, onset at birth, visual acuity 1.6 logMAR (20/800 Snellen). (**a**) Color fundus photograph of the right eye, showing retinal vessel attenuation, extensive chorioretinal atrophy in the macula (with staphyloma), atrophy outside the arcades with bone spicule pigment deposits, as well as peripapillary atrophy. (**b**) Fundus autofluorescence imaging shows diffuse hypoautofluorescence regions in areas of atrophy (including the macula), with residual autofluorescence in the intervening regions. There is also hyperfluorescence in the residual RPE around the optic nerve head outside the area of peripapillary atrophy. (**c**) Spectral domain-OCT of the macula, showing a staphyloma in the setting of extensive outer retinal atrophy, with loss of the EZ and ONL band as well as the RPE band in some areas.

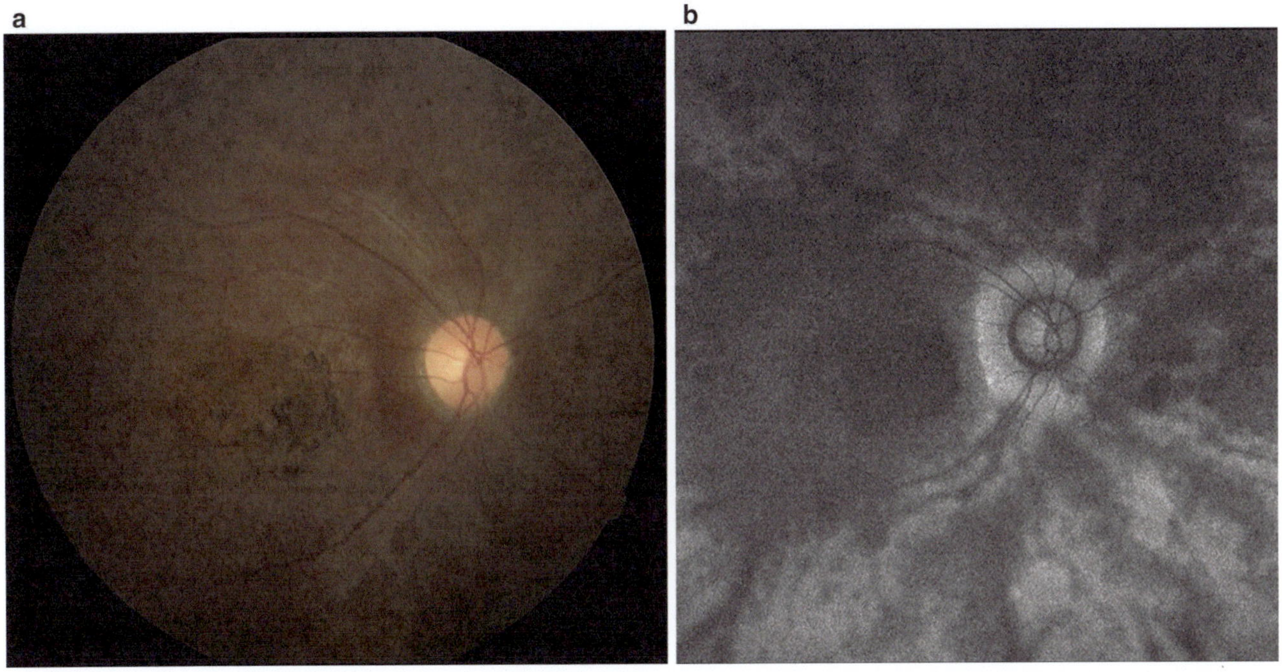

Fig. 65.4 Case summary: 3-year-old Hispanic female (CEI24625). (**a**) Color fundus photograph of the right eye, showing retinal vessel attenuation, macular atrophy with pigment deposition, RPE depigmentation and atrophy inside and outside the arcades, and peripapillary atrophy. (**b**) Fundus autofluorescence, showing diffuse hypoautofluorescence regions in areas of atrophy (including the macula), with residual autofluorescence in the intervening regions. Again, there is hyperautofluorescence at the border of the residual RPE around the optic nerve head surrounding the area of hypoautofluorescent peripapillary atrophy.

References

1. Janecke AR, Thompson DA, Utermann G, Becker C, Hübner CA, Schmid E, et al. Mutations in RDH12 encoding a photoreceptor cell retinol dehydrogenase cause childhood-onset severe retinal dystrophy. Nat Genet. 2004;36(8):850–4.
2. Perrault I, Hanein S, Gerber S, Barbet F, Ducroq D, Dollfus H, et al. Retinal dehydrogenase 12 (RDH12) mutations in leber congenital amaurosis. Am J Hum Genet. 2004;75(4):639–46.
3. Thompson DA, Janecke AR, Lange J, Feathers KL, Hübner CA, McHenry CL, et al. Retinal degeneration associated with RDH12 mutations results from decreased 11-cis retinal synthesis due to disruption of the visual cycle. Hum Mol Genet. 2005;14(24):3865–75.
4. Benayoun L, Spiegel R, Auslender N, Abbasi AH, Rizel L, Hujeirat Y, et al. Genetic heterogeneity in two consanguineous families segregating early onset retinal degeneration: the pitfalls of homozygosity mapping. Am J Med Genet A. 2009;149A(4):650–6.
5. Avila-Fernandez A, Cantalapiedra D, Aller E, Vallespín E, Aguirre-Lambán J, Blanco-Kelly F, et al. Mutation analysis of 272 Spanish families affected by autosomal recessive retinitis pigmentosa using a genotyping microarray. Mol Vis. 2010;16:2550–8.
6. Sodi A, Caputo R, Passerini I, Bacci GM, Menchini U. Novel RDH12 sequence variations in Leber congenital amaurosis. J AAPOS. 2010;14(4):349–51.
7. Walia S, Fishman GA, Jacobson SG, Aleman TS, Koenekoop RK, Traboulsi EI, et al. Visual acuity in patients with Leber's congenital amaurosis and early childhood-onset retinitis pigmentosa. Ophthalmology. 2010;117(6):1190–8.
8. Valverde D, Pereiro I, Vallespin E, Ayuso C, Borrego S, Baiget M. Complexity of phenotype-genotype correlations in Spanish patients with RDH12 mutations. Invest Ophthalmol Vis Sci. 2009;50(3):1065–8.
9. Schuster A, Janecke AR, Wilke R, Schmid E, Thompson DA, Utermann G, et al. The phenotype of early-onset retinal degeneration in persons with RDH12 mutations. Invest Ophthalmol Vis Sci. 2007;48(4):1824–31.
10. Mackay DS, Dev Borman A, Moradi P, Henderson RH, Li Z, Wright GA, et al. RDH12 retinopathy: novel mutations and phenotypic description. Mol Vis. 2011;17:2706–16.
11. Sun W, Gerth C, Maeda A, Lodowski DT, Van Der Kraak L, Saperstein DA, et al. Novel RDH12 mutations associated with Leber congenital amaurosis and cone-rod dystrophy: biochemical and clinical evaluations. Vis Res. 2007;47(15):2055–66.
12. Fingert JH, Oh K, Chung M, Scheetz TE, Andorf JL, Johnson RM, et al. Association of a novel mutation in the retinol dehydrogenase 12 (RDH12) gene with autosomal dominant retinitis pigmentosa. Arch Ophthalmol. 2008;126(9):1301–7.

66 RDH5

RDH5 encodes retinol dehydrogenase, which catalyzes the conversion of 11-cis retinol to 11-cis retinal in the final step in the synthesis 11-cis retinaldehyde, the chromophore in visual pigments. Mutations in *RDH5* cause fundus albipunctatus (FA), which follows an autosomal recessive pattern of inheritance.

Initial symptoms start in early childhood and usually begin with complaints of impaired dark adaptation and nyctalopia [1]. Most patients have good visual acuities, which are usually 20/30 or better. Fundus examination reveals the presence of extensive fine white dots extending to the mid-periphery of the retina, usually excluding the macula (Fig. 66.1a) [2–4]. Cone and macular dystrophies are generally observed in older patients later in the disease course. In one study, however, a 9-year-old patient with FA exhibited symmetric atrophic macular lesions in both eyes [5]. These white dots typically have very discrete borders and may range in size from 50 to 150 μm in diameter. In general, fundus autofluorescence imaging varies, sometimes showing a localized crescent or bull's eye pattern with macular hypoautofluorescence (Fig. 66.1d) [6–8]. In younger patients, fundus autofluorescence imaging may reveal hyperautofluorescent spots, which correlate with the retinal white dots, though not all fundoscopic white dots autofluoresce [5]. Some patients may also have a ring of hyperautofluorescence surrounding the fovea [6]. It is important to note that the overall autofluorescence signal is lower than in that of control patients, which may reflect reduced lipofuscin in the outer retina as a result of the pathway defect in *RDH5* mutations, similar to LCA caused by mutations in *RPE65, LRAT* or vitamin A deficiency [6, 8]. Given this limitation, infrared reflectance (IR) imaging has been reported to be useful in revealing greater detail. IR imaging has been reported to better reveal the hyper-reflective dots that correspond to white dots seen on fundoscopy [7]. SD-OCT demonstrates triangular-shaped deposits corresponding to the white dots seen on fundus exam, which extend from the Bruch's membrane through the ellipsoid zone and even the external limiting membrane (Fig. 66.1c, e) [6–8]. These deposits are notably different from the dome-shaped deposits seen in retinitis punctata albescens. ERG responses are usually mildly diminished for both photopic and scotopic parameters, although prolonged dark adaptation will result in improvement of the scotopic responses (Fig. 66.1b) [3, 4, 6, 7, 9]. Scotopic bright flash ERG may have a b:a ratio low enough to be classified as a negative ERG [6]. One study observed that 38% of patients with FA exhibit extensive cone dysfunction and that cone-ERG b-wave amplitudes tend to decline with increasing age [10].

S. Zahid et al., *Retinal Dystrophy Gene Atlas*, https://doi.org/10.1007/978-3-319-10867-4_66

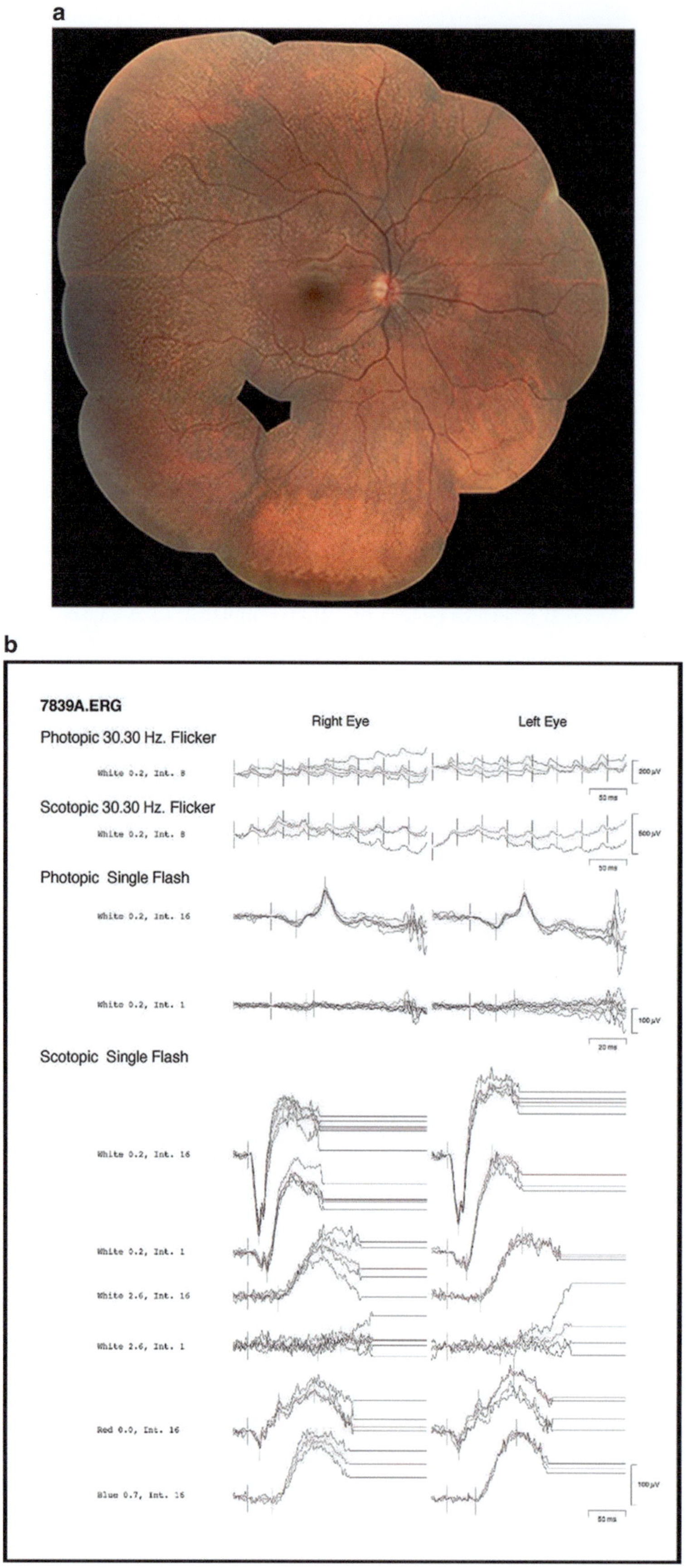

Fig. 66.1 Case summary: 10-year-old female (CEI25381) with fundus albipunctatus. (**a**) Color fundus photograph of the right eye, showing typical findings of fundus albipunctatus, with extensive fine white dots extending from the arcades to the mid-peripheral retina. (**b**) Full-field electroretinogram of the right and left eyes, showing mildly diminished photopic and scotopic parameters.

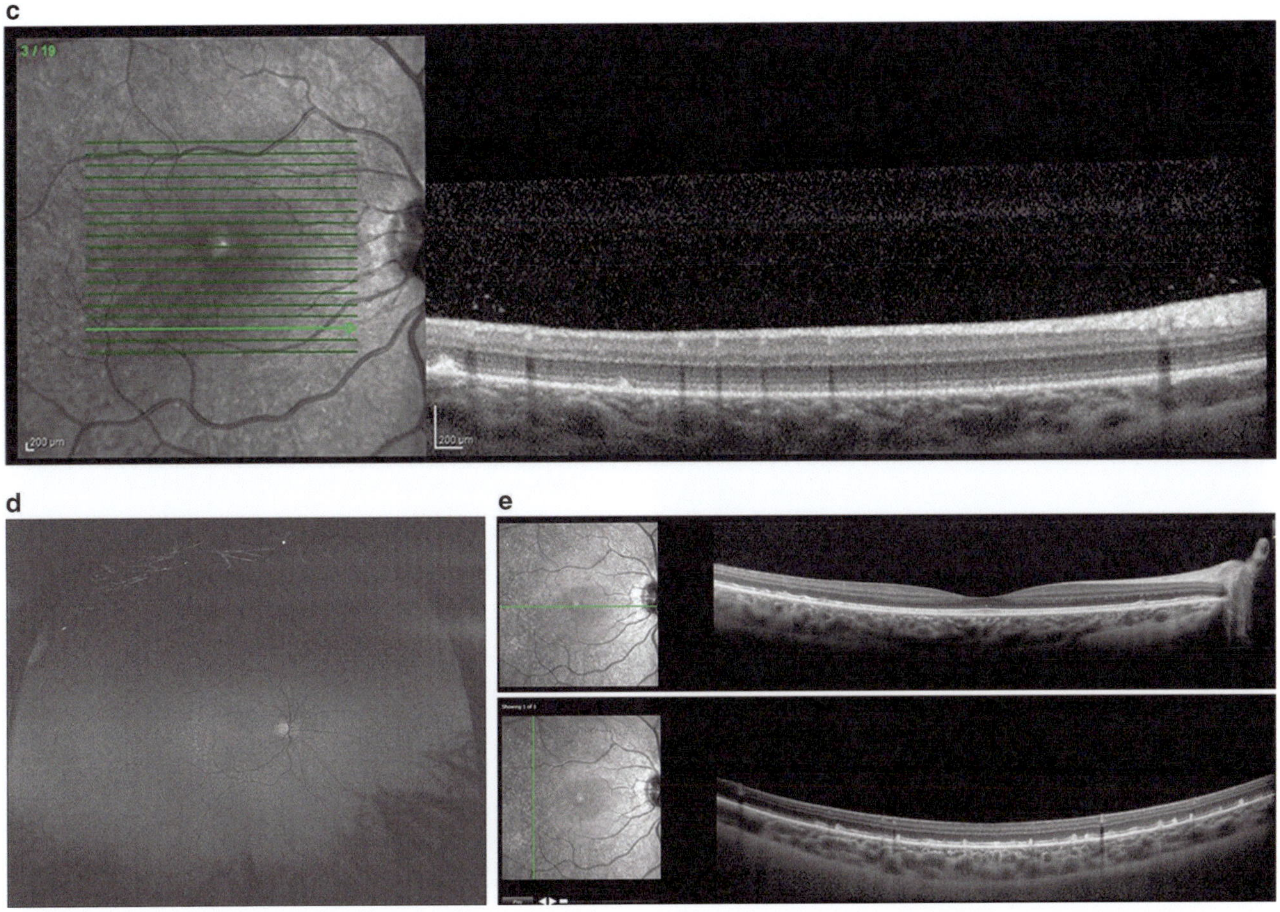

Fig. 66.1 (continued) (**c**) Spectral domain-optical coherence tomography (SD-OCT) of the right eye at age 10, showing the white dots as hyperreflective lesions in the subretinal space. (**d**) Fundus autofluorescence of the right eye at age 12 years, showing overall reduced retinal autofluorescence, with numerous discrete foci of hyperautofluorescence corresponding to the white dots around the vascular arcades. (**e**) Spectral domain-OCT of the right eye at age 15 years, showing subretinal deposits corresponding to the white dots.

References

1. Gonzalez-Fernandez F, Kurz D, Bao Y, Newman S, Conway BP, Young JE, et al. 11-cis retinol dehydrogenase mutations as a major cause of the congenital night-blindness disorder known as fundus albipunctatus. Mol Vis. 1999;5:41.
2. Ajmal M, Khan MI, Neveling K, Khan YM, Ali SH, Ahmed W, et al. Novel mutations in RDH5 cause fundus albipunctatus in two consanguineous Pakistani families. Mol Vis. 2012;18:1558–71.
3. Yamamoto H, Simon A, Eriksson U, Harris E, Berson EL, Dryja TP. Mutations in the gene encoding 11-cis retinol dehydrogenase cause delayed dark adaptation and fundus albipunctatus. Nat Genet. 1999;22(2):188–91.
4. Iannaccone A, Tedesco SA, Gallaher KT, Yamamoto H, Charles S, Dryja TP. Fundus albipunctatus in a 6-year old girl due to compound heterozygous mutations in the RDH5 gene. Doc Ophthalmol. 2007;115(2):111–6.
5. Nakamura M, Miyake Y. Macular dystrophy in a 9-year-old boy with fundus albipunctatus. Am J Ophthalmol. 2002;133(2):278–80.
6. Sergouniotis PI, Sohn EH, Li Z, McBain VA, Wright GA, Moore AT, et al. Phenotypic variability in RDH5 retinopathy (fundus albipunctatus). Ophthalmology. 2011;118(8):1661–70.
7. Wang NK, Chuang LH, Lai CC, Chou CL, Chu HY, Yeung L, et al. Multimodal fundus imaging in fundus albipunctatus with RDH5 mutation: a newly identified compound heterozygous mutation and review of the literature. Doc Ophthalmol Adv Ophthalmol. 2012;125(1):51–62.
8. Schatz P, Preising M, Lorenz B, Sander B, Larsen M, Eckstein C, et al. Lack of autofluorescence in fundus albipunctatus associated with mutations in RDH5. Retina. 2010;30(10):1704–13.
9. Parker RO, Crouch RK. Retinol dehydrogenases (RDHs) in the visual cycle. Exp Eye Res. 2010;91(6):788–92.
10. Niwa Y, Kondo M, Ueno S, Nakamura M, Terasaki H, Miyake Y. Cone and rod dysfunction in fundus albipunctatus with RDH5 mutation: an electrophysiological study. Invest Ophthalmol Vis Sci. 2005;46(4):1480–5.

67 RHO

RHO encodes rhodopsin, which is the visual pigment found in rod photoreceptors. Pathogenic mutations have been associated with autosomal dominant retinitis pigmentosa (ADRP), including sectoral RP, with autosomal dominant congenital stationary night blindness (CSNB), and, rarely, with autosomal recessive RP. *RHO* mutations are the most common cause of ADRP, accounting for 25–30% of ADRP. p.Pro23His is the most frequently identified mutation in *RHO* in the USA [1, 2].

Patients with *RHO*-associated ADRP typically complain of difficulties with night vision and peripheral vision, with onset in the second-to-fourth decades [3, 4]. Fundoscopic features include the typical bone-spicule pigmentation seen in RP, which, when not generalized, is most commonly seen confined to the inferior retina (sectoral RP) (Figs. 67.1a–c, 67.2a, and 67.3a). Sectoral RP is associated with a milder visual deterioration, with patients occasionally being asymptomatic and identified at routine examination [5]. Loss of visual field generally precedes declines in visual acuity [6, 7]. There are over 150 RHO pathogenic variants identified to date [8], with some known genotype-phenotype correlations. For example, the p.Pro23His variant is associated with a relatively mild but variable phenotype [9]. Electroretinography (ERG) usually shows a rod-cone pattern that progresses to broader retinal dysfunction with time. Fundus autofluorescence imaging may exhibit a hyperautofluorescent perifoveal ring that progressively constricts over the course of disease (Figs. 67.2b and 67.3b) [10]. Optical coherence tomography may show cystoid macular edema as well as the extent of outer retinal atrophy (Figs. 67.2c and 67.3c).

Infrequently, autosomal recessive RP may be caused by mutations in *RHO*. Carriers are asymptomatic but have mildly abnormal scotopic ERGs.

Dominantly-inherited CSNB may also be caused by certain mutations in *RHO* [11]. These patients typically experience nyctalopia from infancy but maintain relatively good central visual acuity and color vision. Fundoscopy usually reveals a normal fundus. Patients may have electrophysiological evidence of inner retinal rod system dysfunction (electronegative ERG in response to a bright white flash in the dark-adapted eye, with a reduced b-wave-to-a-wave ratio) in association with normal cone ERGs.

S. Zahid et al., *Retinal Dystrophy Gene Atlas*, https://doi.org/10.1007/978-3-319-10867-4_67

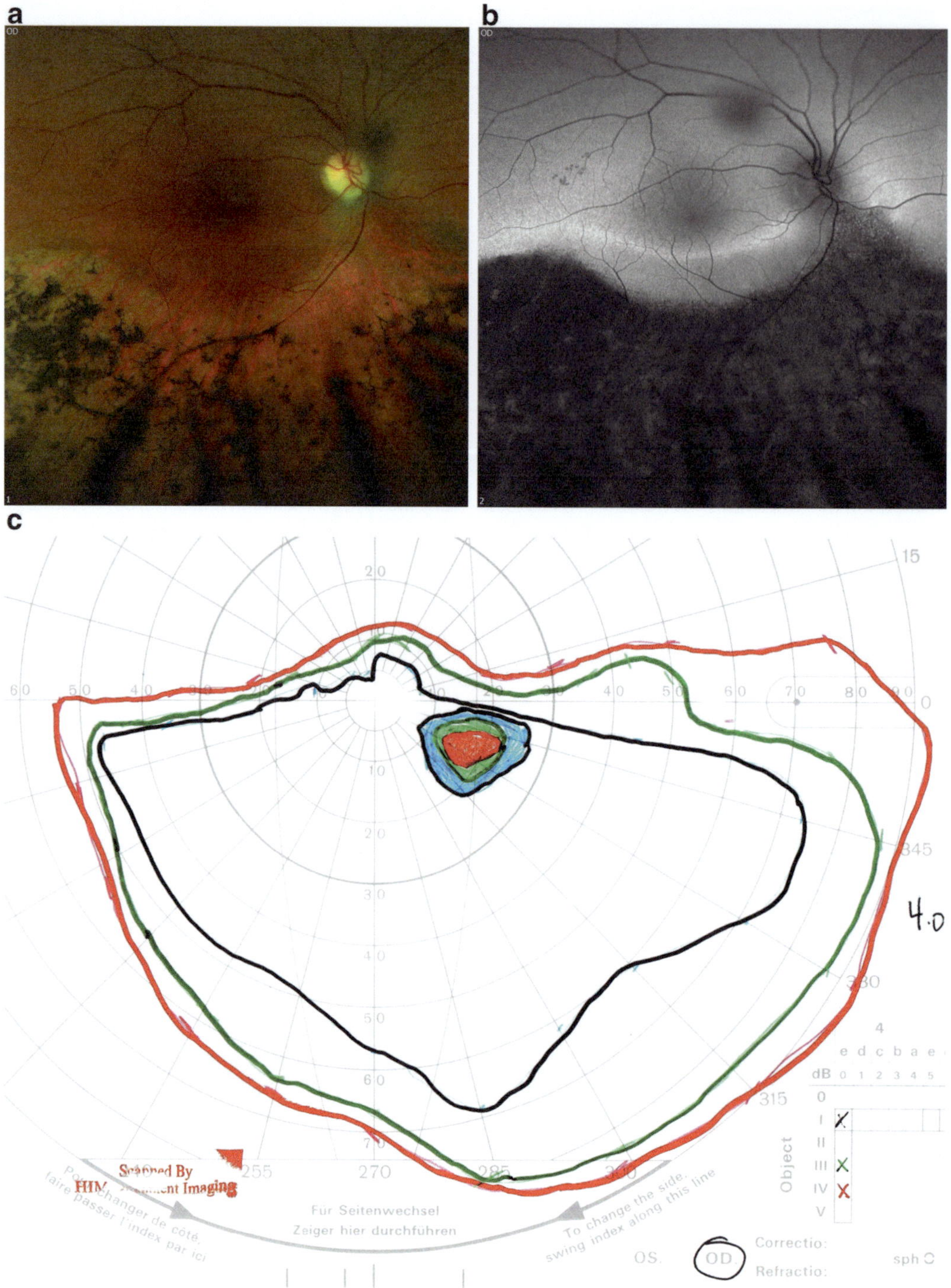

Fig. 67.1 Case summary: Fifty-four-year-old man with sectoral RP. (**a**) Color fundus photograph of the right eye, showing inferior RPE atrophy with bone spicule pigment deposits extending to the inferior arcades. (**b**) Fundus autofluorescence of the right eye, showing hypoautofluorescence in the inferior retina extending peripherally from the inferior arcades; this area corresponds to the area of atrophy and bone spicule pigment deposition. There are also foci of hypoautofluorescence in the temporal and superior macula, as well as a streak of hyperautofluorescence across the inferior macula. (**c**) Goldman visual field testing, showing sectoral loss of visual field.

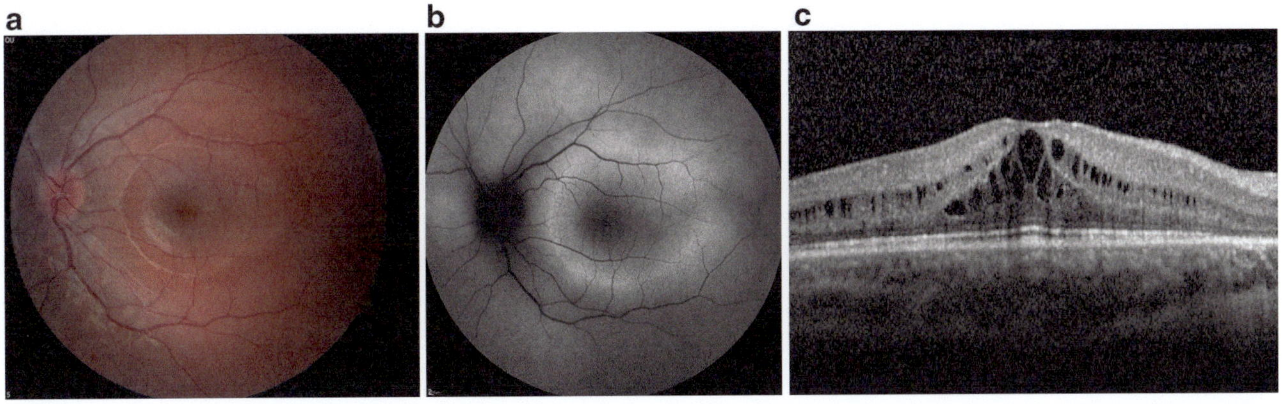

Fig. 67.2 (**a**) Color fundus photograph of the left eye from a 13-year-old boy, showing an essentially unremarkable fundus. (**b**) Fundus autofluorescence of the left eye, showing a macular hyperautofluorescent ring in the parafovea. (**c**) Spectral domain-optical coherence tomography of the macula, showing cystoid macular edema.

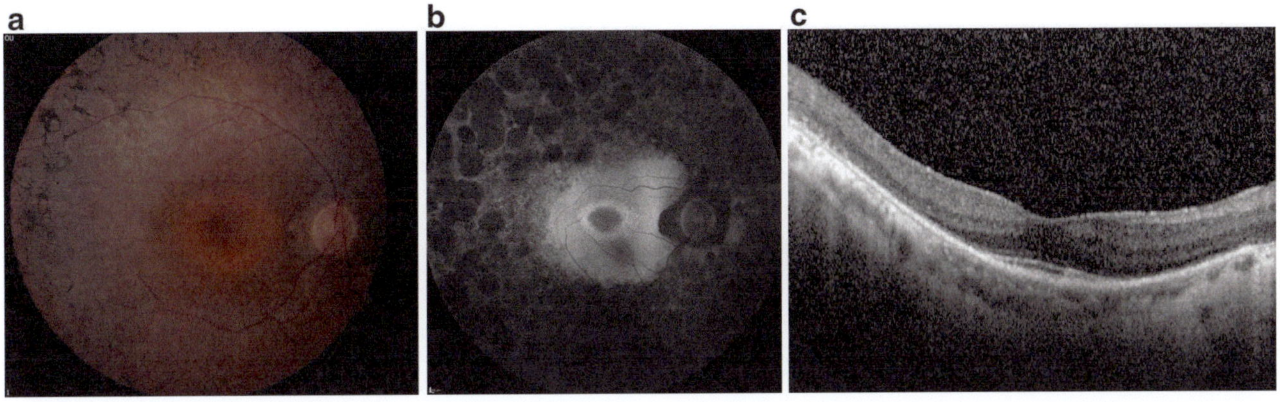

Fig. 67.3 (**a**) Color fundus photograph of the right eye from the 48-year-old father of the 13-year-old boy in Fig. 67.2, showing extensive peripheral atrophy, with bone spicule pigment deposits extending from the periphery to the vascular arcades. There is also abnormal pigmentation without obvious atrophy in a ring surrounding the fovea. (**b**) Fundus autofluorescence of the right eye, showing a macular hyperautofluorescent ring surrrounding the fovea that appears more constricted than that seen in Fig. 67.2b. There are extensive areas of hypoautofluorescence outside the arcades corresponding to the areas of atrophy. (**c**) Spectral domain-OCT, showing loss of the outer nuclear layer and ellipsoid zone, with foveal-sparing.

References

1. Daiger SP, Bowne SJ, Sullivan LS, Blanton SH, Weinstock GM, Koboldt DC, et al. Application of next-generation sequencing to identify genes and mutations causing autosomal dominant retinitis pigmentosa (adRP). Adv Exp Med Biol. 2014;801:123–9.
2. Sung CH, Davenport CM, Nathans J. Rhodopsin mutations responsible for autosomal dominant retinitis pigmentosa. Clustering of functional classes along the polypeptide chain. J Biol Chem. 1993;268(35):26645–9.
3. Andreasson S, Ehinger B, Abrahamson M, Fex G. A six-generation family with autosomal dominant retinitis pigmentosa and a rhodopsin gene mutation (arginine-135-leucine). Ophthalmic Paediatr Genet. 1992;13(3):145–53.
4. Rosenfeld PJ, Cowley GS, McGee TL, Sandberg MA, Berson EL, Dryja TP. A null mutation in the rhodopsin gene causes rod photoreceptor dysfunction and autosomal recessive retinitis pigmentosa. Nat Genet. 1992;1(3):209–13.
5. Berson EL, Rosner B, Weigel-DiFranco C, Dryja TP, Sandberg MA. Disease progression in patients with dominant retinitis pigmentosa and rhodopsin mutations. Invest Ophthalmol Vis Sci. 2002;43(9):3027–36.
6. Berson EL, Rosner B, Sandberg MA, Dryja TP. Ocular findings in patients with autosomal dominant retinitis pigmentosa and a rhodopsin gene defect (Pro-23-His). Arch Ophthalmol. 1991;109(1):92–101.
7. Sandberg MA, Rosner B, Weigel-DiFranco C, Dryja TP, Berson EL. Disease course of patients with X-linked retinitis pigmentosa due to RPGR gene mutations. Invest Ophthalmol Vis Sci. 2007;48(3):1298–304.
8. Athanasiou, Aguila, Bellingham, Li, McCulley, Reeves, Cheetham. The moelcular and cellural basis of rhodopsin retinitis pigmentosa reveals strategies for therapy. Prog Retina Eye Research. Oct 2017.

9. KT O, Weleber RG, Lotery A, Oh DM, Billingslea AM, Stone EM. Description of a new mutation in rhodopsin, Pro23Ala, and comparison with electroretinographic and clinical characteristics of the Pro23His mutation. Arch Ophthalmol. 2000;118(9):1269–76.
10. Robson AG, Tufail A, Fitzke F, Bird AC, Moore AT, Holder GE, et al. Serial imaging and structure-function correlates of high-density rings of fundus autofluorescence in retinitis pigmentosa. Retina. 2011;31(8):1670–9.
11. Dryja TP, Berson EL, Rao VR, Oprian DD. Heterozygous missense mutation in the rhodopsin gene as a cause of congenital stationary night blindness. Nat Genet. 1993;4(3):280–3.

68 *RIMS1*

RIMS1 encodes Rab-3 interacting molecule, which is a photoreceptor synaptic protein involved in regulating vesicle exocytosis. Mutations in *RIMS1* are associated with autosomal dominant cone-rod dystrophy (CORD7) [1, 2].

RIMS1-related CORD7 has a variable age of onset, ranging from the second to the fifth decade of life. Patients initially experience deterioration in central vision, with subsequent nyctalopia. Some patients may experience mild photophobia. Visual acuity varies from 20/20 to 20/400. Fundus changes range from mild RPE disturbance to extensive atrophy and pigmentation in the macula but may also involve the periphery in some patients (Fig. 68.1a). Vessel attenuation and bull's eye maculopathy (BEM) may also be observed (Fig. 68.2a). Fundus autofluorescence (FAF) imaging may reveal (i) areas of reduced FAF corresponding to atrophy seen clinically, (ii) a BEM appearance, and/or (iii) a perifoveal ring of increased FAF (Fig. 68.2b, c) [1]. This ring of increased FAF may enlarge with time, with the size of the ring correlating with age. FAF imaging may be helpful to identify young pre-symptomatic patients. Full-field ERG reveals reduced cone and rod responses, with the cone system affected to a greater extent than the rod system [2, 3].

S. Zahid et al., *Retinal Dystrophy Gene Atlas*, https://doi.org/10.1007/978-3-319-10867-4_68

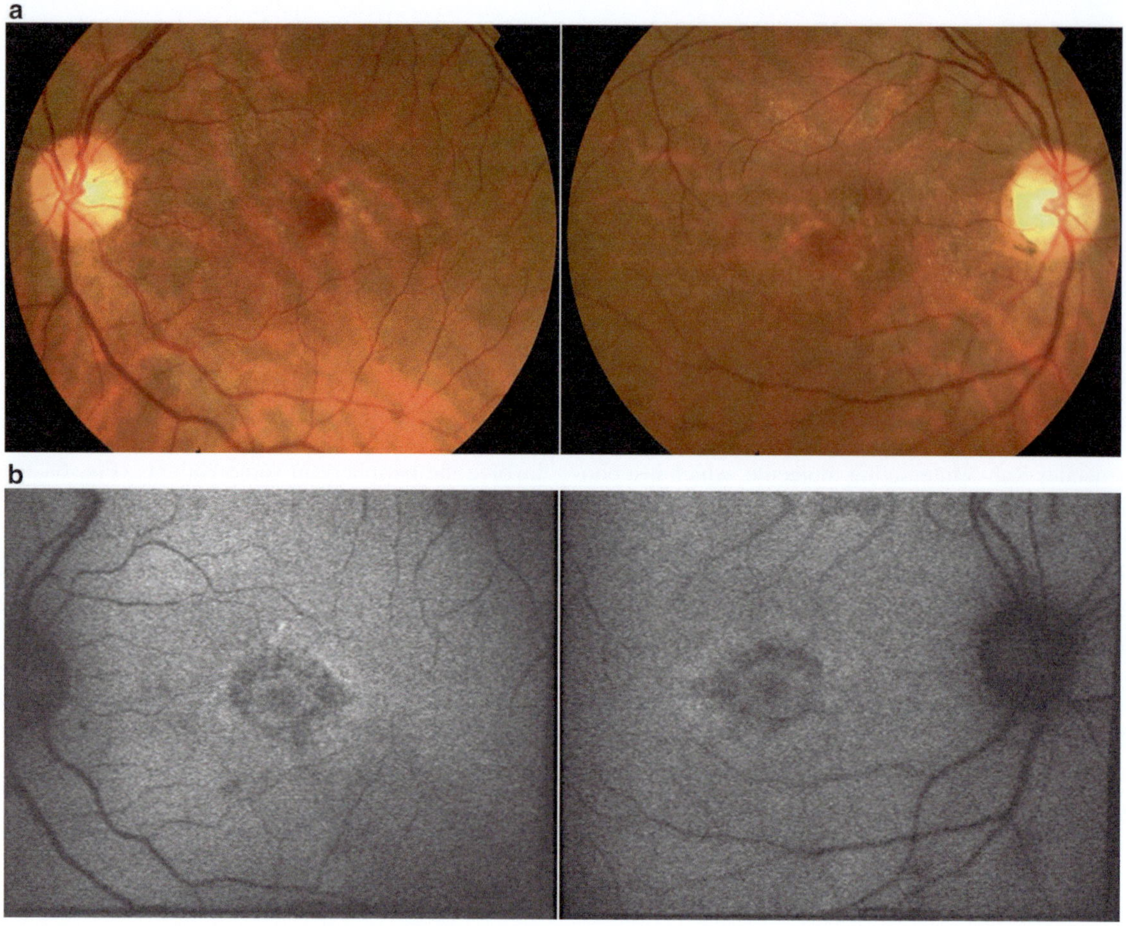

Fig. 68.1 (**a**) Color fundus photos of the right and left eyes, showing macular atrophy and RPE changes in both eyes, with the appearance of bull's eye maculopathy in the left eye. (**b**) Fundus autofluorescence of the right and left eyes, showing patchy hypoautofluorescence surrounding the fovea, corresponding to areas of atrophy, with a surrounding ring of hyperautofluorescence.

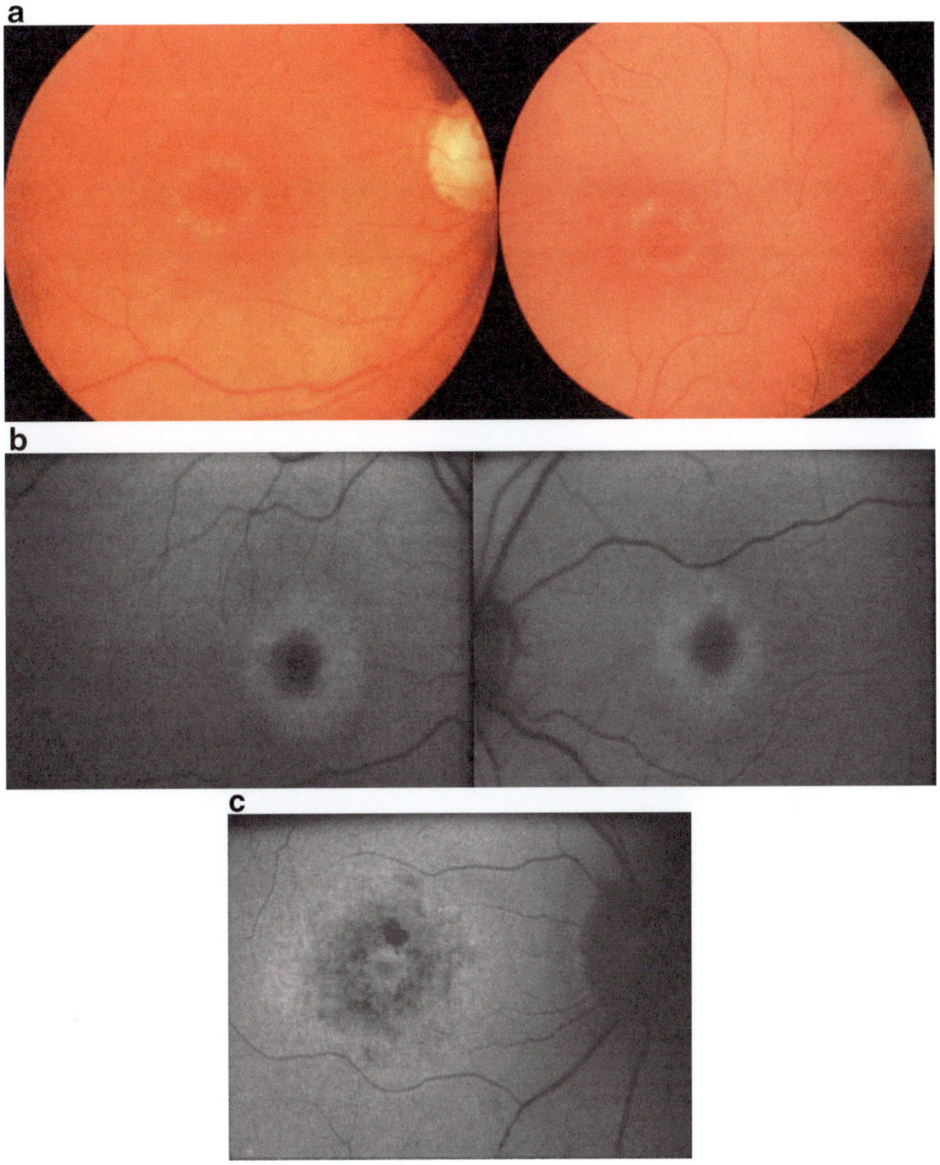

Fig. 68.2 (**a**) Color fundus photos of the right and left eyes in a different patient, showing macular bull's eye atrophy changes. (**b**) Fundus autofluorescence of the right and left eyes, showing hyperautofluorescent rings surrounding the foveae. (**c**) Fundus autofluorescence of the right eye at follow-up, showing foveal hyperautofluorescence with surrounding patchy hypoautofluorescence in areas corresponding to atrophy; a patchy hyperautofluorescent ring surrounding the fovea can still be appreciated.

References

1. Robson AG, Michaelides M, Luong VA, Holder GE, Bird AC, Webster AR, et al. Functional correlates of fundus autofluorescence abnormalities in patients with RPGR or RIMS1 mutations causing cone or cone rod dystrophy. Br J Ophthalmol. 2008;92(1):95–102.
2. Michaelides M, Holder GE, Hunt DM, Fitzke FW, Bird AC, Moore AT. A detailed study of the phenotype of an autosomal dominant cone-rod dystrophy (CORD7) associated with mutation in the gene for RIM1. Br J Ophthalmol. 2005;89(2):198–206.
3. Johnson S, Halford S, Morris AG, Patel RJ, Wilkie SE, Hardcastle AJ, et al. Genomic organisation and alternative splicing of human RIM1, a gene implicated in autosomal dominant cone-rod dystrophy (CORD7). Genomics. 2003;81(3):304–14.

69 RLBP1

RLBP1 (also known as *CRALBP*) encodes cellular retinaldehyde-binding protein, which acts primarily as an acceptor of 11-*cis* retinal during the isomerization step of the visual cycle. Mutations in *RLBP1* cause Bothnia retinal dystrophy, fundus albipunctatus, Newfoundland rod-cone dystrophy, and retinitis punctata albescens [1].

The retinal phenotype is similar to most forms of Retinitis Pigmentosa (RP; rod-cone dystrophy), although there may be marked variation in severity between affected individuals. Three early-onset forms of autosomal recessive RP caused by mutations in the *RLBP1* gene are associated with multiple white deposits at the level of the RPE. One of these is retinitis punctata albescens, while the other two have been described in genetic isolates from North-Eastern Canada (Newfoundland rod-cone dystrophy) and Northern Sweden (Bothnia dystrophy).

RLBP1-related retinitis punctata albescens (RPA) follows an autosomal recessive pattern of inheritance. Patients have early onset (usually in the first decade of life) of nyctalopia. Best corrected visual acuities (BCVA) are typically 20/20 or better [2]. Fundoscopy reveals round punctate white deposits throughout the entire retina (Fig. 69.1a) [2–4]. Pigment mottling, hypopigmentation, arteriole attenuation, waxy disc pallor, and blunted foveal reflexes may also be seen in older patients [2]. Fundus autofluorescence may show a reduction of overall autofluorescence, with hyperautofluorescent foci corresponding to the white subretinal deposits (Fig. 69.1b). Optical coherence tomography (OCT) may reveal diffuse retinal thinning in the macular area, particularly in the outer nuclear layer, and may show subretinal hyperreflective lesions corresponding to the white deposits in the earlier stages of disease (Fig. 69.1c) [4]. Electroretinogram (ERG) may show significantly reduced rod and cone responses, with a predominant loss of rod function [3, 5].

RLBP1-related fundus albipunctatus is characterized by symmetrical white dots in the fundus, with higher concentrations in the mid-periphery, which is similar to the irregular white deposits of RPA (Fig. 69.1a). Initial symptoms begin in early childhood with nyctalopia and dim-light vision difficulties. Visual acuities may vary, ranging from 20/40 to 20/200, but younger patients may be less affected [6, 7]. Fundus photography typically shows multiple round white deposits (about 100–125 μm in diameter) in the mid-peripheral retina. At early ages, the central macula is usually spared of dots, but at later ages the deposits may be prominent in the major vascular arcades (Fig. 69.1a) [7]. In the fifth-to-sixth decades of life, optic disc pallor, arteriole attenuation, bone spicules, and atrophy may also be observed [7]. Electroretinography reveals low or nonrecordable scotopic readings and low photopic responses with slightly prolonged implicit times [6, 7].

Bothnia dystrophy (BD) is an atypical variant of autosomal recessive retinitis pigmentosa (RP). Individuals with *RLBP1*-related BD typically have an onset of nyctalopia in their early childhood [8]. Visual acuities often deteriorate to legal blindness with disease progression. Vision loss often starts in the second decade of life, with evidence of paracentral and central scotomas [8]. Fundoscopy may reveal extensive white-yellow spots similar to those found in retinitis punctata albescens. The midperiphery may have a mottled appearance, and there may be circular confluent atrophic areas (especially in later stages of disease). Macular atrophy reminiscent of central areolar atrophy may also be found in patients after the third decade of life [8]. OCT may show general retinal thinning at the fovea, surrounding the fovea, and in areas of the outer macula; RPA-like deposits are usually visualized at the level of the RPE (Fig. 69.1c) [9, 10]. ERGs typically show non-recordable scotopic responses and prolonged dark adaptation [10, 11].

Newfoundland rod-cone dystrophy (NFRCD) is similar to RPA and BD but with a younger age of onset and a more rapid progression [1]. Nyctalopia is typically present from birth or infancy. From childhood to the second-to-fourth decades of life, patients experience progressive loss of peripheral, central, and color vision, with early maintenance of visual acuity. Goldman visual field testing may reveal a ring scotoma close to fixation instead of in the midperipheral field (where it is often found in typical RP). The ring scotoma

S. Zahid et al., *Retinal Dystrophy Gene Atlas*, https://doi.org/10.1007/978-3-319-10867-4_69

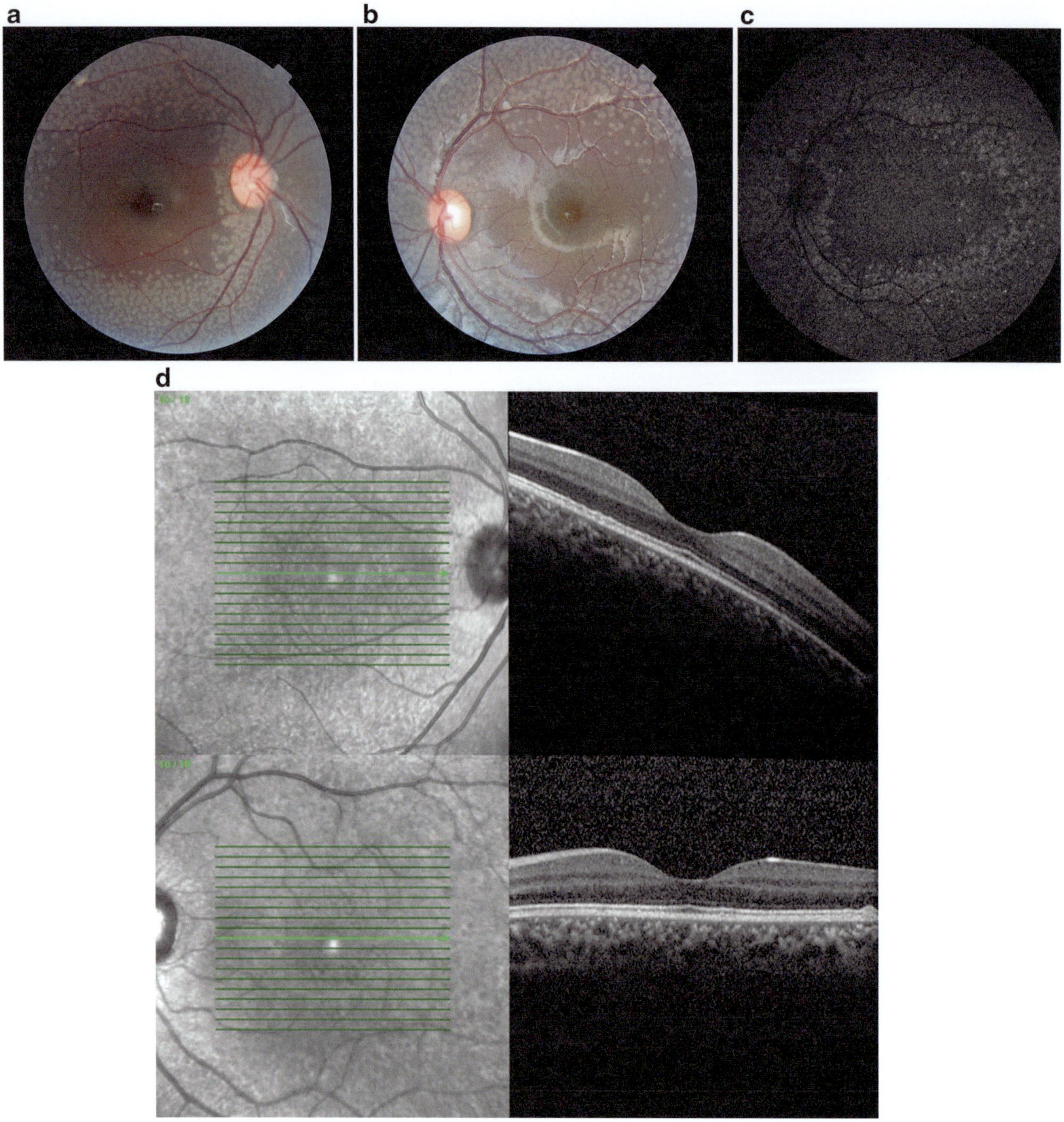

Fig. 69.1 (**a**, **b**) Color fundus photograph of the right eye from a 6-year-old female patient, showing multiple round white deposits around the arcades, with macular-sparing. (**c**) Fundus autofluorescence of the left eye, showing an overall reduction of autofluorescence, with foci of hyperautofluorescence corresponding to the white deposits shown in (**b**). (**d**) Spectral domain-optical coherence tomography of the right and left eyes, showing generally maintained retinal cross-sectional architecture without atrophy, as well as a subretinal hyperreflective lesion in the temporal macula of the left eye.

may become a complete central scotoma with disease progression. Color vision abnormalities may be found initially as mild protanomaly/deutanomaly and/or tritanomaly, but these typically progress to eventual loss of color perception. Funduscopy may reveal a normal fundus or mild arteriolar attenuation until later in the disease progression, when there may be macular atrophy with a "beaten bronze" appearance [1]. In young patients, a perimacular ring of white stippling may be observed, along with scalloped-bordered lacunar atrophy of the midperipheral RPE over time (similar to that seen in gyrate atrophy, but without elevated ornithine levels) [1]. ERG scotopic responses may be low in young patients, while both scotopic and photopic responses may be extinguished later in the disease process.

References

1. Eichers ER, Green JS, Stockton DW, Jackman CS, Whelan J, McNamara JA, et al. Newfoundland rod-cone dystrophy, an early-onset retinal dystrophy, is caused by splice-junction mutations in RLBP1. Am J Hum Genet. 2002;70(4):955–64.
2. Fishman GA, Roberts MF, Derlacki DJ, Grimsby JL, Yamamoto H, Sharon D, et al. Novel mutations in the cellular retinaldehyde-binding protein gene (RLBP1) associated with retinitis punctata albescens: evidence of interfamilial genetic heterogeneity and fundus changes in heterozygotes. Arch Ophthalmol. 2004;122(1):70–5.
3. Demirci FY, Rigatti BW, Mah TS, Gorin MB. A novel compound heterozygous mutation in the cellular retinaldehyde-binding protein gene (RLBP1) in a patient with retinitis punctata albescens. Am J Ophthalmol. 2004;138(1):171–3.
4. Nakamura M, Lin J, Ito Y, Miyake Y. Novel mutation in RLBP1 gene in a Japanese patient with retinitis punctata albescens. Am J Ophthalmol. 2005;139(6):1133–5.
5. Morimura H, Berson EL, Dryja TP. Recessive mutations in the RLBP1 gene encoding cellular retinaldehyde-binding protein in a form of retinitis punctata albescens. Invest Ophthalmol Vis Sci. 1999;40(5):1000–4.
6. Naz S, Ali S, Riazuddin SA, Farooq T, Butt NH, Zafar AU, et al. Mutations in RLBP1 associated with fundus albipunctatus in consanguineous Pakistani families. Br J Ophthalmol. 2011;95(7):1019–24.
7. Katsanis N, Shroyer NF, Lewis RA, Cavender JC, Al-Rajhi AA, Jabak M, et al. Fundus albipunctatus and retinitis punctata albescens in a pedigree with an R150Q mutation in RLBP1. Clin Genet. 2001;59(6):424–9.
8. Burstedt MS, Sandgren O, Holmgren G, Forsman-Semb K. Bothnia dystrophy caused by mutations in the cellular retinaldehyde-binding protein gene (RLBP1) on chromosome 15q26. Invest Ophthalmol Vis Sci. 1999;40(5):995–1000.
9. Burstedt MS, Golovleva I. Central retinal findings in Bothnia dystrophy caused by RLBP1 sequence variation. Arch Ophthalmol. 2010;128(8):989–95.
10. Burstedt M, Jonsson F, Kohn L, Kivitalo M, Golovleva I. Genotype-phenotype correlations in Bothnia dystrophy caused by RLBP1 gene sequence variations. Acta Ophthalmol. 2013;91(5):437–44.
11. Nojima K, Hosono K, Zhao Y, Toshiba T, Hikoya A, Asai T, et al. Clinical features of a Japanese case with Bothnia dystrophy. Ophthalmic Genet. 2012;33(2):83–8.

70 RP1

RP1 encodes oxygen-regulated protein 1, which is involved in photoreceptor development, the organization of photoreceptor outer segments, and the regulation of photoreceptor microtubules. Mutations in *RP1* cause autosomal dominant retinitis pigmentosa (ADRP) (rod-cone dystrophy), often associated with a relatively good prognosis [1–5]. There have also been reports of *RP1* mutations that cause autosomal recessive RP [6–8].

Patients with ADRP often present in their early twenties with complaints of night blindness and/or peripheral field loss, though some patients may present as late as in their 50s. Good visual acuity is usually maintained until late in the disease course. Patients with dyschromatopsia are more likely to exhibit worse visual acuity. Patients may develop cataracts at an earlier age (often posterior subcapsular) or develop cystoid macular edema (CME). Fundus examination usually demonstrates typical findings of RP (Figs. 70.1a–c and 70.2a). Fundus autofluorescence reveals areas of RPE atrophy, which may be present in the periphery outside the arcades or in the macula (sometimes with patchy hypoautofluorescence at the macula). Full-field ERG usually reveals both rod and cone dysfunction, usually in a rod-cone pattern. Multifocal ERG usually shows maintained responses at the centrally-located hexagons. GVF reveals a rod-cone pattern of degeneration with constricted fields. OCT may show maintained macular retinal lamination, although some patients exhibit thinning at the macula, loss of the outer nuclear layer (ONL), or cystoid macular edema (CME) (Fig. 70.2b). Incomplete penetrance and variable expressivity have been reported in patients with *RP1* mutations and result in phenotypic variability with respect to disease onset, fundus features, visual acuity, visual fields, and ERG findings (Figs. 70.1a–c and 70.2a) [3, 9, 10]. Monocular disease, with the contralateral eye exhibiting a completely normal fundus and full-field ERG, has been reported in one patient with a mutation in *RP1* [11].

Patients with certain homozygous or compound heterozygous mutations in *RP1* may exhibit autosomal recessive retinitis pigmentosa [6, 7]. These patients typically present early in childhood with nyctalopia and rapidly lose vision by the second decade of life. Fundus findings may feature optic disc pallor, vessel attenuation, macular stippling, and bone-spicule deposits in the mid-periphery, but these are not universal findings. The full-field ERG is often non-recordable or shows severe loss of both rod and cone function. Carriers of these mutations usually have no symptoms or signs of disease.

Of note, homozygosity of the p.N985Y variant at the *RP1* locus has been associated with an elevated risk of hypertriglyceridemia, though the mechanism and clinical significance of this association are unknown [12].

S. Zahid et al., *Retinal Dystrophy Gene Atlas*, https://doi.org/10.1007/978-3-319-10867-4_70

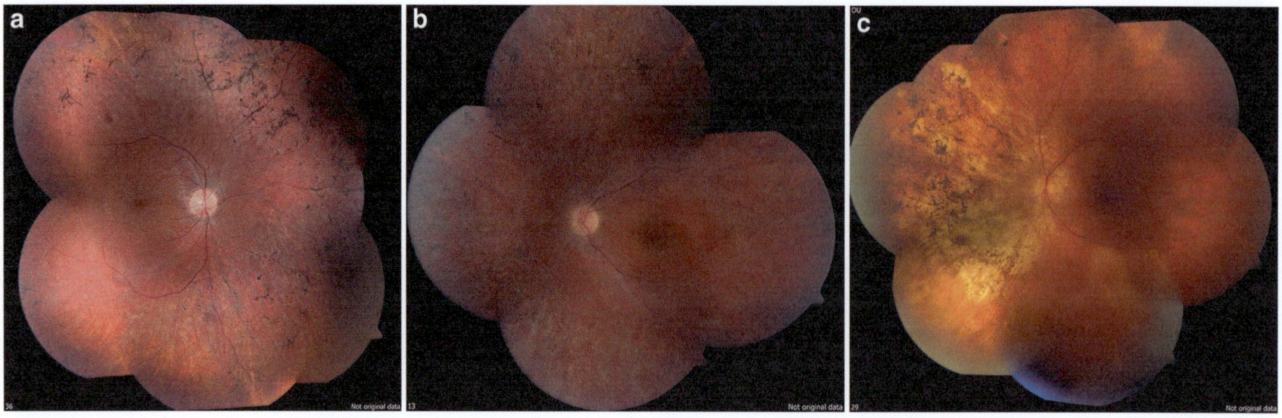

Fig. 70.1 Color fundus photographs from three different patients with *RP1* mutations, showing different variations and degrees of typical findings of retinitis pigmentosa (RP), including optic nerve pallor, retinal vascular attenuation, and peripheral atrophy with bone spicule pigment deposits. (**a**) Right eye from a 23-year-old male patient. (**b**) Left eye from a 24-year-old female patient. (**c**) Left eye from a 56-year-old male patient.

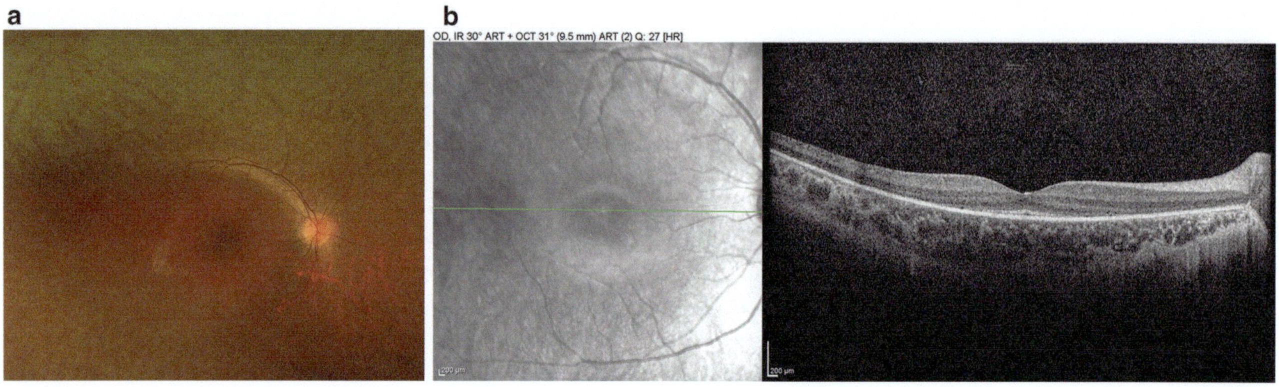

Fig. 70.2 Case summary: 6-year-old boy with compound heterozygous mutations and early-onset RP. (**a**) Color fundus photograph of the right eye, showing typical findings of RP. (**b**) Spectral domain-optical coherence tomography at age 7, showing foveal preservation and outer retinal degeneration (loss of the ellipsoid zone and outer nuclear layer) outside the fovea.

References

1. Pierce EA, Quinn T, Meehan T, McGee TL, Berson EL, Dryja TP. Mutations in a gene encoding a new oxygen-regulated photoreceptor protein cause dominant retinitis pigmentosa. Nat Genet. 1999;22(3):248–54.
2. Sullivan LS, Heckenlively JR, Bowne SJ, Zuo J, Hide WA, Gal A, et al. Mutations in a novel retina-specific gene cause autosomal dominant retinitis pigmentosa. Nat Genet. 1999;22(3):255–9.
3. Bowne SJ, Daiger SP, Hims MM, Sohocki MM, Malone KA, McKie AB, et al. Mutations in the RP1 gene causing autosomal dominant retinitis pigmentosa. Hum Mol Genet. 1999;8(11):2121–8.
4. Guillonneau X, Piriev NI, Danciger M, Kozak CA, Cideciyan AV, Jacobson SG, et al. A nonsense mutation in a novel gene is associated with retinitis pigmentosa in a family linked to the RP1 locus. Hum Mol Genet. 1999;8(8):1541–6.
5. Audo I, Mohand-Said S, Dhaenens CM, Germain A, Orhan E, Antonio A, et al. RP1 and autosomal dominant rod-cone dystrophy: novel mutations, a review of published variants, and genotype-phenotype correlation. Hum Mutat. 2012;33(1):73–80.
6. Khaliq S, Abid A, Ismail M, Hameed A, Mohyuddin A, Lall P, et al. Novel association of RP1 gene mutations with autosomal recessive retinitis pigmentosa. J Med Genet. 2005;42(5):436–8.
7. Riazuddin SA, Zulfiqar F, Zhang Q, Sergeev YV, Qazi ZA, Husnain T, et al. Autosomal recessive retinitis pigmentosa is associated with mutations in RP1 in three consanguineous Pakistani families. Invest Ophthalmol Vis Sci. 2005;46(7):2264–70.
8. Chen LJ, Lai TY, Tam PO, Chiang SW, Zhang X, Lam S, et al. Compound heterozygosity of two novel truncation mutations in RP1 causing autosomal recessive retinitis pigmentosa. Invest Ophthalmol Vis Sci. 2010;51(4):2236–42.
9. Berson EL, Grimsby JL, Adams SM, McGee TL, Sweklo E, Pierce EA, et al. Clinical features and mutations in patients with dominant retinitis pigmentosa-1 (RP1). Invest Ophthalmol Vis Sci. 2001;42(10):2217–24.
10. Jacobson SG, Cideciyan AV, Iannaccone A, Weleber RG, Fishman GA, Maguire AM, et al. Disease expression of RP1 mutations causing autosomal dominant retinitis pigmentosa. Invest Ophthalmol Vis Sci. 2000;41(7):1898–908.
11. Mukhopadhyay R, Holder GE, Moore AT, Webster AR. Unilateral retinitis pigmentosa occurring in an individual with a germline mutation in the RP1 gene. Arch Ophthalmol. 2011;129(7):954–6.
12. Fujita Y, Ezura Y, Emi M, Ono S, Takada D, Takahashi K, et al. Hypertriglyceridemia associated with amino acid variation Asn985Tyr of the RP1 gene. J Hum Genet. 2003;48(6):305–8.

71 RP2

RP2 encodes a protein that localizes to the base of photoreceptor cilia and is thought to be involved in cellular transport regulation. *RP2* mutations are responsible for 10–20% of X-linked retinitis pigmentosa (XLRP) [1, 2].

Broadly, XLRP has an earlier onset than dominant or recessive RP [3]. Patients present within the first decade of life with night blindness and reduced visual acuity [2, 4]. Visual acuity typically deteriorates to worse than 20/200 as early as the third decade. Several studies have noted high myopia [4, 5]. Funduscopic findings usually show more severe disease at the macula than at the peripheral retina when compared to retinitis pigmentosa caused by other genes. The appearance of the macula varies greatly: it may be normal or may show granular changes, bull's-eye atrophy, perimacular atrophy, or generalized macular atrophy (Figs. 71.1, 71.2, 71.3, 71.4, and 71.5) [4, 6]. Optic disc pallor and atrophy (either peripapillary or temporal) are often observed (Figs. 71.1 and 71.2). The peripheral retina may exhibit granularity, depigmentation, variable degrees of pigment deposits, or chorioretinal atrophy (Figs. 71.1 and 71.2). Tapetal sheen, which is commonly seen in *RPGR* mutations, has not been reported in patients with *RP2* mutations. ERG usually exhibits a rod-cone pattern of degeneration, although a cone-rod pattern has been reported [4]. GVF reveals central scotomata in up to 50% of patients and is often observed in patients younger than 12. Most patients exhibit constricted peripheral fields. Superior field loss (also seen in patients with *RHO* mutations) has been reported as well. Studies comparing the phenotype to *RPGR* have shown that patients with *RP2* mutations generally have worse visual acuity when adjusted for age but no significant difference in dark adaptation thresholds, visual field area, or ERG [7].

Some patients have been reported to exhibit choroideremia-like peripheral retinal atrophy with no pigment deposits (Figs. 71.1 and 71.4) [4].

Manifesting carriers may also exhibit a wide range of signs of disease, including myopia, macular atrophy, reduced visual acuity, asymmetrical disease, and central scotomas [4].

S. Zahid et al., *Retinal Dystrophy Gene Atlas*, https://doi.org/10.1007/978-3-319-10867-4_71

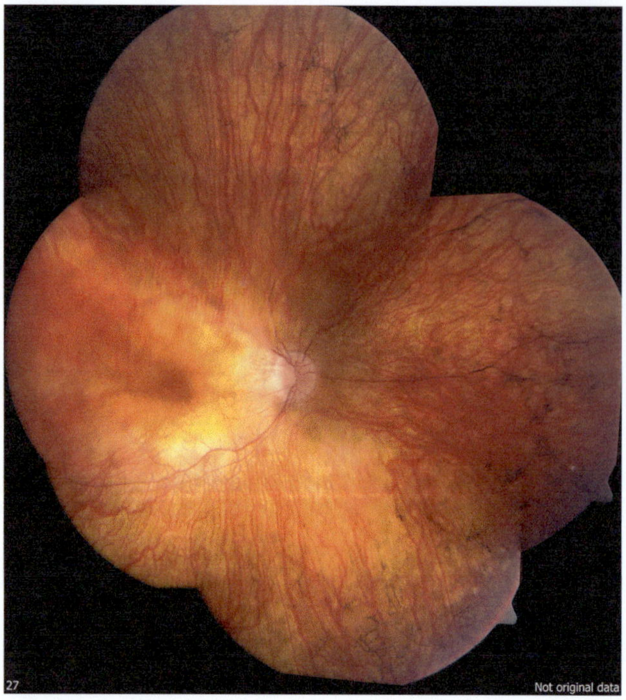

Fig. 71.1 Color fundus photography of the right eye from a 13-year-old male patient, showing peripheral atrophy with bone spicule pigment deposits and peripapillary atrophy in the context of a choroideremia-like appearance.

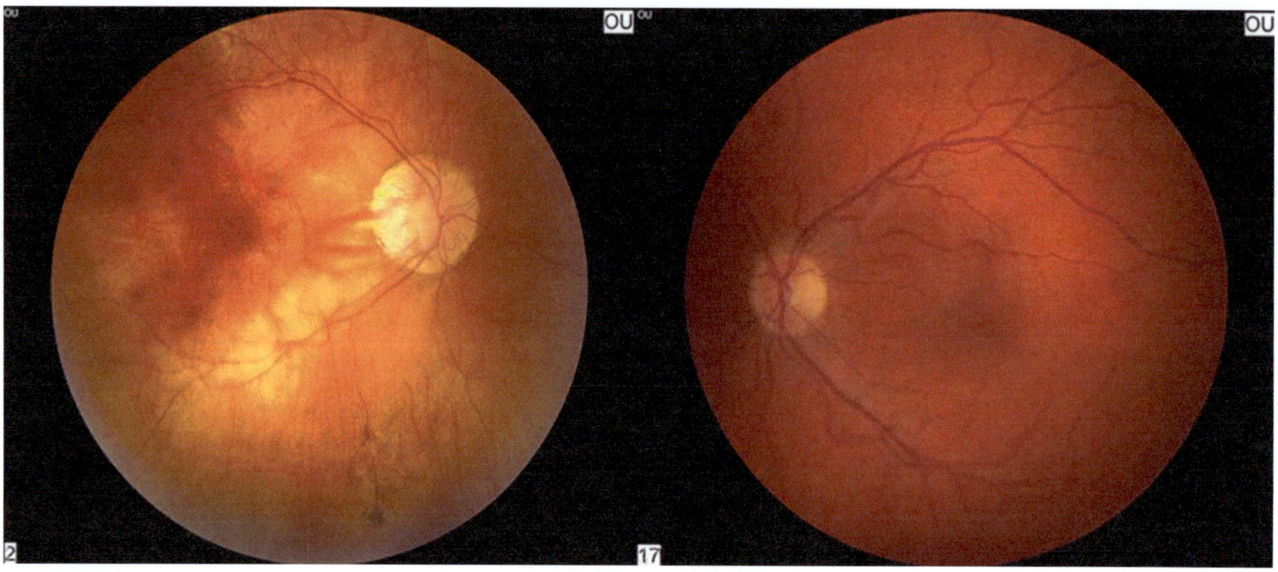

Fig. 71.2 Color fundus photographs of the right and left eyes from a 41-year-old woman with an *RP2* mutation, showing asymmetric disease burden, with the left eye having an essentially unremarkable fundus and the right eye demonstrating peripheral atrophy with bone spicule pigment deposits and peripapillary atrophy.

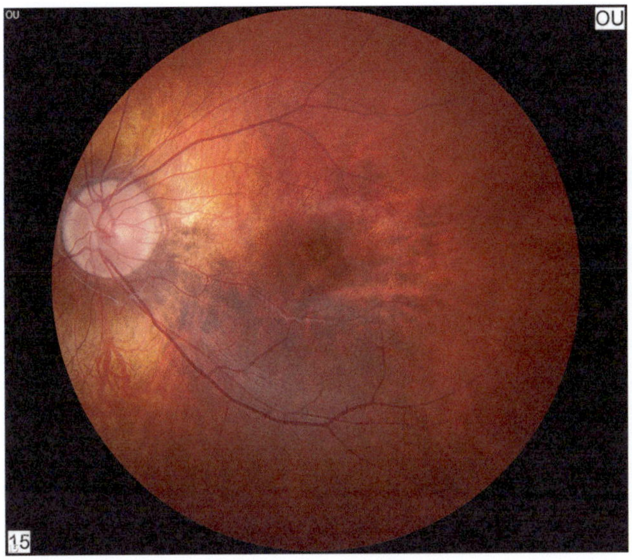

Fig. 71.3 Color fundus photographs of the left eye from the 5-year-old son of the patient from Fig. 71.2, showing macular atrophy.

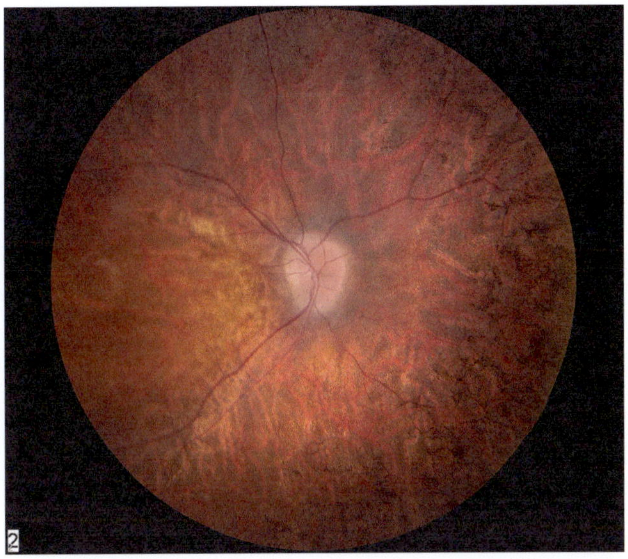

Fig. 71.5 Color fundus photographs of the right eye from a 13-year-old male patient, showing peripapillary atrophy and peripheral bone spicule pigment deposits.

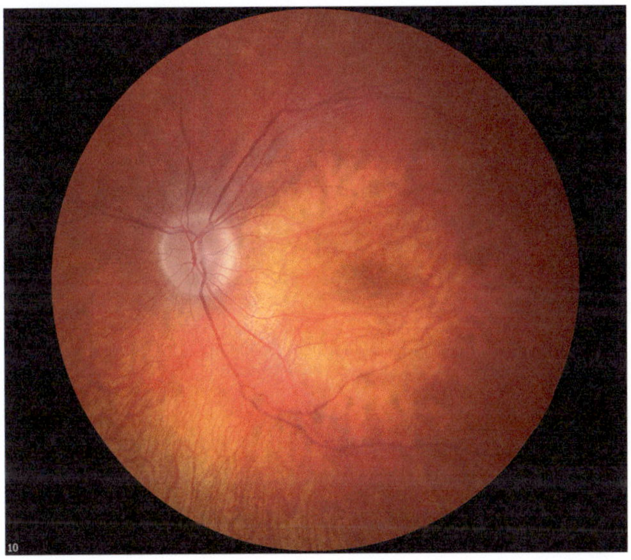

Fig. 71.4 Color fundus photographs of the left eye from a 13-year-old male with macular atrophy in the context of a choroideremia-like fundus.

References

1. Branham K, Othman M, Brumm M, Karoukis AJ, Atmaca-Sonmez P, Yashar BM, et al. Mutations in RPGR and RP2 account for 15% of males with simplex retinal degenerative disease. Invest Ophthalmol Vis Sci. 2012;53(13):8232–7.
2. Sharon D, Sandberg MA, Rabe VW, Stillberger M, Dryja TP, Berson EL. RP2 and RPGR mutations and clinical correlations in patients with X-linked retinitis pigmentosa. Am J Hum Genet. 2003;73(5):1131–46.
3. Hartong DT, Berson EL, Dryja TP. Retinitis pigmentosa. Lancet. 2006;368(9549):1795–809.
4. Jayasundera T, Branham KE, Othman M, Rhoades WR, Karoukis AJ, Khanna H, et al. RP2 phenotype and pathogenetic correlations in X-linked retinitis pigmentosa. Arch Ophthalmol. 2010;128(7):915–23.
5. Ji Y, Wang J, Xiao X, Li S, Guo X, Zhang Q. Mutations in RPGR and RP2 of Chinese patients with X-linked retinitis pigmentosa. Curr Eye Res. 2010;35(1):73–9.
6. Jin ZB, Liu XQ, Hayakawa M, Murakami A, Nao i N. Mutational analysis of RPGR and RP2 genes in Japanese patients with retinitis pigmentosa: identification of four mutations. Mol Vis. 2006;12:1167–74.

72 RPE65

RPE65 encodes retinoid isomerase, which generates (and regenerates) 11-*cis* retinal in the RPE as part of the canonical retinoid visual pathway [1]. Mutations in *RPE65* cause early-onset autosomal recessive retinitis pigmentosa (rod-cone dystrophy), Leber Congenital Amaurosis (LCA), and Severe Early Childhood Onset Retinal Dystrophy (SECORD) [2]. *RPE65* mutations may also cause dominantly inherited RP [3]. Sequence variants in *RPE65* have also been identified in patients with a retinal appearance similar to Fundus Albipunctatus [4].

RPE65 mutations account for 3–16% of LCA and SECORD, with LCA characterized by poor vision beginning within the first year of life and SECORD before age 5 [5, 6]. Patients with LCA tend to exhibit poor visual pursuit, roving eye movements, reduced or absent pupillary responses, and nystagmus. Night blindness may be noted in some infants. Patients with LCA exhibit poor visual acuity from infancy. The fundus may be normal at birth, but patients may exhibit RPE mottling or granularity at the macula or periphery, RPE thinning, vessel attenuation, and peripapillary loss of pigmentation; some patients may exhibit macular atrophy later in life (Figs. 72.1, 72.2, 72.3a, and 72.4). The ERG is usually non-recordable in LCA, and GVF reveals gradual concentric loss of peripheral fields. The full-field stimulus test (FST) can detect sensitivity to specific light stimuli and determine the presence of residual rod and cone function in patients [10–12]. Fundus autofluorescence usually reveals hypoautofluorescence due to lack of production of chromophores [13, 14], though some studies have reported reduced autofluorescence in patients with hypomorphic mutations [9]. Foveal hyperautofluorescence may also be observed (Fig. 72.3b).

Two percent of recessive RP is caused by mutations in *RPE65* [2]. This diagnosis is part of a spectrum that includes LCA and has been given to those presenting in early childhood (Severe Early Childhood Onset Retinal Dystrophy) but not as early as LCA. Many of the symptoms described above may be present in these patients as well. Night blindness is a prominent symptom early in life in these patients, and they generally have better visual acuity (20/50 to LP; median 20/80) than those with LCA [15–17]. Patients with SECORD retain measurable visual acuity in the first/second decades and sometimes beyond, with slow progressive loss over time [7]. Several studies have reported improvement in visual acuity for a period of time in association with SECORD [7, 8]. Nystagmus early in life is common; photophobia is uncommon in these patients, though some patients may develop it later in life [7, 18]. Fundus findings range from RPE granularity to optic disc pallor, peripapillary hypopigmentation, retinal vascular attenuation, and peripheral circular patches of atrophy and macular atrophy. Bone spicule deposits may be observed but are uncommon in these patients (Fig. 72.4). Weleber et al. [8] reported that some patients with *RPE65* mutations display discrete intraretinal fine white dots with chorioretinal atrophy. The ERG may reveal a rod-cone pattern of degeneration in patients with a recordable full-field ERG. One study described a patient who presented within the first year of life with poor vision, nystagmus, and non-recordable ERG, suggestive of a diagnosis of LCA, who maintained good central visual acuity into their late teens, highlighting the overlap between these two disease entities [8]. A milder phenotype may be associated with residual activity from hypomorphic alleles [9]. One study showed that the majority of loss of visual acuity and field occurs during the mid-teenage years (Fig. 72.3c) [7].

A dominantly-acting *RPE65* mutation was reported in a family with RP with involvement of the choroid [3]. Patients in this family presented in their second-to-fifth decades with night blindness and poor dark adaptation. As the disease progressed, peripheral vision was gradually lost. Fundus findings ranged from mid-peripheral bone-spicule or nummular pigment deposits and RPE thinning to diffuse outer retinal atrophy. The ERG showed a rod-cone pattern of degeneration.

S. Zahid et al., *Retinal Dystrophy Gene Atlas*, https://doi.org/10.1007/978-3-319-10867-4_72

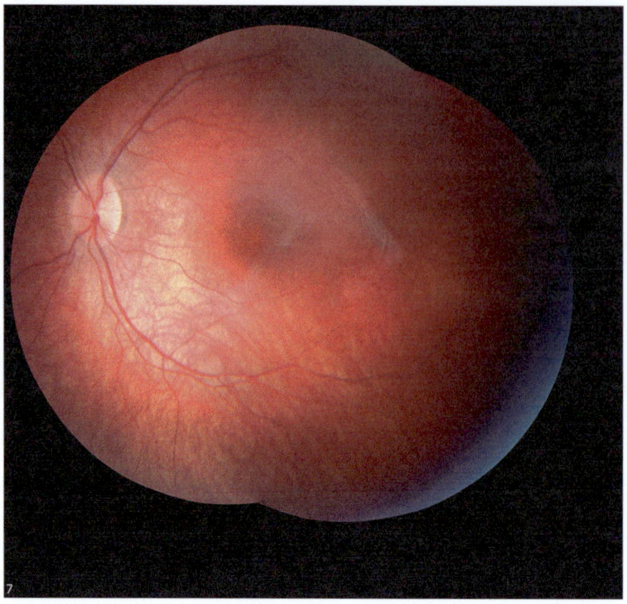

Fig. 72.1 Color fundus photograph of the left eye from a 2-year-old girl with Leber congenital amaurosis (LCA), showing macular retinal pigment epithelium (RPE) granularity and a choroideremia-like fundus.

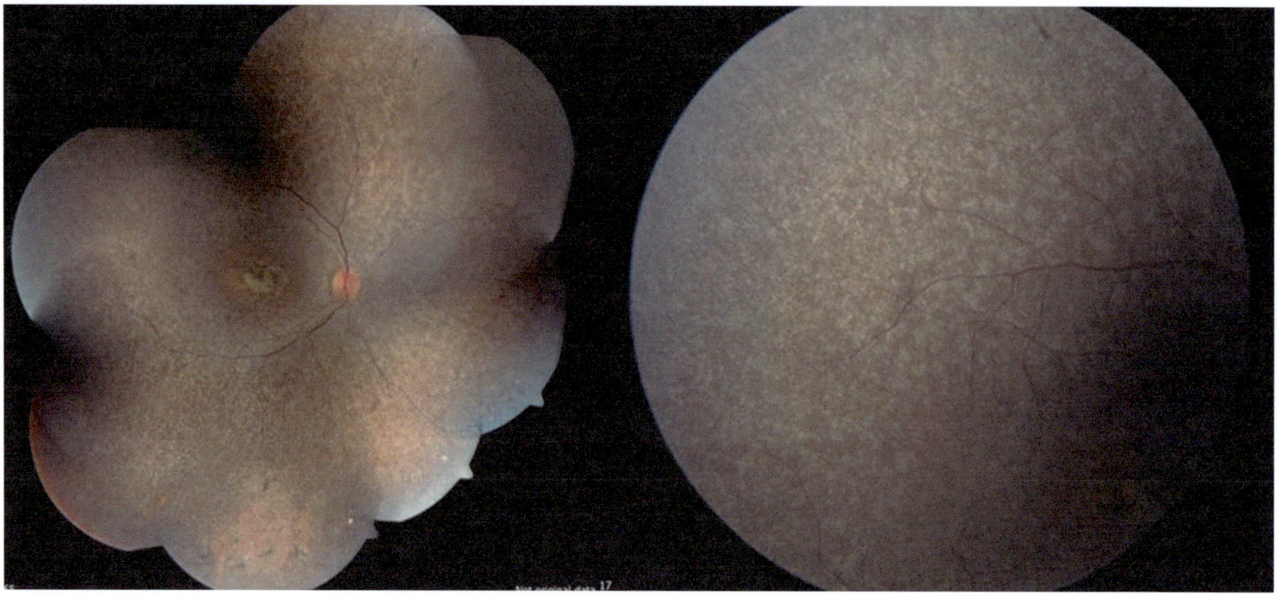

Fig. 72.2 Color fundus photograph of the right eye from a 22-year-old woman diagnosed with Severe Early Childhood Onset Retinal Dystrophy (SECORD) at the age of 3. Fundus images show intraretinal white dots in the periphery, macular atrophy, and midperipheral RPE granularity, with sparse bone spicule pigment deposits in the periphery.

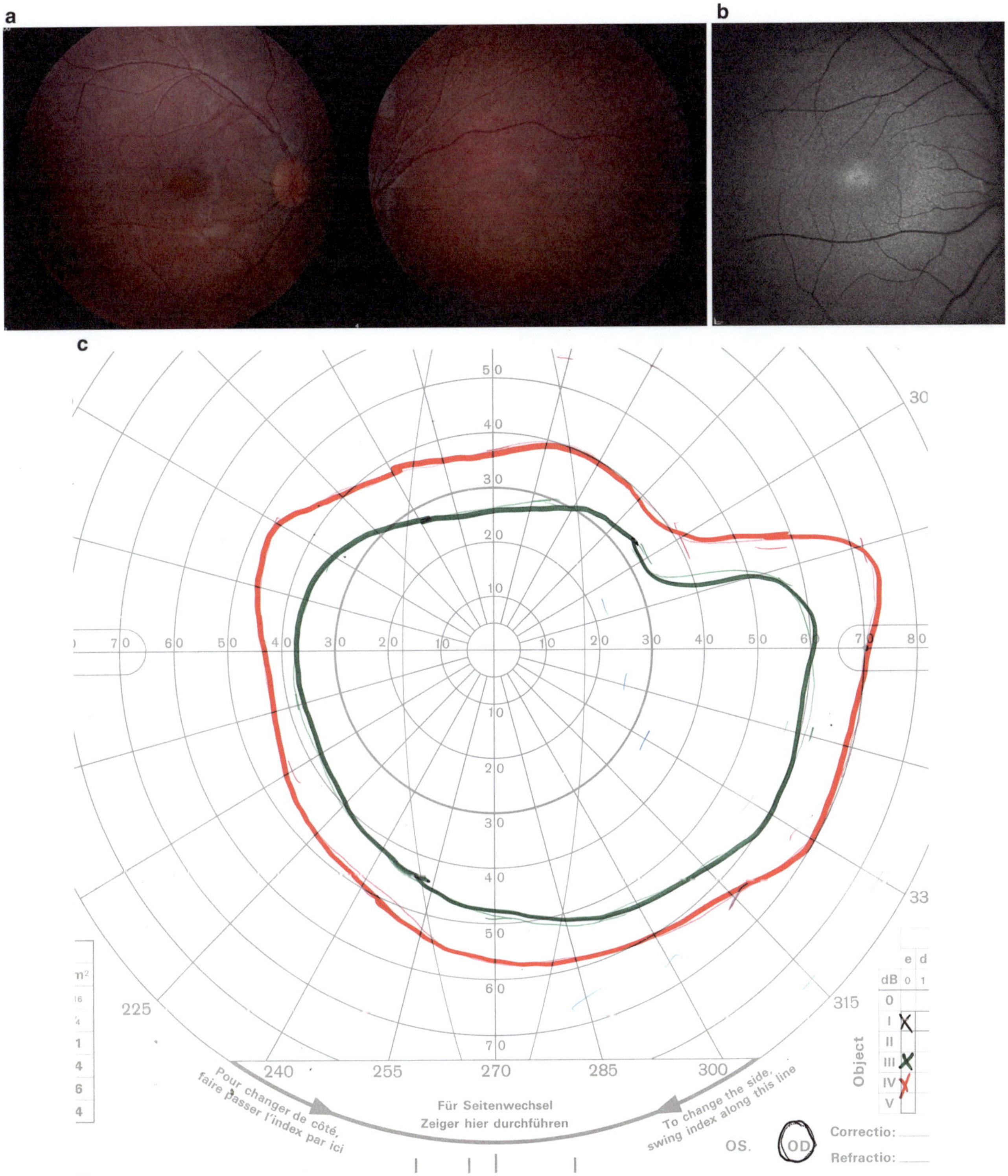

Fig. 72.3 Case summary: 5-year-old with LCA. (**a**) Color fundus photograph of the right eye, showing RPE granularity. (**b**) Fundus autofluorescence of the right eye, showing foveal hyperautofluorescence. (**c**) Goldmann visual field of the right eye, showing mildly constricted visual fields.

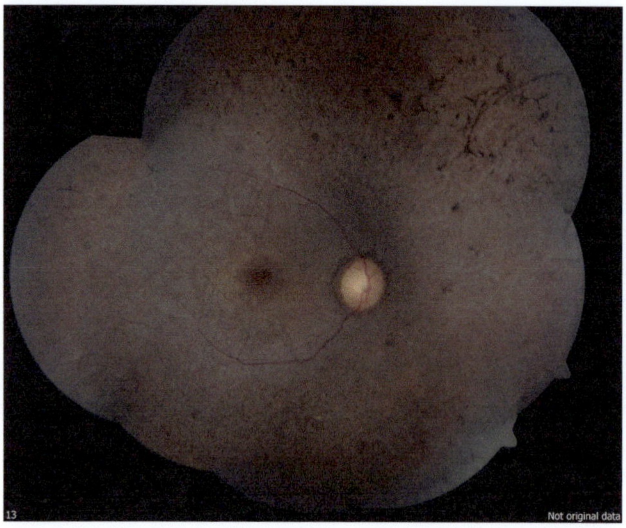

Fig. 72.4 Color fundus photograph of the right eye from a 23-year-old female with LCA, showing diffuse RPE granularity with mid-peripheral atrophy and bone spicule pigment deposits.

References

1. Moiseyev G, Chen Y, Takahashi Y, Wu BX, Ma JX. RPE65 is the isomerohydrolase in the retinoid visual cycle. Proc Natl Acad Sci U S A. 2005;102(35):12413–8.
2. Morimura H, Fishman GA, Grover SA, Fulton AB, Berson EL, Dryja TP. Mutations in the RPE65 gene in patients with autosomal recessive retinitis pigmentosa or leber congenital amaurosis. Proc Natl Acad Sci U S A. 1998;95(6):3088–93.
3. Bowne SJ, Humphries MM, Sullivan LS, Kenna PF, Tam LC, Kiang AS, et al. A dominant mutation in RPE65 identified by whole-exome sequencing causes retinitis pigmentosa with choroidal involvement. Eur J Hum Genet. 2011;19(10):1074–81.
4. Schatz P, Preising M, Lorenz B, Sander B, Larsen M, Rosenberg T. Fundus albipunctatus associated with compound heterozygous mutations in RPE65. Ophthalmology. 2011;118(5):888–94.
5. Weleber RG, Francis PJ, Trzupek KM, Beattie C. Leber congenital Amaurosis. In: Pagon RA, Adam MP, Bird TD, Dolan CR, Fong CT, Stephens K, editors. GeneReviews. Seattle: University of Washington; 1993–2017. Updated 2013.
6. Zernant J, Kulm M, Dharmaraj S, den Hollander AI, Perrault I, Preising MN, et al. Genotyping microarray (disease chip) for Leber congenital amaurosis: detection of modifier alleles. Invest Ophthalmol Vis Sci. 2005;46(9):3052–9.
7. Paunescu K, Wabbels B, Preising MN, Lorenz B. Longitudinal and cross-sectional study of patients with early-onset severe retinal dystrophy associated with RPE65 mutations. Graefes Arch Clin Exp Ophthalmol. 2005;243(5):417–26.
8. Weleber RG, Michaelides M, Trzupek KM, Stover NB, Stone EM. The phenotype of severe early childhood onset retinal dystrophy (SECORD) from mutation of RPE65 and differentiation from Leber congenital amaurosis. Invest Ophthalmol Vis Sci. 2011;52(1):292–302.
9. Lorenz B, Poliakov E, Schambeck M, Friedburg C, Preising MN, Redmond TM. A comprehensive clinical and biochemical functional study of a novel RPE65 hypomorphic mutation. Invest Ophthalmol Vis Sci. 2008;49(12):5235–42.
10. Jacobson SG, Aleman TS, Cideciyan AV, Roman AJ, Sumaroka A, Windsor EA, et al. Defining the residual vision in leber congenital amaurosis caused by RPE65 mutations. Invest Ophthalmol Vis Sci. 2009;50(5):2368–75.
11. Roman AJ, Cideciyan AV, Aleman TS, Jacobson SG. Full-field stimulus testing (FST) to quantify visual perception in severely blind candidates for treatment trials. Physiol Meas. 2007;28(8):N51–6.
12. Roman AJ, Schwartz SB, Aleman TS, Cideciyan AV, Chico JD, Windsor EA, et al. Quantifying rod photoreceptor-mediated vision in retinal degenerations: dark-adapted thresholds as outcome measures. Exp Eye Res. 2005;80(2):259–72.
13. Wabbels B, Demmler A, Paunescu K, Wegscheider E, Preising MN, Lorenz B. Fundus autofluorescence in children and teenagers with hereditary retinal diseases. Graefes Arch Clin Exp Ophthalmol. 2006;244(1):36–45.
14. Lorenz B, Wabbels B, Wegscheider E, Hamel CP, Drexler W, Preising MN. Lack of fundus autofluorescence to 488 nanometers from childhood on in patients with early-onset severe retinal dystrophy associated with mutations in RPE65. Ophthalmology. 2004;111(8):1585–94.
15. Perrault I, Rozet JM, Ghazi I, Leowski C, Bonnemaison M, Gerber S, et al. Different functional outcome of RetGC1 and RPE65 gene mutations in Leber congenital amaurosis. Am J Hum Genet. 1999;64(4):1225–8.
16. Walia S, Fishman GA, Jacobson SG, Aleman TS, Koenekoop RK, Traboulsi EI, et al. Visual acuity in patients with Leber's congenital amaurosis and early childhood-onset retinitis pigmentosa. Ophthalmology. 2010;117(6):1190–8.
17. Xu F, Dong Q, Liu L, Li H, Liang X, Jiang R, et al. Novel RPE65 mutations associated with Leber congenital amaurosis in Chinese patients. Mol Vis. 2012;18:744–50.
18. Lorenz B, Gyurus P, Preising M, Bremser D, Gu S, Andrassi M, et al. Early-onset severe rod-cone dystrophy in young children with RPE65 mutations. Invest Ophthalmol Vis Sci. 2000;41(9):2735–42.

73 RPGR

RPGR encodes retinitis pigmentosa GTPase regulator, which plays a role in photoreceptor ciliary function. Mutations in *RPGR* are inherited in an X-linked manner and have been shown to cause X-linked retinitis pigmentosa (XLRP), cone/cone-rod dystrophy, and macular dystrophy [1, 2]. Sequence variants in *RPGR* account for approximately 70–80% of XLRP. *RPGR* exhibits significant phenotypic variability, which partly results from two predominant alternatively-spliced isoforms [Exons 1–14 and Open Reading Frame 15 (ORF15)] that can each harbor mutations [3]. However, the vast majority of mutations are located in ORF15.

XLRP has an earlier onset and more rapidly progressive natural history than many other forms of retinitis pigmentosa (RP). Studies have shown that patients with mutations in *RPGR* experience a more rapid deterioration than patients with mutations in *RHO* [4]. Broadly, studies have suggested that mutations in ORF15 are associated with greater phenotypic variability than are mutations in other regions of *RPGR* [4–6]. Male patients usually present in childhood with nyctalopia and reduced peripheral vision. This progresses over time to involve central vision, with severe visual acuity loss between ages 30 and 50 [7]. Many patients exhibit myopia. Male patients have typical fundus findings of RP. Fundoscopically, this corresponds to mid-peripheral bone-spicule deposits that progressively increase with time with increasing peripheral atrophy; retinal vascular attenuation, tapetal reflex, and optic disc pallor are also commonly observed (Fig. 73.1a) [8]. Patients often show severely reduced or absent full-field electroretinography (ERG) at presentation. Carrier females are usually asymptomatic. Although some carriers may be mildly affected, they are rarely severely affected. Carrier status can often be determined with clinical examination, fundus autofluorescence imaging, or electrophysiological testing.

There is some degree of genotype-phenotype correlation, with sequence variants at the 3′-end of *RPGR-ORF15* more often associated with a cone/cone-rod phenotype and 5′ variants associated with a rod-cone phenotype. Patients with cone-rod dystrophy present with reduced visual acuity, abnormal color vision, and photophobia [9]. They experience progressive deterioration in central vision over time, with later rod involvement, nyctalopia (occurring 5–10 years after onset of initial reduced visual acuity), and peripheral visual field loss. In contrast, patients with cone dystrophy have isolated cone dysfunction [9–11]—a far less frequently observed phenotype, since the vast majority of patients develop rod involvement over time, resulting in significant overlap between cone dystrophy and cone-rod dystrophy [12]. Fundus abnormalities are typically confined to the macula, ranging from mild retinal pigment epithelium (RPE) changes to bull's-eye maculopathy and macular atrophy (Fig. 73.2). Peripheral changes are less common, but they have been observed in older patients, consisting of typical signs associated with RP. A parafoveal ring of increased autofluorescence on fundus autofluorescence imaging can be observed in both RP and cone-rod dystrophy associated with *RPGR* (Fig. 73.1b). This hyperautofluorescent ring has been shown to constrict over time in rod-cone dystrophy and expand over time in cone-rod dystrophy, allowing it to be a marker of disease progression with prognostic implications [11, 13, 14]. Optical coherence tomography is helpful in visualizing the extent and distribution of photoreceptor and RPE loss (Fig. 73.1c).

RPGR mutations have also been reported to cause "atrophic macular degeneration" [15]. Patients present in their 20s to 40s with reduced visual acuity without symptoms of peripheral visual field loss or nyctalopia. Myopia is commonly observed. Fundoscopy is characterized by localized macular RPE atrophy in both eyes with normal peripheral retina and vasculature. Full-field ERG is usually within normal limits, although it may be reduced in a minority of patients. Goldmann visual field testing exhibits a central scotoma with normal peripheral fields.

RPGR mutations may be associated with significant intra- and inter-familial phenotypic heterogeneity [7, 11, 16, 17]. Walia et al. and Zahid et al. described siblings who exhibited discordant phenotypes (cone-rod vs. rod-cone) despite

S. Zahid et al., *Retinal Dystrophy Gene Atlas*, https://doi.org/10.1007/978-3-319-10867-4_73

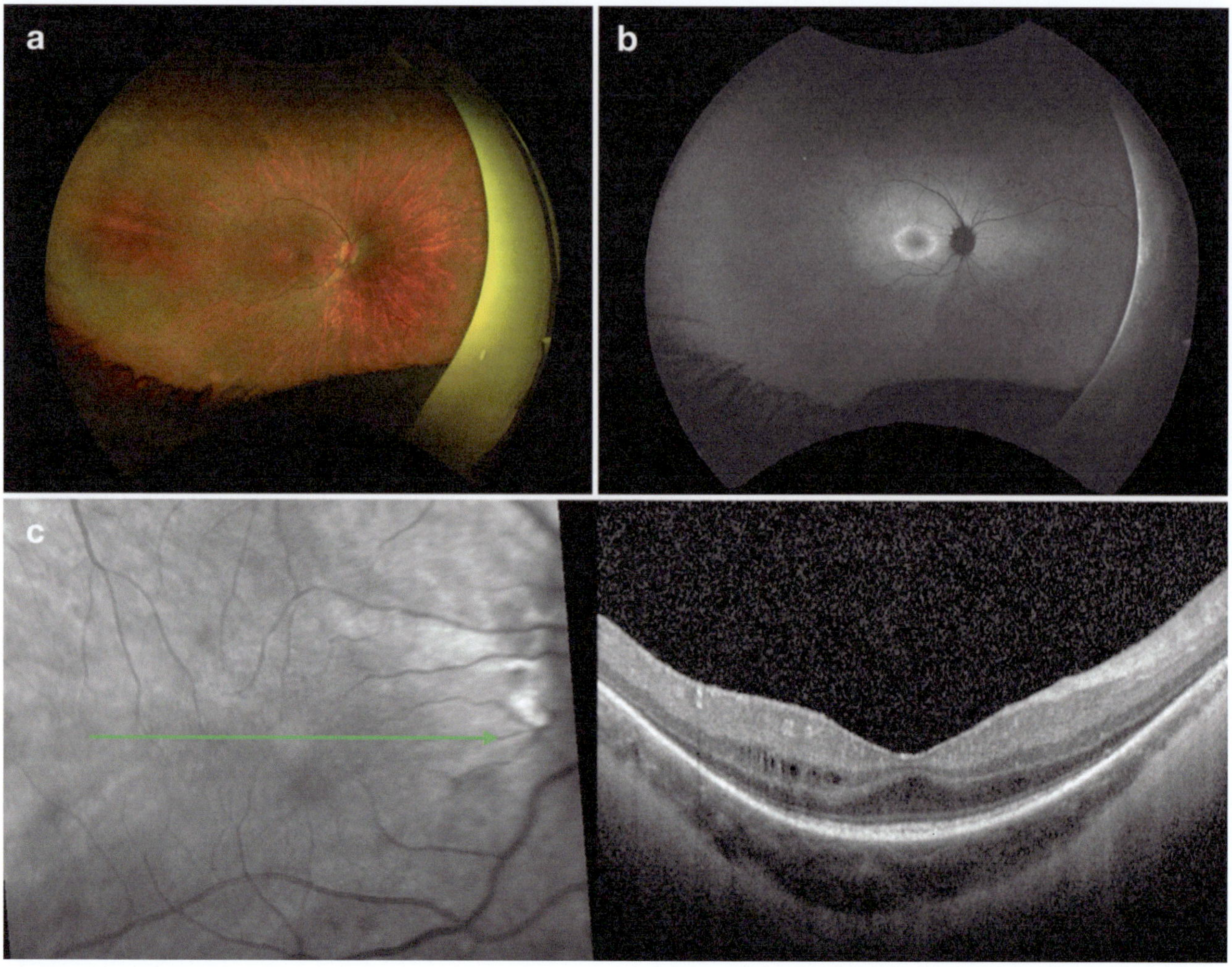

Fig. 73.1 Case summary: 8-year-old male with X-linked retinitis pigmentosa (XLRP) associated with a mutation in *RPGR*. (**a**) Widefield color fundus photo of the right eye, showing diffuse retinal atrophy. (**b**) Widefield fundus autofluorescence imaging of the right eye, demonstrating a hyperautofluorescent ring centered in the macula. (**c**) Spectral Domain Optical Coherence Tomography of the right eye, showing loss of the ellipsoid zone perifoveally and presence of microcysts.

harboring the same mutation [18, 19]. Some studies have reported *RPGR* mutations in families thought to have dominantly-inherited disease, highlighting the importance of considering X-linked inheritance even when females are also affected [20]. X-linked inheritance should be considered in both isolated male cases and in any family where males are more severely affected than females. *RPGR* variants can also be associated with syndromic inherited retinal disease, with signs and symptoms of systemic ciliary dysfunction, including respiratory problems, deafness, and infertility [21, 22].

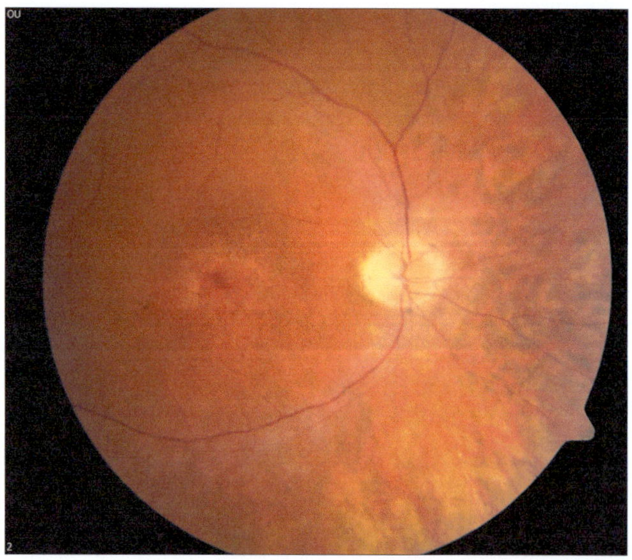

Fig. 73.2 Color fundus photography of the right eye from a patient with macular atrophy.

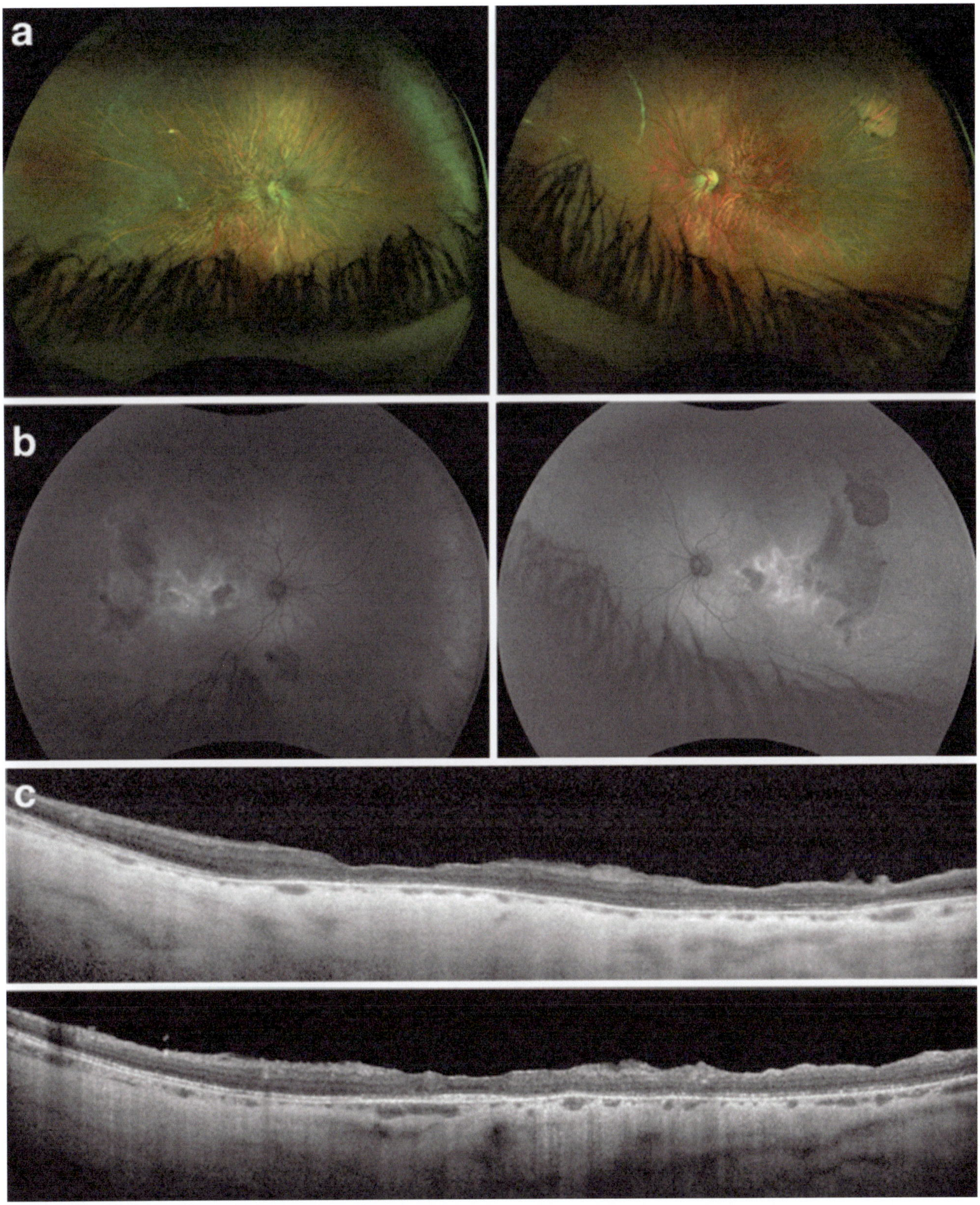

Fig. 73.3 (**a**) Widefield color fundus photos of both eyes, showing retinal atrophy in the posterior pole, extending temporally. (**b**) Widefield fundus autofluorescence of both eyes, demonstrating patches of hyperautofluorescence surrounded by areas of hypoautofluorescence corresponding to the areas of retinal atrophy. (**c**) Spectral Domain Optical Coherence tomography of both eyes, showing diffuse retinal and choroidal atrophy.

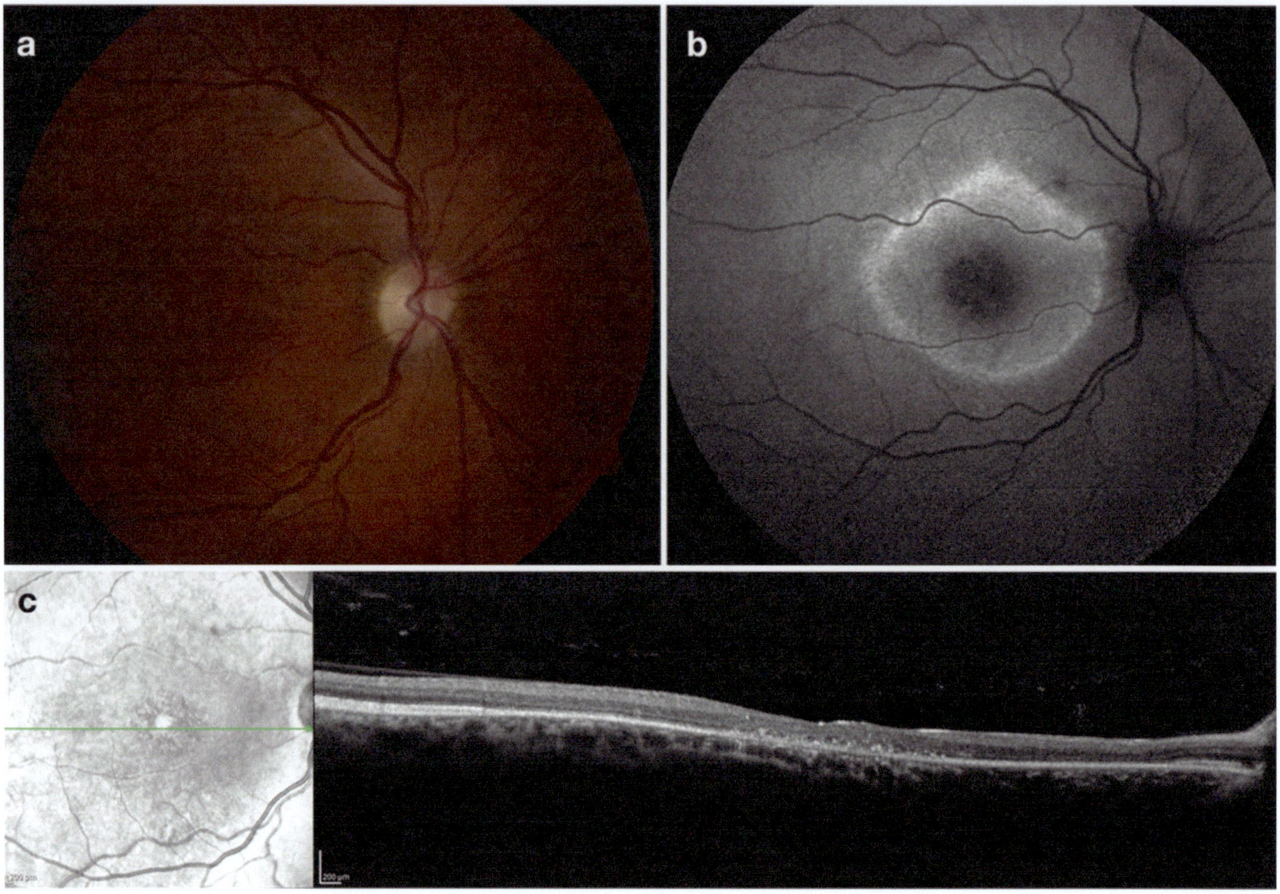

Fig. 73.4 (**a**) Color photo of the right eye, showing a relatively normal fundus. (**b**) Fundus autofluorescence of the right eye, demonstrating a hyperautofluorescent ring centered in the macula. (**c**) Spectral Domain Optical Coherence Tomography of the right eye, showing diffuse disruption of the outer retina, more prominent in the fovea.

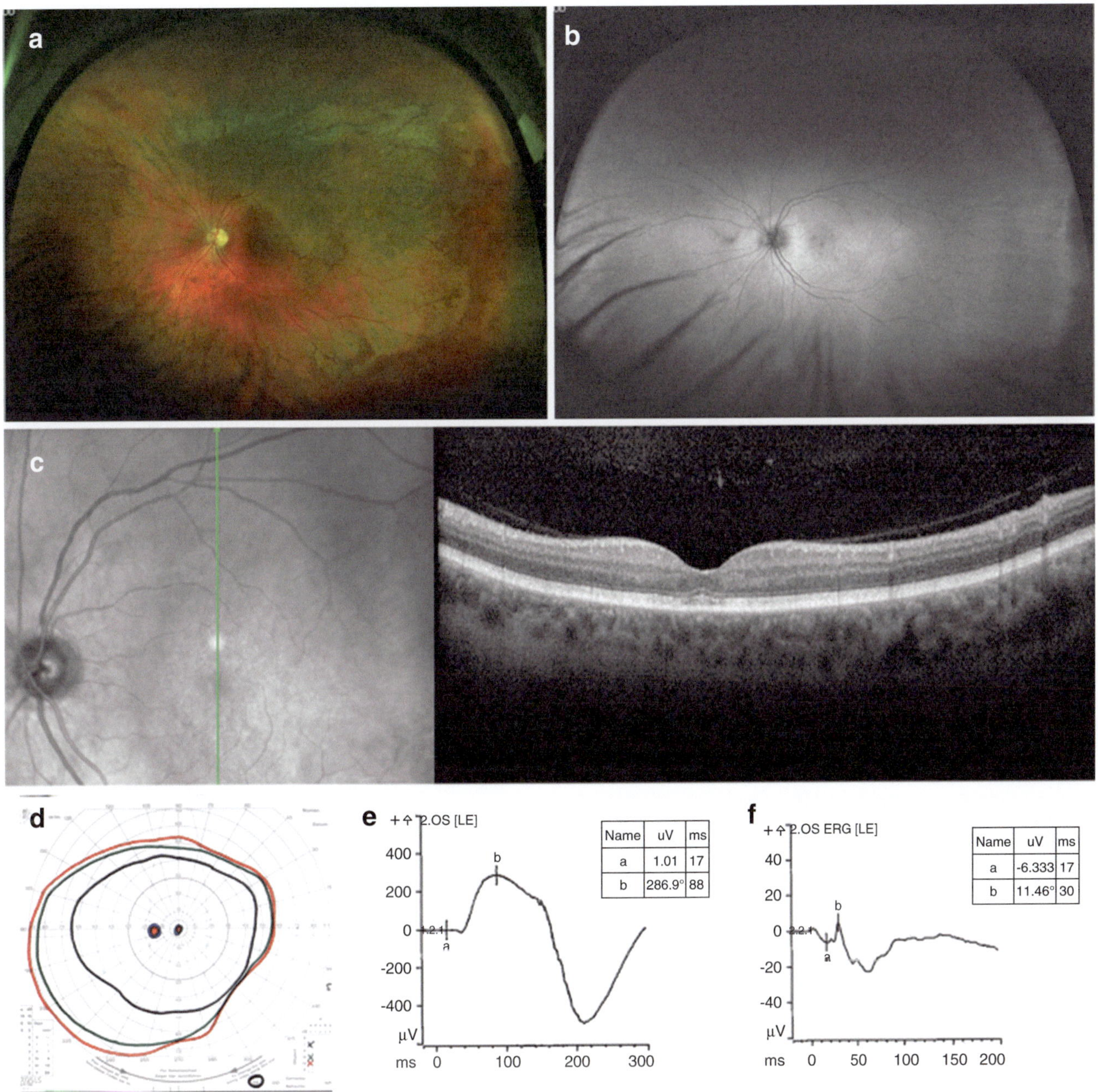

Fig. 73.5 Case summary: 48 year old man with a cone dystrophy. (**a**) Widefield color photograph of the left eye, showing a normal fundus. (**b**) Widefield fundus autofluorescence of the left eye, showing no evident abnormalities. (**c**) Spectral Domain Optical Coherence Tomography of the left eye, showing a subtle disruption of the ellipsoid zone in the fovea. (**d**) Goldman visual field of the left eye, demonstrating a small central scotoma. (**e**) Scotopic full-field electroretinogram of the left eye, showing b-wave with normal amplitude. (**f**) Photopic full-field electroretinogram of the left eye, showing reduced a-wave amplitude.

References

1. Branham K, Othman M, Brumm M, Karoukis AJ, Atmaca-Sonmez P, Yashar BM, et al. Mutations in RPGR and RP2 account for 15% of males with simplex retinal degenerative disease. Invest Ophthalmol Vis Sci. 2012;53(13):8232–7.
2. Hartong DT, Berson EL, Dryja TP. Retinitis pigmentosa. Lancet. 2006;368(9549):1795–809.
3. Bader I, Brandau O, Achatz H, Apfelstedt-Sylla E, Hergersberg M, Lorenz B, et al. X-linked retinitis pigmentosa: RPGR mutations in most families with definite X linkage and clustering of mutations in a short sequence stretch of exon ORF15. Invest Ophthalmol Vis Sci. 2003;44(4):1458–63.
4. Sandberg MA, Rosner B, Weigel-DiFranco C, Dryja TP, Berson EL. Disease course of patients with X-linked retinitis pigmentosa due to RPGR gene mutations. Invest Ophthalmol Vis Sci. 2007;48(3):1298–304.
5. Fahim AT, Bowne SJ, Sullivan LS, Webb KD, Williams JT, Wheaton DK, et al. Allelic heterogeneity and genetic modifier loci contribute to clinical variation in males with X-linked retinitis pigmentosa due to RPGR mutations. PLoS One. 2011;6(8):e23021.
6. Sharon D, Sandberg MA, Rabe VW, Stillberger M, Dryja TP, Berson EL. RP2 and RPGR mutations and clinical correlations in patients with X-linked retinitis pigmentosa. Am J Hum Genet. 2003;73(5):1131–46.
7. Al-Maskari A, O'Grady A, Pal B, McKibbin M. Phenotypic progression in X-linked retinitis pigmentosa secondary to a novel mutation in the RPGR gene. Eye. 2009;23(3):519–21.
8. Jin ZB, Liu XQ, Hayakawa M, Murakami A, Nao-i N. Mutational analysis of RPGR and RP2 genes in Japanese patients with retinitis pigmentosa: identification of four mutations. Mol Vis. 2006;12:1167–74.
9. Demirci FY, Rigatti BW, Wen G, Radak AL, Mah TS, Baic CL, et al. X-linked cone-rod dystrophy (locus COD1): identification of mutations in RPGR exon ORF15. Am J Hum Genet. 2002;70(4):1049–53.
10. Thiadens AA, Soerjoesing GG, Florijn RJ, Tjiam AG, den Hollander AI, van den Born LI, et al. Clinical course of cone dystrophy caused by mutations in the RPGR gene. Graefes Arch Clin Exp Ophthalmol. 2011;249(10):1527–35.
11. Ebenezer ND, Michaelides M, Jenkins SA, Audo I, Webster AR, Cheetham ME, et al. Identification of novel RPGR ORF15 mutations in X-linked progressive cone-rod dystrophy (XLCORD) families. Invest Ophthalmol Vis Sci. 2005;46(6):1891–8.
12. Michaelides M, Hardcastle AJ, Hunt DM, Moore AT. Progressive cone and cone-rod dystrophies: phenotypes and underlying molecular genetic basis. Surv Ophthalmol. 2006;51(3):232–58.
13. Robson AG, Michaelides M, Luong VA, Holder GE, Bird AC, Websteret AR, et al. Functional correlates of fundus autofluorescence abnormalities in patients with RPGR or RIMS1 mutations causing cone or cone rod dystrophy. Br J Ophthalmol. 2008;92(1):95–102.
14. Robson AG, Michaelides M, Saihan Z, Bird AC, Webster AR, Moore AT, et al. Functional characteristics of patients with retinal dystrophy that manifest abnormal parafoveal annuli of high density fundus autofluorescence; a review and update. Doc Ophthalmol. 2008;116(2):79–89.
15. Ayyagari R, Demirci FY, Liu J, Bingham EL, Stringham H, Kakuk LE, et al. X-linked recessive atrophic macular degeneration from RPGR mutation. Genomics. 2002;80(2):166–71.
16. Koenekoop RK, Loyer M, Hand CK, Al Mahdi H, Dembinska O, Beneish R, et al. Novel RPGR mutations with distinct retinitis pigmentosa phenotypes in French-Canadian families. Am J Ophthalmol. 2003;136(4):678–87.
17. Andreasson S, Ponjavic V, Abrahamson M, Ehinger B, Wu W, Fujita R, et al. Phenotypes in three Swedish families with X-linked retinitis pigmentosa caused by different mutations in the RPGR gene. Am J Ophthalmol. 1997;124(1):95–102.
18. Walia S, Fishman GA, Swaroop A, Branham KE, Lindeman M, Othman M, et al. Discordant phenotypes in fraternal twins having an identical mutation in exon ORF15 of the RPGR gene. Arch Ophthalmol. 2008;126(3):379–84.
19. Zahid S, Khan N, Branham K, Othman M, Karoukis AJ, Sharma N, et al. Phenotypic conservation in patients with x-linked retinitis pigmentosa caused by RPGR mutations. JAMA Ophthalmol. 2013;131(8):1016–25.
20. Churchill JD, Bowne SJ, Sullivan LS, Lewis RA, Wheaton DK, Birch DG, et al. Mutations in the X-linked retinitis pigmentosa genes RPGR and RP2 found in 8.5% of families with a provisional diagnosis of autosomal dominant retinitis pigmentosa. Invest Ophthalmol Vis Sci. 2013;54(2):1411–6.
21. Moore A. RPGR is mutated in patients with a complex X linked phenotype combining primary ciliary dyskinesia and retinitis pigmentosa. Journal of Medical Genetics. 2005;43(4):326–33.
22. Zito I. RPGR mutation associated with retinitis pigmentosa, impaired hearing, and sinorespiratory infections. Journal of Medical Genetics 2003;40(8):609–15.

74 RPGRIP1

RPGRIP1 encodes X-linked retinitis pigmentosa GTPase regulator-interacting protein 1, which is important for the function of RPGR and plays a role in photoreceptor disc morphogenesis. Autosomal recessive mutations in *RPGRIP1* cause about 5% of Leber congenital amaurosis (LCA) as well as cone-rod dystrophy [1–4].

Patients with LCA usually present within the first year of life with poor vision, nystagmus, roving eye movements, poor fixation to light, and the oculo-digital sign [5]. Photophobia is more common than night blindness at an early age [5–7]. In a cohort of four Pakistani families with mutations in *RPGRIP1*, night blindness and photoaversion were reported in 38% and 31% of patients, respectively [8]. Patients are often hyperopic [6, 7]. Cataracts and keratoconus are usually observed in older patients [5, 7, 8]. Visual acuity may range from 20/400 to CF [6], but it often deteriorates to LP or NLP within the first decade [7]. McKibbin et al. [5] reported a visual acuity range of 20/200 to LP in four families [8]. The full-field ERG is usually nonrecordable at an early age. Fundus abnormalities may be limited to mild vessel attenuation at an early age, but they eventually include optic disc pallor, RPE mottling, and peripheral pigment deposits in the second or third decade (often in a bone-spicule pattern, but may be nummular) [5, 9]. White drusen-like deposits have been reported in some patients [7]. The foveal structure may be normal in younger patients [7, 8]. Macular atrophy develops later in the disease course, often not until the third decade [8]. FAF may show macular loss of autofluorescence [5]. OCT imaging may reveal normal retinal architecture or show maintained thickness at the fovea and peripheral retina with reduced thickness in the parafovea [9]. Developmental delay has been reported in some patients with LCA caused by *RPGRIP1* mutations [5].

In keeping with other genetic loci causing LCA, there is phenotypic variability in LCA caused by *RPGRIP1* mutations. Some patients may have an early-onset rod-cone dystrophy. One patient reported visual difficulties since childhood but experienced more nyctalopia and peripheral vision loss along with loss of visual acuity [10]. The patient had horizontal nystagmus and a fundus characterized by optic disc pallor, attenuated vessels, and peripheral pigmentary changes. GVF revealed only central islands of vision remaining (rod-cone pattern). OCT in this patient showed maintained foveal architecture with atrophy in the para- and perifoveal regions. In another study, visual acuity of 0.1 (≈ 20/25) at age 15 was reported in a patient with an onset of 2 years of age and a history of nyctalopia and poor color vision. This patient exhibited macular atrophy and a severely reduced ERG [4].

RPGRIP1 mutations have also been reported to cause autosomal recessive cone-rod dystrophy in two consanguineous Pakistani families [3]. These patients experienced photophobia beginning early in childhood, with color blindness and gradual loss of central vision. Hameed et al. [3] report a rapid loss of visual acuity to 20/1200 in the mid-teenage years. Fundus features include granularity and macular atrophy (sometimes in a bull's-eye pattern). Full-field ERG revealed a cone-rod pattern of degeneration (Fig. 74.1).

S. Zahid et al., *Retinal Dystrophy Gene Atlas*, https://doi.org/10.1007/978-3-319-10867-4_74

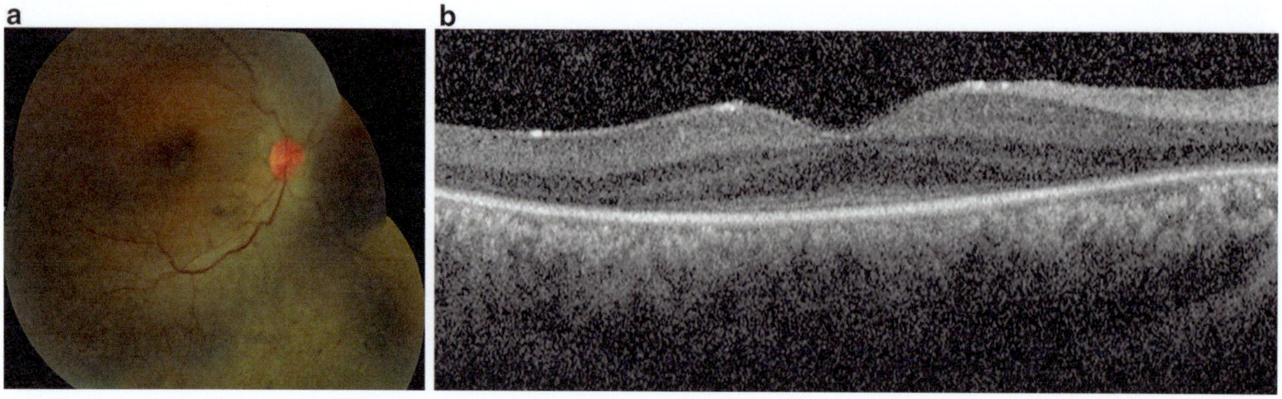

Fig. 74.1 Case summary: 17-year-old patient with *RPGRIP1*-associated Leber congenital amaurosis, onset at birth, and hand motion visual acuity. (**a**) Color fundus photograph of the right eye, showing a hyperemic disc, attenuated vessels, peripheral pigmentary changes, and retinal pigment epithelium atrophy most prominent along and outside the arcades. (**b**) Spectral domain-optical coherence tomography, showing a preserved ellipsoid zone (EZ) at the fovea with EZ and outer nuclear layer loss outside the fovea.

References

1. Dryja TP, Adams SM, Grimsby JL, McGee TL, Hong DH, Li T, et al. Null RPGRIP1 alleles in patients with Leber congenital amaurosis. Am J Hum Genet. 2001;68(5):1295–8.
2. Gerber S, Perrault I, Hanein S, Barbet F, Ducroq D, Ghazi I, et al. Complete exon-intron structure of the RPGR-interacting protein (RPGRIP1) gene allows the identification of mutations underlying Leber congenital amaurosis. Eur J Hum Genet. 2001;9(8):561–71.
3. Hameed A, Abid A, Aziz A, Ismail M, Mehdi SQ, Khaliq S. Evidence of RPGRIP1 gene mutations associated with recessive cone-rod dystrophy. J Med Genet. 2003;40(8):616–9.
4. Booij JC, Florijn RJ, ten Brink JB, Loves W, Meire F, van Schooneveld MJ, et al. Identification of mutations in the AIPL1, CRB1, GUCY2D, RPE65, and RPGRIP1 genes in patients with juvenile retinitis pigmentosa. J Med Genet. 2005;42(11):e67.
5. Khan AO, Abu-Safieh L, Eisenberger T, Bolz HJ, Alkuraya FS. The RPGRIP1-related retinal phenotype in children. Br J Ophthalmol. 2013;97(6):760–4.
6. Hanein S, Perrault I, Gerber S, Tanguy G, Barbet F, Ducroq D, et al. Leber congenital amaurosis: comprehensive survey of the genetic heterogeneity, refinement of the clinical definition, and genotype-phenotype correlations as a strategy for molecular diagnosis. Hum Mutat. 2004;23(4):306–17.
7. Galvin JA, Fishman GA, Stone EM, Koenekoop RK. Evaluation of genotype-phenotype associations in leber congenital amaurosis. Retina. 2005;25(7):919–29.
8. McKibbin M, Ali M, Mohamed MD, Booth AP, Bishop F, Pal B, et al. Genotype-phenotype correlation for leber congenital amaurosis in Northern Pakistan. Arch Ophthalmol. 2010;128(1):107–13.
9. Fakhratova M. Identification of a novel LCA6 mutation in an Emirati family. Ophthalmic Genet. 2013;34(4):234–7.
10. Jacobson SG, Cideciyan AV, Aleman TS, Sumaroka A, Schwartz SB, Roman AJ, et al. Leber congenital amaurosis caused by an RPGRIP1 mutation shows treatment potential. Ophthalmology. 2007;114(5):895–8.

75 RS1

RS1 encodes retinoschisin, which is expressed in retinal photoreceptors and bipolar cells and plays a role in the organization of retinal architecture and retinal function. Mutations in *RS1* cause X-linked juvenile retinoschisis (XLRS).

Males with mutations in *RS1* may rarely present in infancy with nystagmus, but they more commonly present in childhood with mild loss of central vision. Hyperopia is common. Visual acuity may deteriorate to 20/100, but there is significant variability among patients [1–5]. Visual acuity may remain relatively stable until adulthood [6], but it has been shown to decline with age [3]. Prognosis may be good as long as retinal detachment and vitreous hemorrhage do not occur. The disease usually affects both eyes symmetrically unless complications of the disease (vitreous hemorrhage or retinal detachment) dramatically reduce vision in one eye. Fundoscopy usually reveals foveal schisis, which presents as a characteristic "spoke-wheel" pattern of foveal cysts in the macula (Fig. 75.3a). The macular findings may progress to atrophy in later stages of the disease (Figs. 75.1, 75.2, and 75.4a, b). Peripheral retinal abnormalities, including bilateral schisis cavities (usually infero-temporal), "vitreous veils," vascular closure, inner retinal sheen, and pigmentary retinopathy, are seen in approximately 50% of cases.

There have been reports of some patients who exhibit white flecks [7] and others who exhibit the Mizuo phenomenon (loss of the tapetal reflex with dark-adaptation and recovery with exposure to light) [8]. FAF may provide a better illustration of the "spoke-wheel" pattern, which results from schisis at the fovea and may be associated with increased FAF (Fig. 75.3b) [5]. OCT is the most useful testing modality for diagnosis and reveals cystoid changes in the inner retina, which may wax and wane over time (Figs. 75.3c and 75.4c) [10, 11]. The retinal nerve fiber layer may be thinner in some patients than in controls [12]. Older patients may not exhibit retinoschisis on OCT, but they may have reduced macular thickness and ERM [13]. Full-field ERG testing may reveal a negative ERG, in which the b-wave to a-wave ratio is less than 1 for the scotopic b-wave, or may show prolonged implicit times for the cone flicker parameter [9, 14], while multifocal ERG (mfERG) illustrates the areas of cone dysfunction [15, 16]. Goldmann visual field testing typically shows central visual field loss (Fig. 75.4d). However, several studies have shown that the ERG may be normal, especially early in the disease course [17, 18]. About 5% of cases of XLRS are complicated by vitreous hemorrhage and retinal detachment, and these have been reported as early as the first year of life [19, 20]. Macular holes have also been reported [21].

Female carriers of *RS1* disease alleles usually do not exhibit any signs of structural or functional retinal abnormalities, although some may have abnormalities on mfERG [22], making molecular genetic testing invaluable in confirming carrier status.

S. Zahid et al., *Retinal Dystrophy Gene Atlas*, https://doi.org/10.1007/978-3-319-10867-4_75

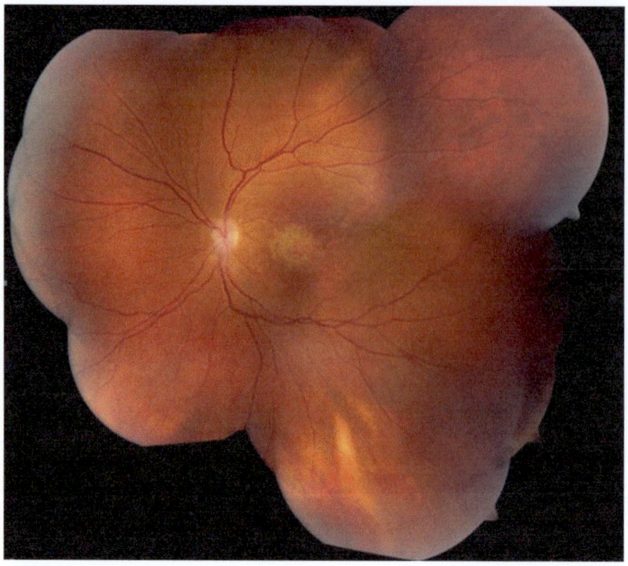

Fig. 75.1 Color fundus photo of the left eye from a 26-year-old man with X-linked juvenile retinoschisis (XLRS), showing macular atrophy.

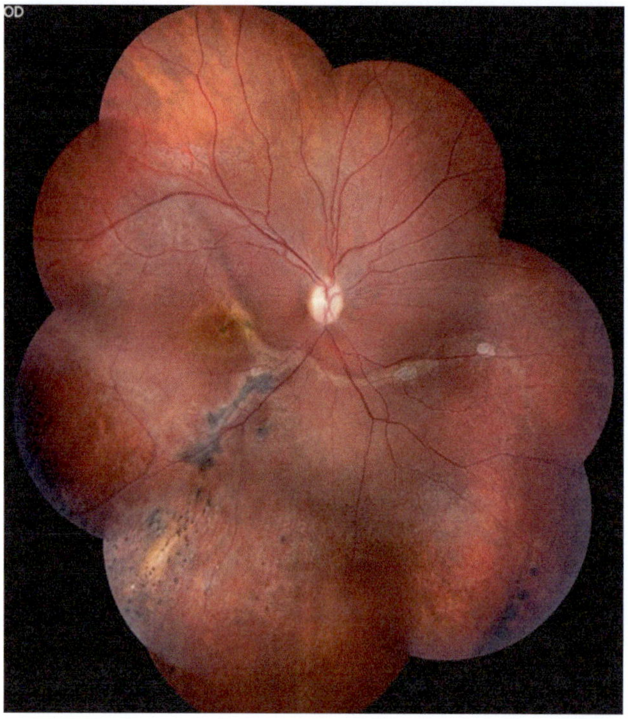

Fig. 75.2 Color fundus photo of the right eye from a 9-year-old boy with XLRS, showing macular atrophy and atrophy with pigmentation along and outside the inferior arcades and retinal periphery.

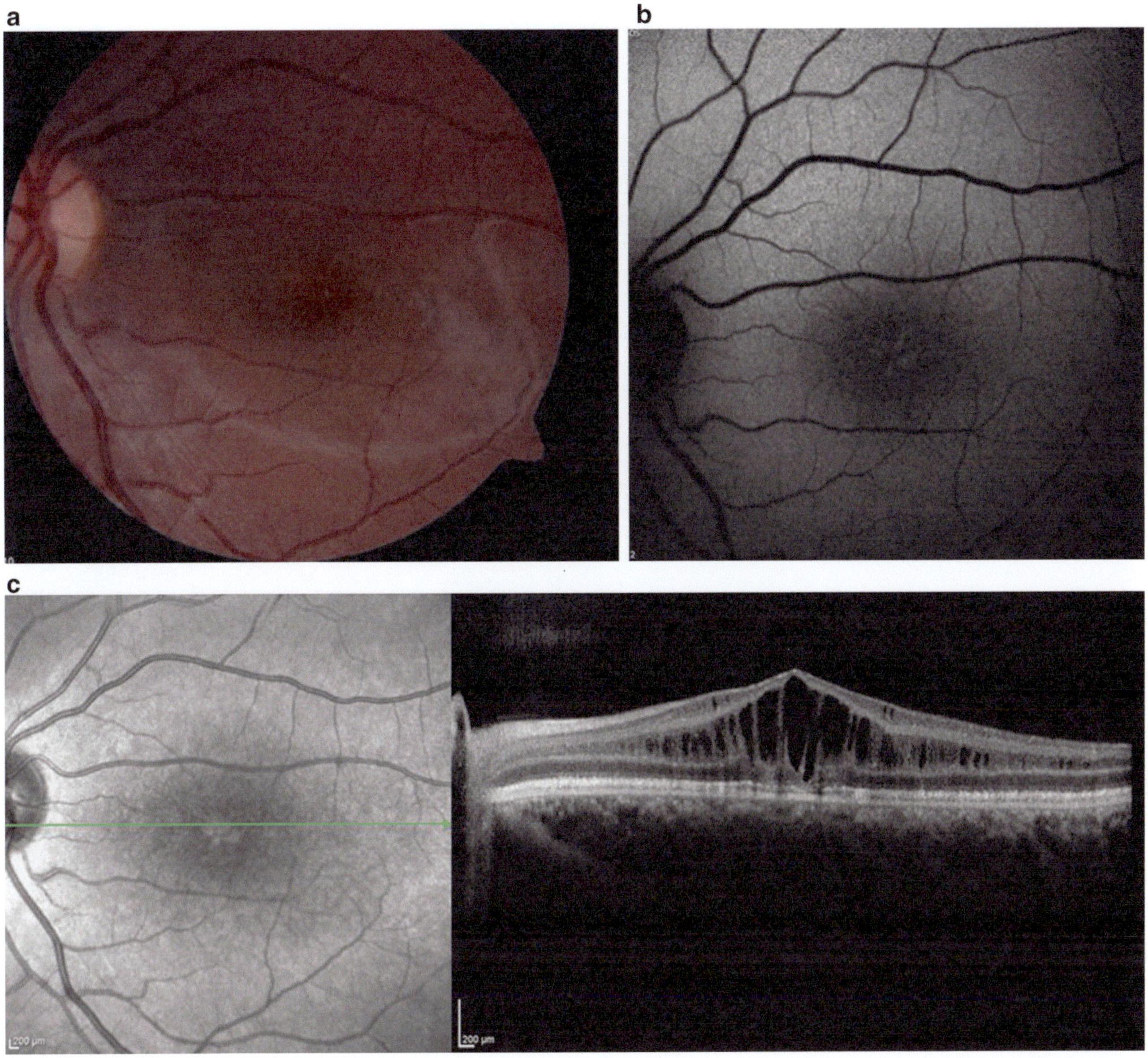

Fig. 75.3 Case summary: 12-year-old boy with a mutation in RS1. (**a**) Color fundus photograph of the left eye, showing macular schisis. (**b**) Fundus autofluorescence of the left eye, showing hyperautofluorescence at the fovea in areas of schisis. (**c**) Spectral domain-optical coherence tomography, showing schisis and segmentation of the inner retinal layers at the fovea.

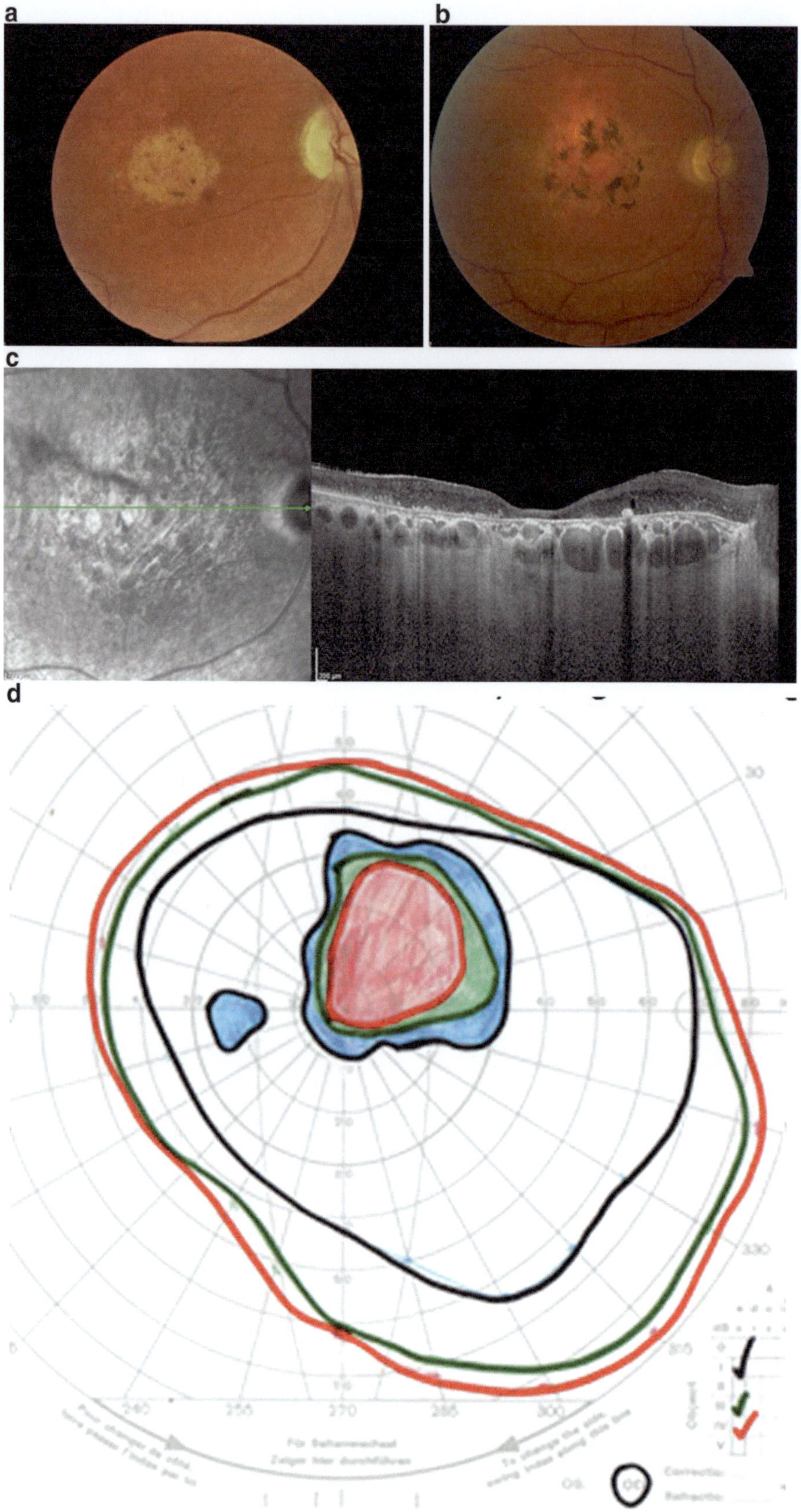

Fig. 75.4 (**a**) Color fundus photograph of the right eye, showing macular atrophy with minimal pigmentary changes at age 48. (**b**) Color fundus photograph of same eye at age 78, showing an increased area of macular atrophy with significant pigment deposits. (**c**) Spectral domain-OCT of the same eye at age 78, showing extensive outer retinal and retinal pigment epithelium atrophy. (**d**) Goldmann visual field of this eye at age 77, showing dense central field loss with all three isopters.

References

1. Molday RS, Kellner U, Weber BH. X-linked juvenile retinoschisis: clinical diagnosis, genetic analysis, and molecular mechanisms. Prog Retin Eye Res. 2012;31(3):195–212.
2. Sieving PA, MacDonald IM, Chan S. X-linked juvenile retinoschisis. In: Pagon RA, Adam MP, Ardinger HH, Wallace SE, Amemiya A, Bean LJH, et al. GeneReviews. Seattle, WA: University of Washington; 1993–2017. Updated 2014.
3. Pimenides D, George ND, Yates JR, Bradshaw K, Roberts SA, Moore AT, et al. X-linked retinoschisis: clinical phenotype and RS1 genotype in 86 UK patients. J Med Genet. 2005;42(6):e35.
4. Riveiro-Alvarez R, Trujillo-Tiebas MJ, Gimenez-Pardo A, Garcia-Hoyos M, Lopez-Martinez MA, Aguirre-Lamban J, et al. Correlation of genetic and clinical findings in Spanish patients with X-linked juvenile retinoschisis. Invest Ophthalmol Vis Sci. 2009;50(9):4342–50.
5. Renner AB, Kellner U, Fiebig B, Cropp E, Foerster MH, Weber BH. ERG variability in X-linked congenital retinoschisis patients with mutations in the RS1 gene and the diagnostic importance of fundus autofluorescence and OCT. Doc Ophthalmol. 2008;116(2):97–109.
6. Apushkin MA, Fishman GA, Rajagopalan AS. Fundus findings and longitudinal study of visual acuity loss in patients with X-linked retinoschisis. Retina. 2005;25(5):612–8.
7. Hotta Y, Nakamura M, Okamoto Y, Nomura R, Terasaki H, Miyake Y. Different mutation of the XLRS1 gene causes juvenile retinoschisis with retinal white flecks. Br J Ophthalmol. 2001;85(2):238–9.
8. Vincent A, Shetty R, Yadav NK, Shetty BK. Foveal schisis with Mizuo phenomenon: etio-pathogenesis of tapetal reflex in X-linked retinoschisis. Eye (Lond). 2009;23(5):1240–1.
9. Eksandh LC, Ponjavic V, Ayyagari R, Bingham EL, Hiriyanna KT, Andréasson S, et al. Phenotypic expression of juvenile X-linked retinoschisis in Swedish families with different mutations in the XLRS1 gene. Arch Ophthalmol. 2000;118(8):1098–104.
10. Dhingra S, Patel CK. Diagnosis and pathogenesis of congenital X-linked retinoschisis with optical coherence tomography. J Pediatr Ophthalmol Strabismus. 2010;47(2):105–7.
11. Apushkin MA, Fishman GA, Janowicz MJ. Correlation of optical coherence tomography findings with visual acuity and macular lesions in patients with X-linked retinoschisis. Ophthalmology. 2005;112(3):495–501.
12. Genead MA, Fishman GA, Walia S. Efficacy of sustained topical dorzolamide therapy for cystic macular lesions in patients with X-linked retinoschisis. Arch Ophthalmol. 2010;128(2):190–7.
13. Menke MN, Feke GT, Hirose T. Effect of aging on macular features of X-linked retinoschisis assessed with optical coherence tomography. Retina. 2011;31(6):1186–92.
14. Renner AB, Kellner U, Cropp E, Foerster MH. Dysfunction of transmission in the inner retina: incidence and clinical causes of negative electroretinogram. Graefes Arch Clin Exp Ophthalmol. 2006;244(11):1467–73.
15. Sen P, Roy R, Maru S, Ravi P. Evaluation of focal retinal function using multifocal electroretinography in patients with X-linked retinoschisis. Can J Ophthalmol. 2010;45(5):509–13.
16. Piao CH, Kondo M, Nakamura M, Terasaki H, Miyake Y. Multifocal electroretinograms in X-linked retinoschisis. Invest Ophthalmol Vis Sci. 2003;44(11):4920–30.
17. Sieving PA, Bingham EL, Kemp J, Richards J, Hiriyanna K. Juvenile X-linked retinoschisis from XLRS1 Arg213Trp mutation with preservation of the electroretinogram scotopic b-wave. Am J Ophthalmol. 1999;128(2):179–84.
18. Eksandh L, Andreasson S, Abrahamson M. Juvenile X-linked retinoschisis with normal scotopic b-wave in the electroretinogram at an early stage of the disease. Ophthalmic Genet. 2005;26(3):111–7.
19. Prasad A, Wagner R, Bhagat N. Vitreous hemorrhage as the initial manifestation of X-linked retinoschisis in a 9-month-old infant. J Pediatr Ophthalmol Strabismus. 2006;43(1):56–8.
20. Lee JJ, Kim JH, Kim SY, Park SS, Yu YS. Infantile vitreous hemorrhage as the initial presentation of X-linked juvenile retinoschisis. Korean J Ophthalmol. 2009;23(2):118–20.
21. Brasil OF, da Cunha AL, de Castro MB, Japiassu RM. Macular hole secondary to X-linked juvenile retinoschisis. Ophthalmic Surg Lasers Imaging. 2011;42 Online:e4–5.
22. Kim LS, Seiple W, Fishman GA, Szlyk JP. Multifocal ERG findings in carriers of X-linked retinoschisis. Doc Ophthalmol. 2007;114(1):21–6.

76 SAG

SAG, also known as *S-antigen or S-arrestin,* encodes a rod photoreceptor protein involved in the recovery phase of light transduction. It is present in the retina and pineal gland and plays an inhibitory role in the activated phototransduction cascade [1, 2]. Mutations are responsible for Oguchi disease and for retinitis pigmentosa (RP).

SAG mutations are responsible for the majority of cases of Oguchi disease in the Japanese population and have an autosomal recessive pattern of inheritance. The most frequent mutation in this population is c.926delA; p.N309Tfs*12 (previously reported as 1147delA) [2, 3]. Hayashi et al. (2010) reported that 5 out of 6 Japanese patients with Oguchi disease are homozygous for the c.926delA mutation [3]. Oguchi is a form of congenital stationary night blindness (CSNB) where the only symptom is generally a childhood-onset of nyctalopia [4]. Visual acuity, visual field, and color vision are usually all within normal range. A characteristic feature of Oguchi is the diffuse golden yellow or gray discoloration of the fundus, which disappears after prolonged dark-adaptation and reappears almost immediately upon re-exposure to light (called the Mizuo-Nakamura phenomenon) [2–4]. Full-field electroretinogram (ERG) is non-recordable after 30 minutes of dark adaptation, but cone and flicker ERG recordings are essentially normal. Combined rod-cone ERG responses show a significantly reduced a-wave, a non-detectable b-wave, and well-preserved oscillatory potentials [3, 4].

SAG mutations have variable expressivity. Some patients have Oguchi disease only [2] and some manifest symptoms RP along with the Mizuo-Nakamura phenomenon [4]. There is a report of a patient with autosomal recessive RP with a homozygous c.926delA mutation in *SAG* who has pigmentary retinal degeneration and retinal pigment epithelium (RPE) atrophy along the vascular arcades. This patient has constricted visual fields and paracentral visual field defects and also exhibits the Mizuo-Nakamura phenomenon [3].

More recently, Sullivan et al. described a dominantly-acting mutation in *SAG* (c.440G>T; p.Cys147Phe) that is reponsible for 36% of the autosomal dominant retinitis pigmentosa in Hispanic patients in the United States. All these patients demonstrated classic fundus features of retinitis pigmentosa with a rod-cone pattern of ERG loss; none demonstrated the Mizuo-Nakamura phenomenon [5].

References

1. O'Neill MJF. S-Antigen; SAG. OMIM. 181031. 1990 (updated 2013). http://omim.org/entry/181031. Accessed 6 Mar 2017.
2. Waheed NK, Qavi AH, Malik SN, Maria M, Riaz M, Cremers FP, et al. A nonsense mutation in S-antigen (p.Glu306*) causes Oguchi disease. Mol Vis. 2012;18:1253–9.
3. Hayashi T, Tsuzuranuki S, Kozaki K, Urashima M, Tsuneoka H. Macular dysfunction in oguchi disease with the frequent mutation 1147delA in the SAG gene. Ophthalmic Res. 2011;46(4):175–80.
4. Sonoyama H, Shinoda K, Ishigami C, Tada Y, Ideta H, Ideta R, et al. Oguchi disease masked by retinitis pigmentosa. Doc Ophthalmol. 2011;123(2):127–33.
5. Sullivan LS, Bowne SJ, Koboldt DC, Cadena EL, Heckenlively JR, Branham KE, Wheaton DH, Jones KD, Ruiz RS, Pennesi ME, Yang P, Davis-Boozer D, Northrup H, Gurevich VV, Chen R, Xu M, Li Y, Birch DG, Daiger SP. A Novel Dominant Mutation in, the Arrestin-1 Gene, Is a Common Cause of Retinitis Pigmentosa in Hispanic Families in the Southwestern United States. Investigative Opthalmology & Visual Science. 2017;58(5):2774.

S. Zahid et al., *Retinal Dystrophy Gene Atlas*, https://doi.org/10.1007/978-3-319-10867-4_76

77 *SEMA4A*

SEMA4A encodes semaphorin-4A, a cell surface receptor involved in cell-to-cell signaling, which plays a role in adaptive immunity as well as in inhibition of angiogenesis and axonal growth. One study showed that mutations in *SEMA4A* result in RPE cell susceptibility to light, oxidative, and endoplasmic reticulum stress *in vitro* [1]. Mutations in *SEMA4A* have been shown to cause autosomal recessive and autosomal dominant retinitis pigmentosa (rod-cone dystrophy) and recessive cone-rod dystrophy [2].

Patients with dominant or recessive rod-cone dystrophy present initially with night blindness and progressive peripheral vision loss, with central vision loss later in the disease process. Fundus findings include peripheral and mid-peripheral bone spicule pigmentation with vascular attenuation; macular involvement is typically found in older patients. Optical coherence tomography may reveal foveal-sparing of photoreceptors (Fig. 77.1b).

Cone-rod dystrophy is typified by early loss of visual acuity and dyschromatopsia, with nyctalopia and peripheral vision loss occurring later; photophobia and photosensitivity are common in these patients. The fundus appears granular, with macular atrophy and peripheral pigmentation. Fundus autofluorescence may reveal increased macular autofluorescence and patchy areas of hypoautofluorescence in the mid-peripheral retina (Fig. 77.1a).

S. Zahid et al., *Retinal Dystrophy Gene Atlas*, https://doi.org/10.1007/978-3-319-10867-4_77

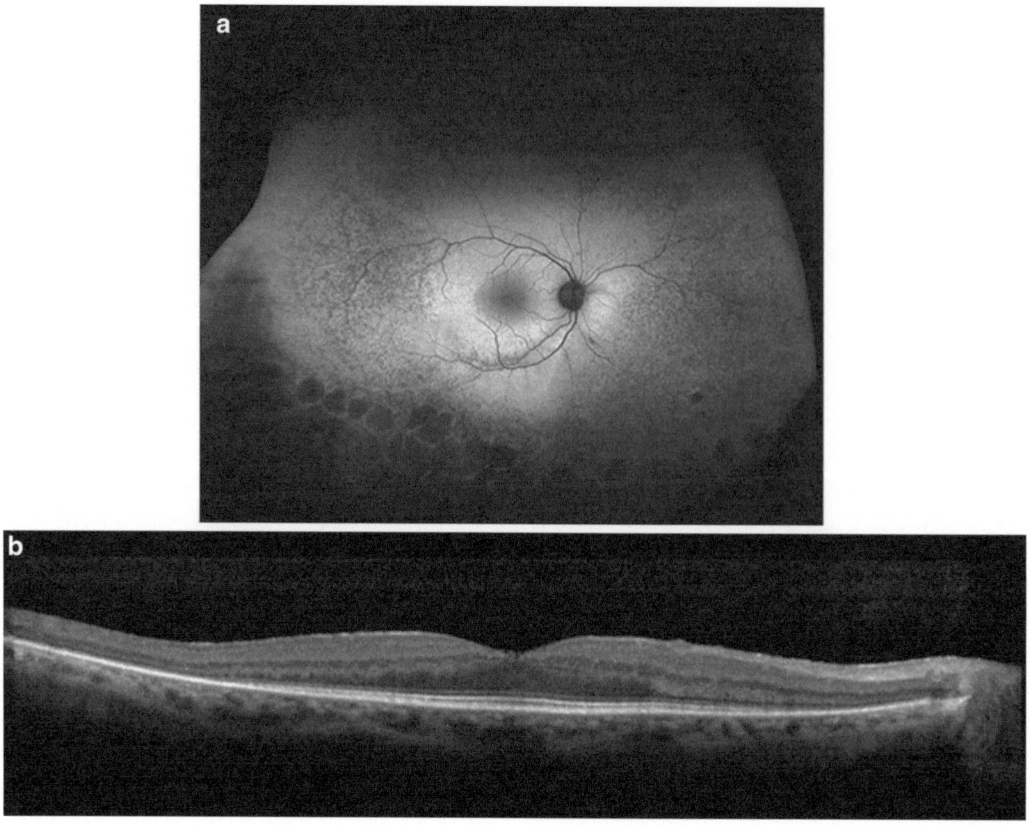

Fig. 77.1 Case summary: 52-year-old Hispanic male (CEI28386) with a family history of dominant retinitis pigmentosa with a mutation in *SEMA4A*. (**a**) Wide-field fundus autofluorescence of the right eye, showing increased macular autofluorescence, with patchy areas of hypoautofluorescence in the mid-peripheral retina. There are also circular areas of hypoautofluorescence corresponding to RPE atrophy in the inferior retina. (**b**) Spectral domain optical coherence tomography of the right eye, showing extrafoveal ellipsoid zone and outer nuclear layer loss.

References

1. Tsuruma K, Nishimura Y, Kishi S, Shimazawa M, Tanaka T, Hara H. SEMA4A mutations lead to susceptibility to light irradiation, oxidative stress, and ER stress in retinal pigment epithelial cells. Invest Ophthalmol Vis Sci. 2012;53(10):6729–37.
2. Abid A, Ismail M, Mehdi SQ, Khaliq S. Identification of novel mutations in the SEMA4A gene associated with retinal degenerative diseases. J Med Genet. 2006;43(4):378–81.

78 SNRNP200

SNRNP200 (also known as *ASCC3L1*) encodes hBrr2, an RNA helicase essential for pre-mRNA splicing. Mutations in this gene have been associated with autosomal dominant retinitis pigmentosa (RP) [1–3].

Patients with *SNRNP200*-related RP typically present with nyctalopia, with an onset in the late first to early second decades of life. Patients exhibit a gradual decline in visual acuity and narrowing of visual fields with age, leading to eventual peripheral field loss with relatively conserved central vision. Fundoscopy may reveal waxy pallor of the optic disc, arteriolar attenuation, bone-spicule pigmentary changes in the mid-periphery, and atrophy of the retinal pigment epithelium, which typically increases with age (Figs. 78.1 and 78.2) [1–3]. Macular atrophy may be seen in some older patients [2]. In one study, two patients in their 40s were also diagnosed with angle-closure glaucoma [1]. Full-field scotopic rod electroretinogram (ERG) may reveal reduced or non-recordable responses. In severe cases, both rod and cone function may be reduced, but in younger patients, cone cell function may be better preserved. Multi-focal ERG may display reduced signals over the entire test field or show reduction in the peripheral macula [1–3].

S. Zahid et al., *Retinal Dystrophy Gene Atlas*, https://doi.org/10.1007/978-3-319-10867-4_78

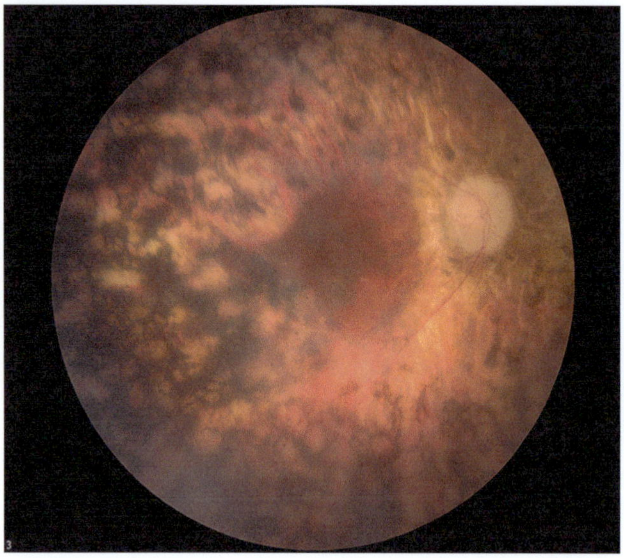

Fig. 78.1 Color fundus photograph from a 59-year-old woman with rod-cone dystrophy, showing typical findings of bone spicule pigmentary changes, waxy pallor of the optic nerve, and attenuation of the retinal vessels.

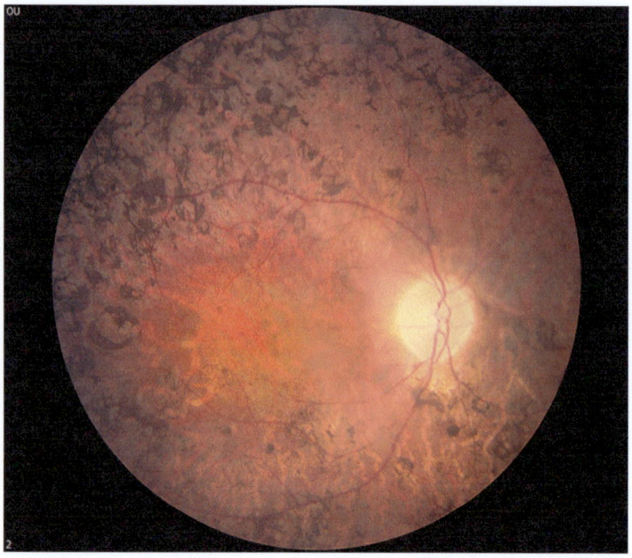

Fig. 78.2 Color fundus photograph from a 45-year-old man with rod-cone dystrophy, showing typical findings of retinitis pigmentosa.

References

1. Liu T, Jin X, Zhang X, Yuan H, Cheng J, Lee J, et al. A novel missense SNRNP200 mutation associated with autosomal dominant retinitis pigmentosa in a Chinese family. PLoS One. 2012;7(9):e45464.
2. Zhao C, Lu S, Zhou X, Zhang X, Zhao K, Larsson C. A novel locus (RP33) for autosomal dominant retinitis pigmentosa mapping to chromosomal region 2cen-q12.1. Hum Genet. 2006;119(6):617–23.
3. Li N, Mei H, MacDonald IM, Jiao X, Hejtmancik JF. Mutations in ASCC3L1 on 2q11.2 are associated with autosomal dominant retinitis pigmentosa in a Chinese family. Invest Ophthalmol Vis Sci. 2010;51(2):1036–43.

79 SPATA7

SPATA7 encodes spermatogenesis-associated protein, whose retinal function is poorly defined. Autosomal recessive mutations in *SPATA7* are associated with Leber congenital amaurosis (LCA) and retinitis pigmentosa (RP).

SPATA7 mutations are a rare cause (1–2%) of autosomal recessive LCA. Patients with *SPATA7*-related LCA may have an early onset of visual symptoms, typically beginning in infancy. Similar to LCA caused by other genes, infants exhibit poor visual fixation and pupillary reflex, nystagmus, nyctalopia, hyperopic astigmatism, and transient photophobia [1–3]. In one study of 10 patients with *SPATA7* mutations, keratoconus was present in one patient, and mild cataracts were present in two patients under the age of 21 [1]. Visual acuity may present as poor as hand movements or worse, and Goldmann visual fields show less than 5° central field preservation within the first decade of life [1]. Fundus examination of patients may reveal a normal fundus at an early age or a gradually deteriorating "salt-and-pepper" appearance with atrophic retinal changes and pigment migration, with arteriolar attenuation and optic disc pallor [1, 3]. Fundus autofluorescence imaging often shows a hyperautofluorescent parafoveal ring, with hypoautofluorescence from the mid-periphery to the periphery as well as along the arterioles. SD-OCT shows diffuse retinal thinning and preservation of the ellipsoid zone at the foveal region. ERGs in younger patients may reveal normal/subnormal rod-ERG b-wave amplitudes, but by the first decade of life, the rod ERG tends to become completely undetectable [1].

SPATA7-related early-onset retinal dystrophy has an autosomal recessive pattern of inheritance and is rare. Phenotypes are very similar to *SPATA7*-related LCA but tend to exhibit less severe disease [2]. Onset of symptoms occurs in early childhood, with complaints of vision loss and nyctalopia. Visual fields may be reduced to 5° within the first decade of life [2]. Visual acuities are normal at an early age but deteriorate over time to 20/200 to hand motion vision. Fundus examination reveals widespread RPE degeneration, arteriolar narrowing, optic disc pallor, and bone-spicule like pigmentary changes, typical of classical RP (Fig. 79.1a). Older patients may exhibit a maculopathy. Full-field ERG is typically non-recordable at an early age in both rod and cone parameters [4]. Fundus autofluorescence may show a ring of hyperautofluorescence in the macula (Fig. 79.1b), and optical coherence tomography is helpful to visualize the extent of photoreceptor and retinal pigment epithelium loss.

S. Zahid et al., *Retinal Dystrophy Gene Atlas*, https://doi.org/10.1007/978-3-319-10867-4_79

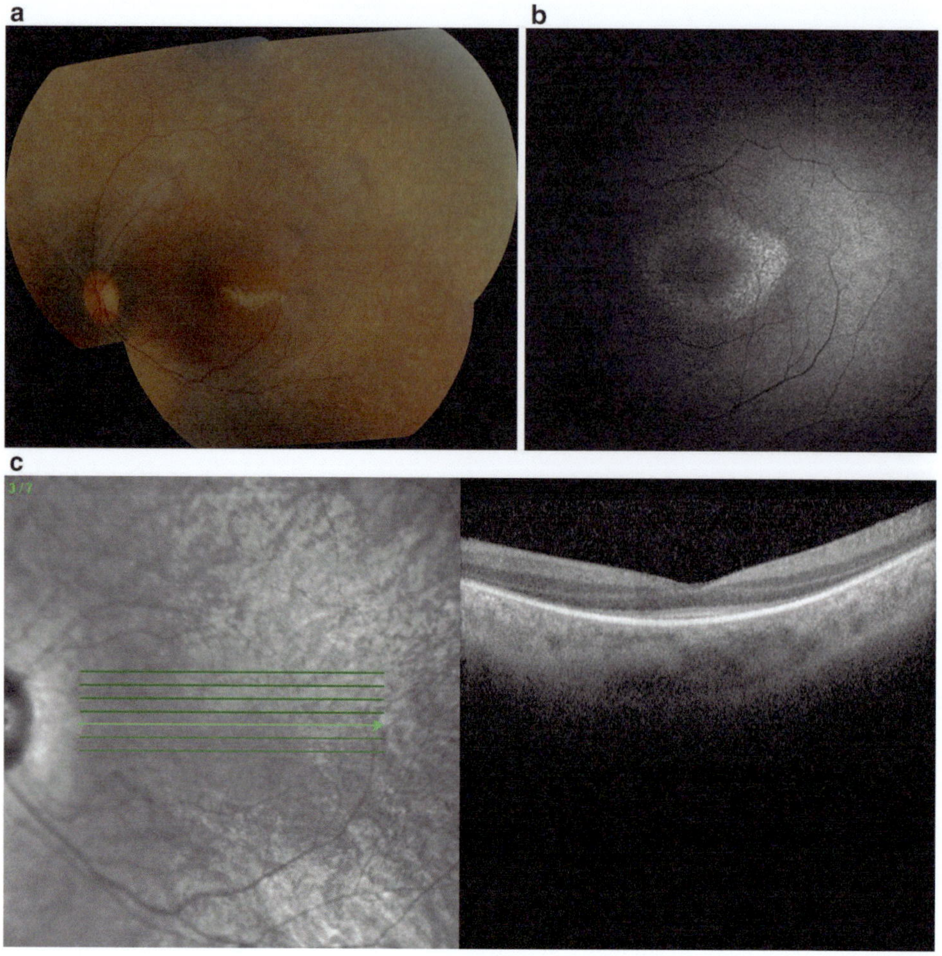

Fig. 79.1 Case summary: 17-year-old with *SPATA7*-associated Leber congenital amaurosis, onset at birth, hand movement visual acuity. (**a**) Color fundus photograph of the left eye, showing attenuated vessels, peripheral retinal pigment epithelium atrophy, and white retinal dots/deposits. (**b**) Fundus autofluorescence, showing a macular ring of hyperautofluorescence surrounding the fovea. (**c**) Spectral domain-optical coherence tomography, showing a broadened foveal pit with perifoveal macular loss of the ellipsoid zone and outer nuclear layer.

References

1. Mackay DS, Ocaka LA, Borman AD, Sergouniotis PI, Henderson RH, Moradi P, et al. Screening of SPATA7 in patients with Leber congenital amaurosis and severe childhood-onset retinal dystrophy reveals disease-causing mutations. Invest Ophthalmol Vis Sci. 2011;52(6):3032–8.
2. Wang H, den Hollander AI, Moayedi Y, Abulimiti A, Li Y, Collin RW, et al. Mutations in SPATA7 cause Leber congenital amaurosis and juvenile retinitis pigmentosa. Am J Hum Genet. 2009;84(3):380–7.
3. Perrault I, Hanein S, Gerard X, Delphin N, Fares-Taie L, Gerber S, et al. Spectrum of SPATA7 mutations in Leber congenital amaurosis and delineation of the associated phenotype. Hum Mutat. 2010;31(3):E1241–50.
4. Kannabiran C, Palavalli L, Jalali S. Mutation of SPATA7 in a family with autosomal recessive early-onset retinitis pigmentosa. J Mol Genet Med. 2012;6:301–3.

80 *TIMP3*

Mutations in *TIMP3*, which encodes an inhibitor of matrix metalloproteinase, have been shown to cause Sorsby fundus dystrophy, an autosomal dominant macular degeneration [1–4].

Patients usually present in their 40s to 50s with a sudden loss of central vision that results from choroidal neovascularization and subretinal fluid [5, 6]. Some patients experience nyctalopia before central visual deficits, but most patients are asymptomatic before sudden central vision loss. In one study, median ages of visual acuity deterioration to below 20/200 were 45 and 59 for the first and second eyes [5]. Choroidal neovascularization (CNV) tends to cause vision loss earlier than macular atrophy, occurring as early as age 45 in the first eye [4]. Some patients may not show CNV in the fellow eye until 3-5 years later [5]. Fundoscopic examination often reveals a normal fundus in patients younger than 20 years, but most patients exhibit drusen-like deposits at the posterior pole by the third decade, which may not affect visual acuity [5, 7]. These deposits are usually not visualized on fluorescein angiography, although patchy hypofluorescence is observed throughout the retina. Macular atrophy may occur with or without CNV and can result in visual acuity less than 20/200 in the 50s (Figs. 80.1 and 80.2). Some studies have shown that drusen-like deposits may precede CNV by three to twelve years, though CNV can occur in the absence of these deposits [5]. CNV occurs in both eyes in 50% of patients, occurring as early as 37 years and as late as 61 years [5]. CNV has been reported to be recurrent and multifocal in patients with certain mutations [5]. Peripheral atrophy is rare.

S. Zahid et al., *Retinal Dystrophy Gene Atlas*, https://doi.org/10.1007/978-3-319-10867-4_80

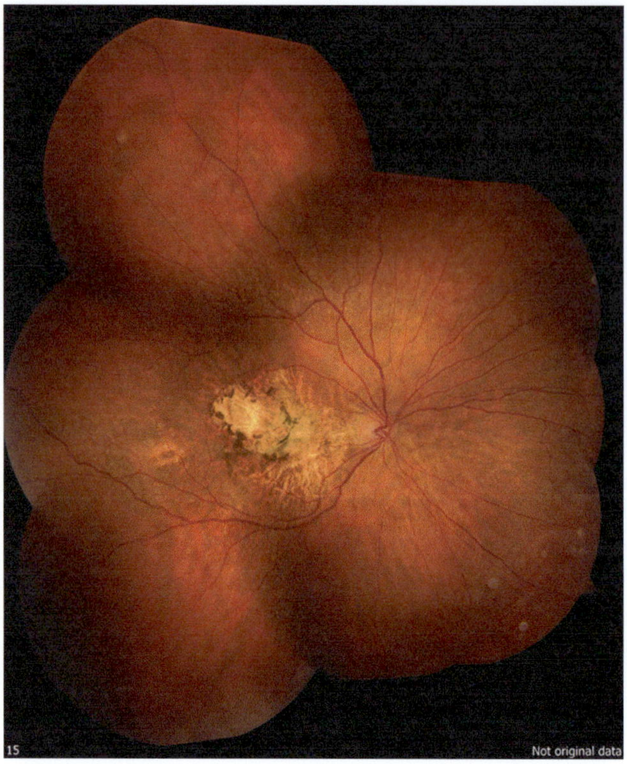

Fig. 80.1 Color fundus photo of the right eye of a 54-year-old woman with Sorsby Fundus Dystrophy, showing drusen along the arcades and macular chorioretinal atrophy with scarring and pigmentation. This patient had a history of neovascularization that led to the macular findings.

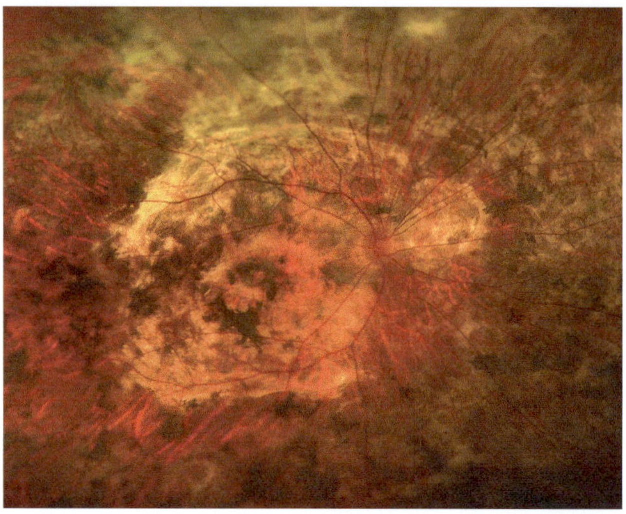

Fig. 80.2 Color fundus photo of the right eye of another 54-year-old woman with Sorsby Fundus Dystrophy, showing extensive chorioretinal atrophy, with scarring and pigmentation involving the macula and extending to outside the arcades. There is also atrophy in the retinal periphery, with dense pigmentary changes.

References

1. Langton KP, McKie N, Curtis A, Goodship JA, Bond PM, Barker MD, et al. A novel tissue inhibitor of metalloproteinases-3 mutation reveals a common molecular phenotype in Sorsby's fundus dystrophy. J Biol Chem. 2000;275(35):27027–31.
2. Weber BH, Vogt G, Pruett RC, Stöhr H, Felbor U. Mutations in the tissue inhibitor of metalloproteinases-3 (TIMP3) in patients with Sorsby's fundus dystrophy. Nat Genet. 1994;8(4):352–6.
3. Felbor U, Stohr H, Amann T, Schonherr U, Weber BH. A novel Ser156Cys mutation in the tissue inhibitor of metalloproteinases-3 (TIMP3) in Sorsby's fundus dystrophy with unusual clinical features. Hum Mol Genet. 1995;4(12):2415–6.
4. Schoenberger SD, Agarwal A. A novel mutation at the N-terminal domain of the TIMP3 gene in Sorsby fundus dystrophy. Retina. 2013;33(2):429–35.
5. Sivaprasad S, Webster AR, Egan CA, Bird AC, Tufail A. Clinical course and treatment outcomes of Sorsby fundus dystrophy. Am J Ophthalmol. 2008;146(2):228–34.
6. Stöhr H, Anand-Apte B. A review and update on the molecular basis of pathogenesis of Sorsby fundus dystrophy. Adv Exp Med Biol. 2012;723:261–7.
7. Barbazetto IA, Hayashi M, Klais CM, Yannuzzi LA, Allikmets R. A novel TIMP3 mutation associated with Sorsby fundus dystrophy. Arch Ophthalmol. 2005;123(4):542–3.

81 TOPORS

TOPORS encodes E3 ubiquitin-protein ligase Topors, which is an enzyme involved in the proteasomal degradation pathway. Mutations in *TOPORS* cause 1% of autosomal dominant retinitis pigmentosa (adRP) (rod-cone dystrophy) [1–3]. Patients typically present between 10 and 50 years of age with night blindness and peripheral vision loss, although some affected patients may be asymptomatic [1, 2]. Visual acuity is usually maintained until late in the disease process (range: 20/20 to CF). The fundus is characterized by RPE atrophy located uniquely around the retinal vessels ("perivascular cuff of RPE atrophy") in very young patients, which progresses with age to diffuse pigment deposits with atrophy (Figs. 81.1 and 81.2) [1]. Patients may also exhibit optic disc pallor and macular RPE atrophy [2]. The full-field ERG reveals a rod-cone pattern of degeneration but exhibits variability [1, 2]. Some patients who carry the mutation may exhibit a normal fundus, even in the context of abnormal ERG parameters [1]. GVF also exhibits a rod-cone pattern, but the extent of visual field loss may vary within the same family [1]. Static perimetry may show loss of sensitivity beyond 10° of eccentricity, with preservation of foveal sensitivities [2]. It has been suggested that the pathogenicity of truncating mutations results from haploinsufficiency [1, 2].

One missense *TOPORS* mutation has been reported to cause autosomal dominant pericentral retinal dystrophy in a family [4, 5]. These patients may be asymptomatic or report central vision defects or pericentral scotomas. Nyctalopia generally begins after age 25 but may not occur until as late as age 50. Color vision abnormalities are uncommon. Fundus findings feature bone spicule deposits near the vascular arcades rather than the mid-periphery, minimal vessel attenuation, and a normal optic disc. Full-field ERG is usually abnormal but is less severely affected than in rod-cone dystrophy as described above and with other forms of adRP. Multifocal ERG usually reveals reduced amplitudes in the macula. Dark-adaptation thresholds may be minimally elevated. GVF reveals a ring scotoma within 30 degrees that spares the fovea. One patient in this family progressed to a clinical picture identical to rod-cone dystrophy, with peripheral bone-spicule deposits and atrophy, vessel attenuation, and eventual involvement of the macula [4].

S. Zahid et al., *Retinal Dystrophy Gene Atlas*, https://doi.org/10.1007/978-3-319-10867-4_81

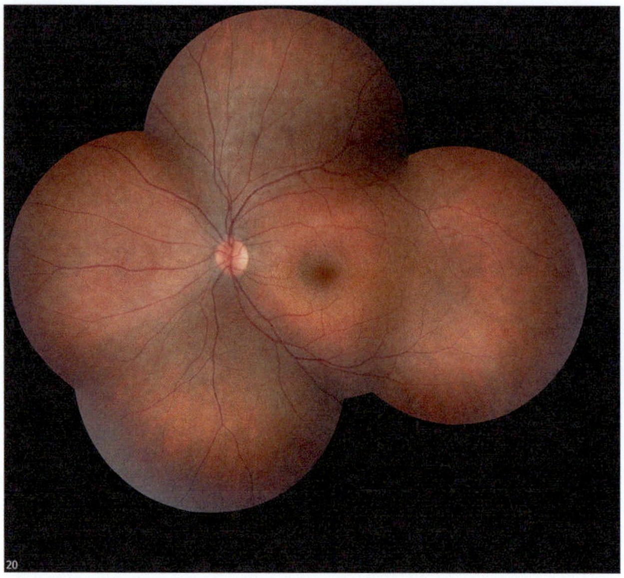

Fig. 81.1 Color fundus photograph of the left eye of a 27-year-old female patient, showing an unremarkable fundus exam, with only subtle retinal pigment epithelium (RPE) changes and without significant bone spicule pigmentation or atrophy.

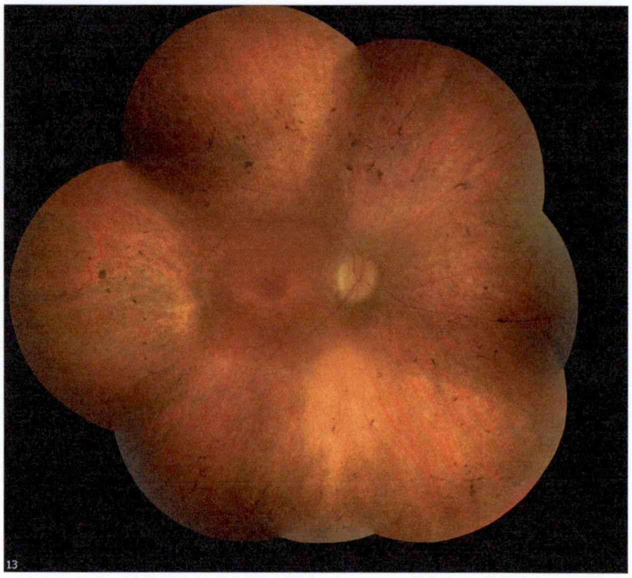

Fig. 81.2 Color fundus photograph of the right eye of a 56-year-old patient (father of patient in Fig. 81.1), showing midperipheral RPE atrophy with bone spicule pigment deposits. Some of these deposits and atrophy are near the retinal vasculature. There is also macular RPE depigmentation in the parafovea.

References

1. Chakarova CF, Papaioannou MG, Khanna H, Lopez I, Waseem N, Shah A, et al. Mutations in TOPORS cause autosomal dominant retinitis pigmentosa with perivascular retinal pigment epithelium atrophy. Am J Hum Genet. 2007;81(5):1098–103.
2. Bowne SJ, Sullivan LS, Gire AI, Birch DG, Hughbanks-Wheaton D, Heckenlively JR, et al. Mutations in the TOPORS gene cause 1% of autosomal dominant retinitis pigmentosa. Mol Vis. 2008;14:922–7.
3. Schob C, Orth U, Gal A, Kindler S, Chakarova CF, Bhattacharya SS, et al. Mutations in TOPORS: a rare cause of autosomal dominant retinitis pigmentosa in continental Europe? Ophthalmic Genet. 2009;30(2):96–8.
4. Selmer KK, Grondahl J, Riise R, Brandal K, Braaten O, Bragadottir R, et al. Autosomal dominant pericentral retinal dystrophy caused by a novel missense mutation in the TOPORS gene. Acta Ophthalmol. 2010;88(3):323–8.
5. Sandberg MA, Gaudio AR, Berson EL. Disease course of patients with pericentral retinitis pigmentosa. Am J Ophthalmol. 2005;140(1):100–6.

82 TULP1

TULP1 encodes tubby-like protein 1, which is a retina-specific protein involved in trafficking of proteins and transport of rhodopsin in photoreceptors. Recessive mutations in *TULP1* cause a range of diseases from Leber congenital amaurosis (LCA) and early-onset retinitis pigmentosa to classic rod-cone dystrophy [1–4].

In one study, Hanein et al. found that mutations in *TULP1* cause 1.7% of LCA. *TULP1*-related LCA patients may show signs of nystagmus, profound visual deficits, and nonrecordable ERGs within the first few months of life. Within their first and second years, patients generally experience nyctalopia more commonly than photophobia. Peripheral visual fields are also reduced [3].

Mutations in *TULP1* cause less than 1% of autosomal recessive retinitis pigmentosa. Patients may exhibit nystagmus (pendular, vertical, or horizontal) shortly after birth as well as visual field loss, poor visual acuity, and night blindness within the first decade of life. Patients may also experience nyctalopia, photoaversion, and head bobbing at early ages. Some patients may have exotropia or early-onset cataracts. Fundus findings may include arteriolar attenuation and typical bone spicule pigmentation in the midperipheral retina (Figs. 82.1a and 82.2a). RPE mottling, posterior staphyloma, and Fuch's spots have also been reported. Optic disc pallor may also be seen in older patients; one study also found cellophane reflexes from the macula in two patients [5]. Typically, patients exhibit visual acuities less than 20/200 in their 30s and exhibit rod-cone ERG and GVF patterns [1]. Some patients demonstrate non-recordable ERGs for both rod and cone parameters at a younger age. Visual field constriction may progress to absolute scotoma later in the disease process [2, 4, 6–9]. Fundus autofluorescence may show a macular ring of hyperautofluorescence and show hypoautofluorescence in areas of retinal pigment epithelium (RPE) atrophy (Fig. 82.2b). Optical coherence tomography is helpful in demonstrating areas of macular RPE and photoreceptor loss (Fig. 82.1b).

One study described two unrelated patients with a homozygous mutation (p.Arg420Ser) in *TULP1* (inherited through maternal uniparental isodisomy) [10]. While *TULP1* mutations are predominantly associated with rod-mediated diseases, these patients had significant cone dysfunction. They both exhibited progressive loss of visual acuity and bull's-eye maculopathy along with significant loss of cone ERG parameters and central scotomas.

S. Zahid et al., *Retinal Dystrophy Gene Atlas*, https://doi.org/10.1007/978-3-319-10867-4_82

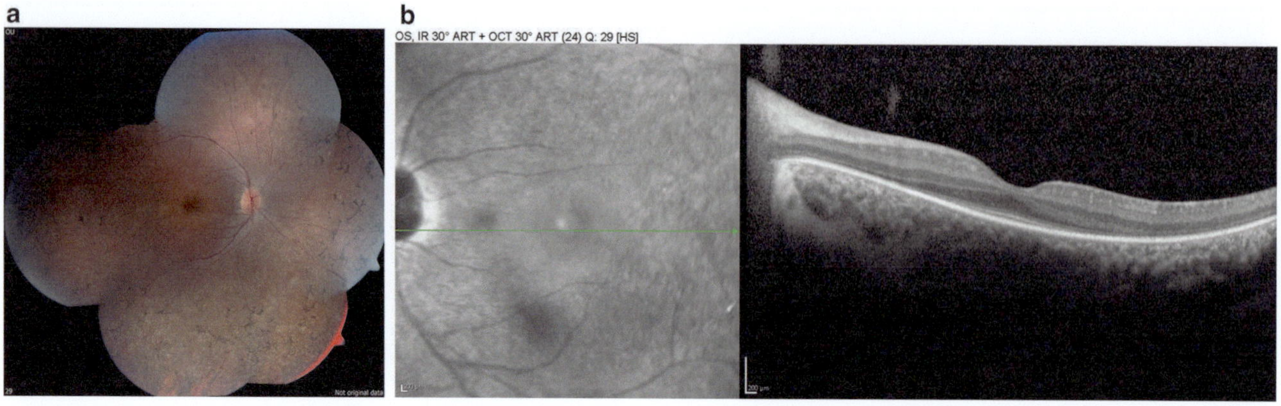

Fig. 82.1 Case summary: 17-year-old with early-onset retinitis pigmentosa. (**a**) Color fundus photograph of the right eye, showing peripheral retinal atrophy with bone spicule pigment deposits in the midperipheral retina with apparent relative macular sparing. (**b**) Spectral domain-optical coherence tomography (SD-OCT), showing loss of the macular ellipsoid zone (EZ) and outer nuclear layer, with a small residual band at the fovea.

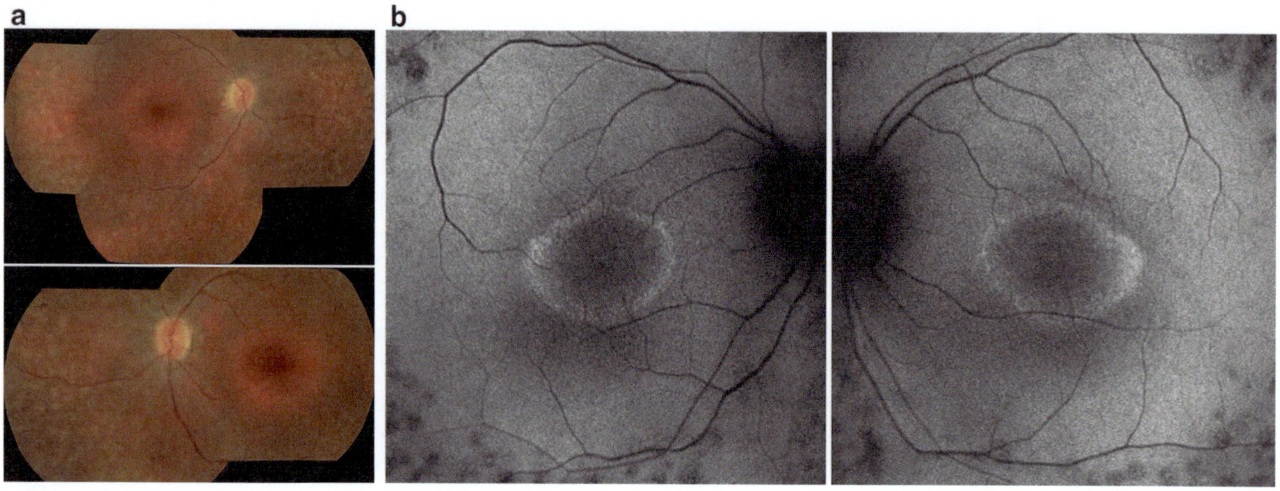

Fig. 82.2 Case summary: 21-year-old with Leber congenital amaurosis, onset at birth, visual acuity 0.4 logMAR in the right eye and 0.78 logMAR in the left eye. (**a**) Color fundus photograph of the right and left eyes, showing macular retinal pigment epithelium (RPE) depigmentation in a ring surrounding the fovea, with midperipheral patchy RPE atrophy and scant pigment deposits in both eyes. (**b**) Fundus autofluorescence of the right and left eyes, showing a ring of hyperautoflourescence with spots of hypoautofluorescence corresponding to RPE atrophy outside the arcades.

References

1. Hagstrom SA, North MA, Nishina PL, Berson EL, Dryja TP. Recessive mutations in the gene encoding the tubby-like protein TULP1 in patients with retinitis pigmentosa. Nat Genet. 1998;18(2):174–6.
2. den Hollander AI, Lopez I, Yzer S, Zonneveld MN, Janssen IM, Strom TM, et al. Identification of novel mutations in patients with Leber congenital amaurosis and juvenile RP by genome-wide homozygosity mapping with SNP microarrays. Invest Ophthalmol Vis Sci. 2007;48(12):56908.
3. Hanein S, Perrault I, Gerber S, Tanguy G, Barbet F, Ducroq D, et al. Leber congenital amaurosis: comprehensive survey of the genetic heterogeneity, refinement of the clinical definition, and genotype-phenotype correlations as a strategy for molecular diagnosis. Hum Mutat. 2004;23(4):306–17.
4. Paloma E, Hjelmqvist L, Bayes M, García-Sandoval B, Ayuso C, Balcells S, et al. Novel mutations in the TULP1 gene causing autosomal recessive retinitis pigmentosa. Invest Ophthalmol Vis Sci. 2000;41(3):656–9.
5. Kannabiran C, Singh H, Sahini N, Jalali S, Mohan G. Mutations in TULP1, NR2E3, and MFRP genes in Indian families with autosomal recessive retinitis pigmentosa. Mol Vis. 2012;18:1165–74.
6. Iqbal M, Naeem MA, Riazuddin SA, Ali S, Farooq T, Qazi ZA, et al. Association of pathogenic mutations in TULP1 with retinitis pigmentosa in consanguineous Pakistani families. Arch Ophthalmol. 2011;129(10):1351–7.

7. Abbasi AH, Garzozi HJ, Ben-Yosef T. A novel splice-site mutation of TULP1 underlies severe early-onset retinitis pigmentosa in a consanguineous Israeli Muslim Arab family. Mol Vis. 2008;14: 675–82.
8. Mataftsi A, Schorderet DF, Chachoua L, Boussalah M, Nouri MT, Barthelmes D, et al. Novel TULP1 mutation causing leber congenital amaurosis or early onset retinal degeneration. Invest Ophthalmol Vis Sci. 2007;48(11):5160–7.
9. den Hollander AI, van Lith-Verhoeven JJ, Arends ML, Strom TM, Cremers FP, Hoyng CB. Novel compound heterozygous TULP1 mutations in a family with severe early-onset retinitis pigmentosa. Arch Ophthalmol. 2007;125(7):932–5.
10. Roosing S, van den Born LI, Hoyng CB, Thiadens AA, de Baere E, Collin RW, et al. Maternal Uniparental Isodisomy of chromosome 6 reveals a TULP1 mutation as a novel cause of cone dysfunction. Ophthalmology. 2013;120(6):1239–46.

USH2A

83

USH2A encodes usherin. Mutations in *USH2A* are the most common cause of autosomal recessive non-syndromic retinitis pigmentosa (10–15%) [1, 2] and of Usher syndrome type 2 (RP and hearing impairment) [3–6].

In patients with non-syndromic RP, visual acuity is usually maintained until relatively late in the disease course [1, 7–9]. Fundus findings show mild or no pigment deposits, peripheral retinal pigment epithelial atrophy or depigmentation, and cystoid macular edema in some patients (Figs. 83.1a and 83.2). Full-field ERGs and kinetic visual fields are consistent with typical RP. Fundus autofluorescence (FAF) may reveal a peri-macular ring of increased AF (Fig. 83.1b), which constricts over time [8]. Sandberg et al. showed that patients with *USH2A* mutations reach legal blindness (due to either visual field or visual acuity loss) at a median age of 58 and exhibit yearly rates of decline of 2.6%, 7.0%, and 13.2% for visual acuity, visual field area, and 30-Hz flicker amplitude, respectively [10].

USH2A mutations account for about 80% of Usher syndrome type 2. Patients typically present with mild-to-moderate sensorineural hearing loss from birth (more severe for higher frequency sounds), and are otherwise in good health, with normal vestibular responses. There is evidence suggesting that there may be progression of hearing loss with age in some individuals [11, 12]. The ophthalmic manifestations are characterized by nyctalopia and peripheral visual field loss within the first two decades, which progresses with age, though the rates of progression may vary, with significant intra- and interfamilial phenotypic variability [10, 13–16]. Fundoscopy may demonstrate mild or no pigment deposits (Figs. 83.1a and 83.2), peripheral retinal pigment epithelial atrophy, or depigmentation (Fig. 83.3); a macular hyperautofluorescent ring on fundus autofluorescence imaging (Fig. 83.1b); and cystoid macular edema in some patients. The full-field ERG is often non-recordable [17, 18].

One study described a family with three unique pathogenic variants in *USH2A* in which, depending on which two variants were inherited by an individual, that family member had either nonsyndromic RP or Usher syndrome [8]. However, no reliable genotype-phenotype correlations have been found thus far, as there is significant intra- and interfamilial variability [10, 15, 16].

S. Zahid et al., *Retinal Dystrophy Gene Atlas*, https://doi.org/10.1007/978-3-319-10867-4_83

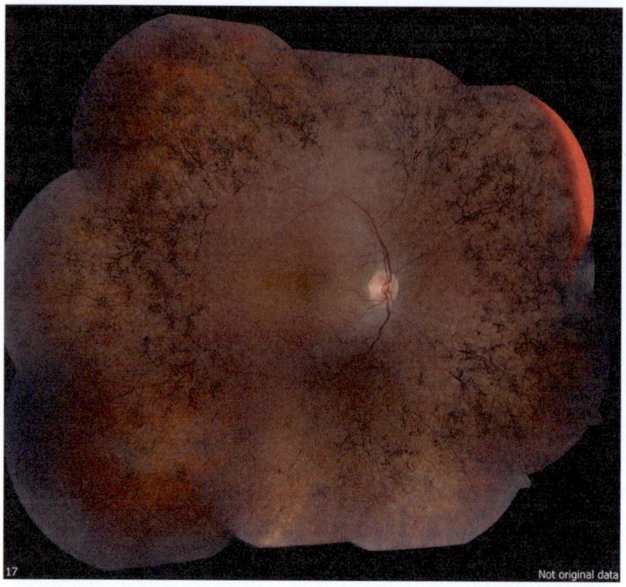

Fig. 83.1 Montage color fundus photograph of the right eye from a 31-year-old man with rod-cone dystrophy, showing typical features of retinitis pigmentosa, with peripheral bone spicule pigmentation in the mid-periphery and retinal vessel attenuation.

a **b**

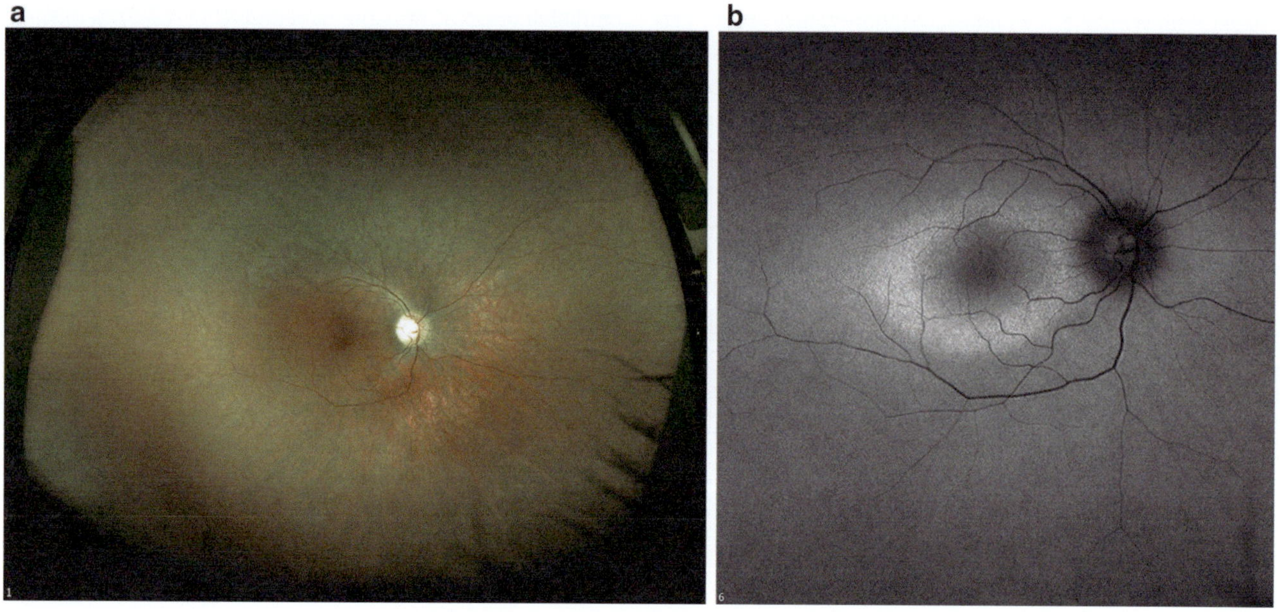

Fig. 83.2 Case summary: 17-year-old female with Usher Syndrome (**a**) Wide-field color fundus photograph of the right eye, showing a blunted foveal reflex and peripapillary atrophy. (**b**) Wide-field fundus autofluorescence, showing a wide hyperautofluorescent ring in the macula.

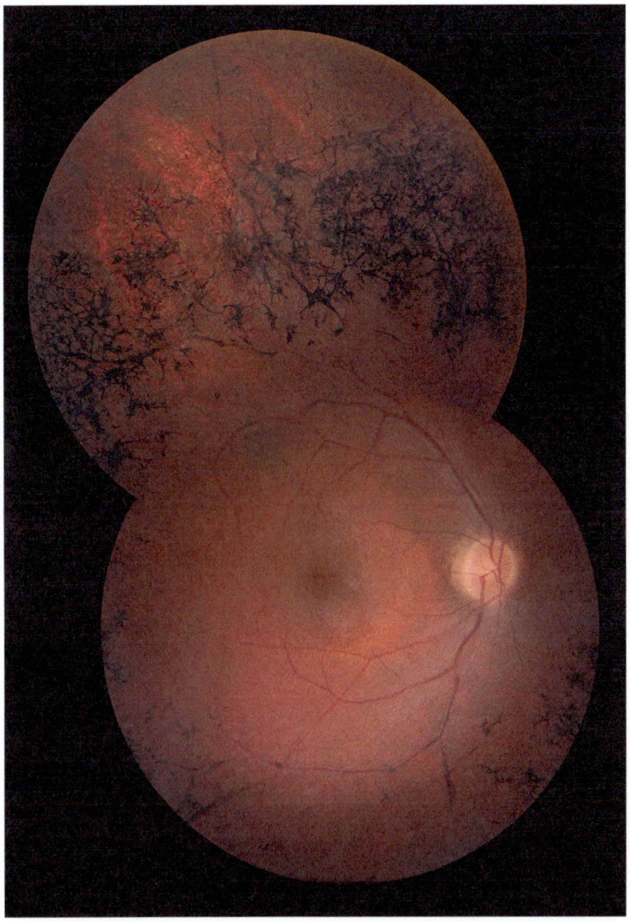

Fig. 83.3 Montage color fundus photograph of the right eye from a 23-year-old woman with Usher Syndrome, showing typical features of retinitis pigmentosa, with dense peripheral bone spicule pigmentation in the mid-periphery and retinal vessel attenuation.

References

1. Rivolta C, Berson EL, Dryja TP. Paternal uniparental heterodisomy with partial isodisomy of chromosome 1 in a patient with retinitis pigmentosa without hearing loss and a missense mutation in the Usher syndrome type II gene USH2A. Arch Ophthalmol. 2002;120(11):1566–71.
2. Seyedahmadi BJ, Rivolta C, Keene JA, Berson EL, Dryja TP. Comprehensive screening of the USH2A gene in Usher syndrome type II and non-syndromic recessive retinitis pigmentosa. Exp Eye Res. 2004;79(2):167–73.
3. Eudy JD, Weston MD, Yao S, Hoover DM, Rehm HL, Ma-Edmonds M, et al. Mutation of a gene encoding a protein with extracellular matrix motifs in Usher syndrome type IIa. Science. 1998;280(5370):1753–7.
4. Weston MD, Eudy JD, Fujita S, Yao S, Usami S, Cremers C, et al. Genomic structure and identification of novel mutations in usherin, the gene responsible for Usher syndrome type IIa. Am J Hum Genet. 2000;66(4):1199–210.
5. Dreyer B, Tranebjaerg L, Rosenberg T, Weston MD, Kimberling WJ, Nilssen O. Identification of novel USH2A mutations: implications for the structure of USH2A protein. Eur J Hum Genet. 2000;8(7):500–6.
6. Aller E, Jaijo T, Beneyto M, Nájera C, Oltra S, Ayuso C, et al. Identification of 14 novel mutations in the long isoform of USH2A in Spanish patients with Usher syndrome type II. J Med Genet. 2006;43(11):e55.
7. Rivolta C, Sweklo EA, Berson EL, Dryja TP. Missense mutation in the USH2A gene: association with recessive retinitis pigmentosa without hearing loss. Am J Hum Genet. 2000;66(6):1975–8.
8. Kaiserman N, Obolensky A, Banin E, Sharon D. Novel USH2A mutations in Israeli patients with retinitis pigmentosa and Usher syndrome type 2. Arch Ophthalmol. 2007;125(2):219–24.
9. Xu W, Dai H, Lu T, Zhang X, Dong B, Li Y. Seven novel mutations in the long isoform of the USH2A gene in Chinese families with nonsyndromic retinitis pigmentosa and Usher syndrome type II. Mol Vis. 2011;17:1537–52.
10. Sandberg MA, Rosner B, Weigel-DiFranco C, McGee TL, Dryja TP, Berson EL. Disease course in patients with autosomal recessive retinitis pigmentosa due to the USH2A gene. Invest Ophthalmol Vis Sci. 2008;49(12):5532–9.
11. Sadeghi M, Cohn ES, Kelly WJ, Kimberling WJ, Tranebjoerg L, Moller C. Audiological findings in Usher syndrome types IIa and II (non-IIa). Int J Audiol. 2004;43(3):136–43.
12. Pennings RJE, Fields RR, Huygen PLM, Deutman AF, Kimberling WJ, Cremers CWRJ. Usher syndrome type III can mimic other types of Usher syndrome. Ann Otol Rhinol Laryngol. 2003;112(6):525–30.
13. Iannaccone A, Kritchevsky SB, Ciccarelli ML, Tedesco SA, Macaluso C, Kimberling WJ, et al. Kinetics of visual field loss in Usher syndrome type II. Invest Ophthalmol Vis Sci. 2004;45(3):784–92.
14. Pennings RJ, Huygen PL, Orten DJ, Wagenaar M, van Aarem A, Kremer H, et al. Evaluation of visual impairment in Usher syndrome 1b and Usher syndrome 2a. Acta Ophthalmol Scand. 2004;82(2):131–9.
15. Bernal S, Medà C, Solans T, Ayuso C, Garcia-Sandoval B, Valverde D, et al. Clinical and genetic studies in Spanish patients with Usher syndrome type II: description of new mutations and evidence for a lack of genotype – phenotype correlation. Clin Genet. 2005;68(3):204–14.
16. Schwartz SB, Aleman TS, Cideciyan AV, Windsor EA, Sumaroka A, Roman AJ, et al. Disease expression in Usher syndrome caused by VLGR1 gene mutation (USH2C) and comparison with USH2A phenotype. Invest Ophthalmol Vis Sci. 2005;46(2):734–43.
17. Nakanishi H, Ohtsubo M, Iwasaki S, Hotta Y, Mizuta K, Mineta H, et al. Identification of 11 novel mutations in USH2A among Japanese patients with Usher syndrome type 2. Clin Genet. 2009;76(4):383–91.
18. Nakanishi H, Ohtsubo M, Iwasaki S, Hotta Y, Usami S, Mizuta K, et al. Novel USH2A mutations in Japanese Usher syndrome type 2 patients: marked differences in the mutation spectrum between the Japanese and other populations. J Hum Genet. 2011;56(7):484–90.

84 VCAN

VCAN encodes four extracellular matrix (ECM) isoforms (due to alternative splicing of introns 7 and 8) that are a component of the vitreous and are likely involved in its maintenance and structural integrity [1, 2]. Mutations, which have only been identified at the splice acceptor region of intron 7 and the splice donor region of intron 8, cause an overexpression of isoforms V2 and V3 and are responsible for Wagner syndrome (WS) [1, 3].

VCAN mutations are responsible for all known cases of Wagner disease, which has an autosomal-dominant pattern of inheritance. The age of onset of the disease is usually during adolescence, but it can also begin during early childhood [4]. Visual acuity and the progression of vision loss has a great deal of inter- and intrafamilial variability [3], but it is generally within normal range for younger patients (ranging from 20 to 50 years [4]) and severely reduced in older patients [5]. Other features include myopia, early-onset cataracts, progressive nyctalopia, and risk for retinal detachment [1, 3, 4]. Seen on slit-lamp examination, the hallmark feature of Wagner is an optically empty vitreous with strands, membranes, or veils [1, 3, 4]. Chorioretinal atrophy with pigment migration into the retina has also been noted [3], in addition to instances of ectopic foveae, inverted papilla, and uveitis without the formation of synechiae [3, 4]. Scotopic and photopic ERG responses are affected to varying degrees, in a family-specific manner, with reductions in both a- and b-wave amplitudes [2, 3]. Visual field shows ring scotomas with eventual loss of central vision [4].

S. Zahid et al., *Retinal Dystrophy Gene Atlas*, https://doi.org/10.1007/978-3-319-10867-4_84

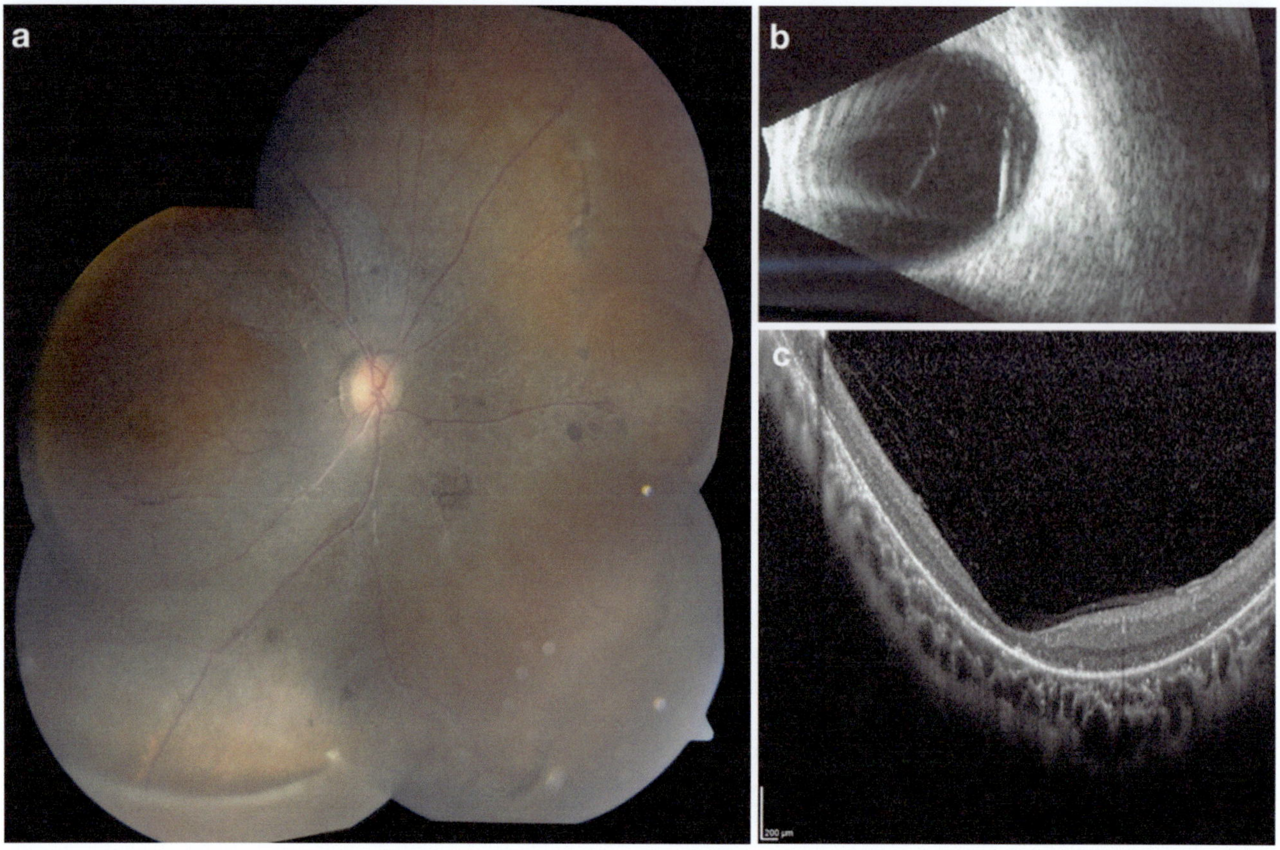

Fig. 84.1 Case Summary: 31 year old woman with *VCAN* mutations. (**a**) Color photograph of the right eye, showing diffuse retinal atrophy, more prosminent adjacent to the vascular arcades and in the fovea. (**b**) B-scan of the right eye, demonstrating vitreous membranes. (**c**) Spectral Domain Optical Coherence Tomography of the right eye, showing diffuse retinal thinning, loss of the ellipsoid zone, and foveal atrophy.

References

1. Kloeckener-Gruissem B, Neidhardt J, Magyar I, Plauchu H, Zech JC, Morlé L, et al. Novel VCAN mutations and evidence for unbalanced alternative splicing in the pathogenesis of Wagner syndrome. Eur J Hum Genet. 2013;21(3):352–6.
2. Kloeckener-Gruissem B, Amstutz C. VCAN-related vitreoretinopathy. 2009 [Updated 2016]. In: Pagon RA, Adam MP, Ardinger HH, et al., editors. GeneReviews® [Internet]. Seattle: University of Washington, Seattle; 1993–2017. Available from: https://www.ncbi.nlm.nih.gov/books/NBK3821/.
3. Rothschild PR, Brézin AP, Nedelec B, Burin d, Roziers C, Ghiotti T, et al. A family with Wagner syndrome with uveitis and a new versican mutation. Mol Vis. 2013;19:2040–9.
4. Meredith SP, Richards AJ, Flanagan DW, Scott JD, Poulson AV, Snead MP. Clinical characterisation and molecular analysis of Wagner syndrome. Br J Ophthalmol. 2007;91(5):655–9.
5. Zech JC, Morlé L, Vincent P, Alloisio N, Bozon M, Gonnet C, et al. Wagner vitreoretinal degeneration with genetic linkage refinement on chromosome 5q13-q14. Graefes Arch Clin Exp Ophthalmol. 1999;237(5):387–93.

Index

S. Zahid et al., *Retinal Dystrophy Gene Atlas*, https://doi.org/10.1007/978-3-319-10867-4

MIX
Papier aus verantwortungsvollen Quellen
Paper from responsible sources
FSC® C105338

If you have any concerns about our products,
you can contact us on
ProductSafety@springernature.com

In case Publisher is established outside the EU,
the EU authorized representative is:
Springer Nature Customer Service Center GmbH
Europaplatz 3, 69115 Heidelberg, Germany

Printed by Libri Plureos GmbH
in Hamburg, Germany